THE POLITICAL ECONOMY OF SOCIAL INEQUALITIES

Consequences for Health and Quality of Life

Edited by
Vicente Navarro

POLICY, POLITICS, HEALTH AND MEDICINE Series
Vicente Navarro, Series Editor

Baywood Publishing Company, Inc.
Amityville, New York

Library of Congress Catalog Number: 00-044494
ISBN: 0-89503-252-X (Paper)
ISBN: 0-89503-220-1 (Cloth)

Library of Congress Cataloging-in-Publication Data

The political economy of social inequalities : consequences for health and quality of life / edited by Vicente Navarro.
p. cm. - - (Policy, politics, health, and medicine series)
Includes bibliographical references and index.
ISBN 0-89503-220-1 (cloth) - - ISBN 0-89503-252-X (paper)
1. Quality of life. 2. Poverty. 3. Equality. 4. Income distribution. 5. Poor- -Medical care. I. Navarro, Vicente. II. Policy, politics, health, and medicine series (Unnumbered)

HN25 .P65 2000
306- -dc21 00-044494

CONTENTS

Introduction

Vicente Navarro

One of the most interesting developments in the scientific literature today is the growing number of studies on the consequences of social inequalities for the health and well-being of populations. This is a new situation. As I describe in the first chapter of this book, in reviewing some of the scholarship on this topic over the last 30 years, the political climate in the United States, United Kingdom, and western Europe during the 1980s was not favorable to these types of studies. And those of us who did conduct such studies labored under extremely difficult conditions. The research funding agencies, both public and private, had an enormous influence in shaping the nature of what could be done, and they clearly discouraged studies of this type. And the academic journals, the majority of which saw themselves as reproducing the conventional wisdom of the times, clearly spurned articles dealing with such topics. Exceptions did exist, however, and the most visible and important of these was the *International Journal of Health Services,* which from its inception more than 30 years ago has focused on the socioeconomic and political determinants of the health and well-being of our populations. It has welcomed all points of view as long as they are presented in a rigorous and scholarly fashion. This book, the first of two volumes, is a collection of updated articles published in that journal.

In the growing body of literature on inequalities and health, one major area has not received the attention it deserves: analyses of the socioeconomic and political reasons for the growth of social inequalities and their consequences for health and well-being. Indeed, in most research on social inequalities and health published in mainstream academic journals and books, the focus has been on the *consequences* of such inequalities for people's health and well-being. Missing from this literature are analyses of *how* and *why* the social inequalities within and among our societies are generated and reproduced, and *how* the socioeconomic and political forces responsible for this situation are affecting the quality of life of our populations. The silence on this topic is largely due to the system of funding of social research in the United States and United Kingdom. The dominant conservative and neoliberal forces that control or have a major influence in the funding agencies—the forces largely responsible for the growth of these inequalities in the first place—have been unwilling to support this type of research. Only recently, since the early 1990s, has a change in the political climate allowed for changes in the research agenda. But even though these funding agencies are now more willing to explore new areas, they still limit themselves to funding research on the *consequences* of social inequalities for health, not on the *causes* of the growth of inequalities and the effects on population health and well-being. As a consequence, there is an enormous scarcity of publications on the political economy of social inequalities and their consequences for health and quality of life—understanding *political economy* in the way both Marx and Adam Smith understood it, as the analysis of how power is realized through our economic, political, and social institutions. Thus the title of this book: *The Political Economy of Social Inequalities.* The contributors to this book analyze how power operates in the world and in our societies and how that power affects the growth of social inequalities and their impact on people's health and well-being.

OVERVIEW OF THE BOOK

The chapters in this book are assembled into six parts. Part I consists of a review of the evolution over the last 30 years of the scholarship on class inequalities and their impact on the quality of life. I gave this personal account on the occasion of the American Public Health Association's celebration of my work at its 1997 annual convention. Chapter 1 can serve as a reminder to younger scholars that others have labored under very difficult conditions, cultivating the fields in which the current research on social inequalities is now blossoming.

Part II includes three chapters in which I focus on the causes of the growing inequalities among and within countries. These causes include deregulation of the financial and labor markets, worldwide concentration of economic and political power, and changes occurring in most of the world's welfare states, changes that have weakened public policies designed to facilitate the redistribution of wealth and income from capital to labor, from high-income to medium- and low-income groups, and from the young to the elderly. In a critique of the neoliberal policies primarily responsible for the growth of these inequalities (Chapter 2), I show empirically how the theses used to sustain neoliberal positions are scientifically unsustainable. I also analyze the flaws in the U.S. economic "miracle" (supposedly based on the New Economy), which is presented as a showcase to be emulated by other countries—including those of the European Union, often criticized for being "eurosclerotic." The data presented in this chapter challenge each thesis of the economic "miracle," questioning that miracle on the grounds of not just social equity but economic efficiency.

Chapter 3 is a critique of the "technocratic," "humanistic," and profoundly "apolitical" discourse used by most international agencies, including the World Health Organization, in their analysis of the growing social inequalities, a discourse that obscures the actual causes of this growth: the power relations among and within countries, as detailed throughout this book. I then analyze the social, economic, and political changes taking place in developed capitalist countries that are affecting their welfare states, in particular the changes in the family, in people's life cycles, in economic and social structures, and, most importantly, in the political contexts (Chapter 4). I show how these changes take place and how the ways in which various countries respond to them depend mainly on the correlation of forces (of which class forces are of great importance) and their expression in the political space. The dominant theoretical frame (promoted by international agencies and many governments) assumes that all governments, regardless of their political coloration, are forced to follow the same policies in order to compete successfully in the globalized economy, where international markets (financial and commercial) determine what governments can and must do. Questioning this economic determinism, I attempt to recover the importance of politics, making politics central to the explanation of what is happening in the welfare states of the developed capitalist countries, including the neoliberal aggression against them.

Part III consists of six chapters that analyze the role of international agencies such as the World Bank, the International Monetary Fund (IMF), and the World Health Organization (WHO) in promoting the neoliberal public policies responsible for the growth of inequalities. Chapter 5, by Gabriel Kolko, is an analysis of the effects of recent IMF structural adjustment programs on the poorest nations, most of which have stagnated or declined economically in spite of (and on occasions because of) such interventions. The IMF's requirement that these countries increase exports despite falling world commodity prices has been a principal cause of their economic malaise. Meanwhile, IMF loan conditions demanding lower government expenditures have led to sharp reductions in general social spending.

In Chapter 6, Adriana Puiggrós analyzes the World Bank's education policy. Neoliberalism does not consider education a strategic investment. The World Bank discourse for Latin America is based on a short-term cost-benefit analysis. Its education policy is determined by "adjustment" of countries' economies so that they can continue to pay their external debts. The goal is to eliminate states' educational expenses by keeping education for the elites, breaking up and privatizing the large public education systems, and nullifying teachers' contracts. Teachers' unions are now at the forefront of opposition to the World Bank's education reforms.

Chapter 7, by Asa Cristina Laurell and Oliva López Arellano, critically evaluates *Investing in Health,* the World Bank's blueprint for a new health policy within the context of structural adjustment. This World Bank document includes a broad range of arguments, but its implicit premises are neoliberal, as can be deduced from its "agenda for action." Health is defined as a private responsibility and health care as a private good; this leads to a health policy based on two complementary principles: reduction of state intervention and public responsibility, and promotion of diversity and competition (i.e., privatization). In this thinking, public institutions should provide only a limited number of public goods and narrowly defined, cost-efficient forms of relief for the poor. All other health-related activities are considered private duties, to be resolved by the market, nongovernmental organizations, or families. The World Bank sees this as the way to achieve fiscal balance, while pushing to recommodify health care and turn health into a terrain for capital accumulation through the selective privatization of health-related financial and "discretionary" services. The World Bank's proposals imply a dismantling of public institutions (the only institutions accessible to the majority) and reject health as a human need and a social right.

Ray Kiely also examines recent World Bank reports on the role of the state in the development process (Chapter 8), with particular reference to the rise of the East Asian newly industrializing countries and the crisis of "governance" in sub-Saharan Africa. He discusses the concepts of "market friendly intervention" and "good governance" and finds them inadequate as explanations for East Asian "success" and African "failure"; he presents an alternative explanation for the rise of the newly industrializing countries, which draws out some of the implications of the developing world.

In Chapter 9, Pilar Vergara evaluates the neoliberal policies in Chile. The economic and social strategies developed by the democratic governments since 1990 have been based on the premise that free-market policies promoting growth and economic stability must continue but should be combined with social policies to promote greater equality. These new policies have produced quick and positive results: strong economic growth and a reduction of poverty. However, not all the government's redistributive efforts have had the same level of success. Inequalities in income distribution are again increasing. Significant segments of society, such as subsistence farmers, rural migrants to cities, women and youth who lack vocational training, and an important segment of the middle class impoverished during the military regime, are being systematically marginalized. Professor Vergara shows that the fundamental problems of current Chilean social policy are rooted in the privatization of social sectors under the military government and the resulting dual model of social welfare.

Debabar Banerji, one of the best known and most respected experts on underdevelopment, analyzes the change in the policies of WHO, UNICEF, and the World Bank, from the Alma-Ata Declaration until today (Chapter 10), showing how these agencies have reproduced the dominant thought in the political, economic, and academic circles of the developed world. According to Professor Banerji, the struggles of the labor and social movements culminated in the Alma-Ata Declaration of self-reliance in health for the peoples of the world. The rich countries, to protect their commercial and political interest, delivered sharp and swift retribution. They "invented" Selective Primary Health Care and used WHO, UNICEF, the World Bank, and other agencies to let loose on poor countries a barrage of "international initiatives" such as global programs on immunization, AIDS, and tuberculosis. Banerji shows how these programs were astonishingly ineffective in concept, design, and implementation, and how the international agencies refused to take note of published criticisms.

The chapters in Part III will undoubtedly give the reader a very different vision and understanding of the international agencies.

The three chapters of Part IV discuss the effects of privatization, deregulation, and profit maximization on the welfare state, and especially on social transfers such as social security and the funding of health care. First, Professor Laurell analyzes the neoliberal reorganization of Mexican society (Chapter 11), taking the social security counterreform of 1997 as her point of reference. This counterreform implied a profound change in the guiding principles of social security, replacing a model based on integrality, solidarity, and redistribution with one based on private administration of funds and services, individualization of entitlement, and reduction of rights. Its economic purpose was to move social services and benefits into the sphere of private capital accumulation. Although these changes involved the entire social security system—old age and disability pensions, health care, childcare, and workers' compensation—they were most immediately evident in the pension scheme: the pay-as-you-go scheme was replaced by privately managed individual retirement accounts that especially favor the big financial groups. Privatization of the social security system required decisive state intervention, with change in the law and a sizable, long-term state subsidy. The supposed positive impact on economic growth and employment remains uncertain. A review of the new law and the estimates of future annuities reveals shrinking pension coverage and inadequate incomes from pensions.

In an analysis of proposals to convert U.S. Medicare to a voucher program (Chapter 12), Jonathan Oberlander argues against the claims that vouchers would increase the health care choices available to Medicare beneficiaries, would reduce the regulatory burden on the federal government, would promote the benefits of fair market competition, and are the only solution to Medicare's short-term financing problems and the long-term "crisis" of the retirement of the baby-boom generation. Implementation of vouchers, says Professor Oberlander, would pose a threat to both the health of beneficiaries and the stability of the Medicare program. Vouchers would not work because of limitations in the risk-adjustment methods and unrealistic assumptions about consumer choice. And the elderly and disabled Medicare population is ill suited to cope in a competitive insurance system. Oberlander discusses the implications of these findings for Medicare reform.

In Chapter 13, Richard B. Du Boff evaluates the current debate among economists on the U.S. Social Security system. Since the 1980s, welfare state protections have been blamed for a host of economic problems. Not until the 1980s could conservatives, who have long disliked Social Security, effectively attack this popular program. They devised a new tactic: warning young people they would never get their "money's worth" from Social Security, which is on the brink of "bankruptcy." The political climate, dominated by a drive to cut back "big government," was also favorable for attempts to destabilize Social Security politically. Negative images of Social Security were thus forced onto the public agenda, and "liberal" economists have uncritically accepted this new set of political "givens."

Part V presents one of the major debates on the pathways of social inequalities and health, the well-known Wilkinson–Muntaner and Lynch debate. In Chapter 14, Carles Muntaner and John Lynch discuss how Wilkinson's "income inequality and social cohesion" model has emerged as a leading research program in social epidemiology, with appealing features for public health scholars and activists working to eliminate social inequalities in health. It provides a sociological alternative to models that emphasized poverty, health behaviors, or the cultural aspects of social relations as determinants of population health. It calls for social explanations, avoids the subjectivist legacy of U.S. functionalist sociology evident in "status" approaches to understanding social inequalities in health, and calls for broad policies of income redistribution. Nevertheless, say Professors Muntaner and Lynch, certain characteristics of Wilkinson's model limit its explanatory power and its ability to inform social policies that address social inequalities in health. It ignores class relations, an approach that might help explain how income inequalities are generated and help account for both relative and absolute deprivation, and it implies that social cohesion rather than political change is the major determinant of population health. Historical evidence, however, suggests that class formation could determine both reductions in social inequalities and increases in social cohesion. Drawing on recent examples, Muntaner and Lynch argue that an emphasis on social cohesion can be used to render communities responsible for their mortality and morbidity rates, as seen in current policy initiatives in the United States and United Kingdom under the New Democrat and New Labor governments.

In his reply (Chapter 15), Richard G. Wilkinson notes that statistical evidence suggests social cohesion provides the link between income inequality and health, but how it does so is unclear. The vagueness of the concept of "cohesion" and the difficulty of seeing how something so apparently ephemeral could exert a major influence on health has led to skepticism about its role in the relation between income distribution and mortality. Professor Wilkinson suggests that social cohesion is indicative of underlying psychosocial risk factors, known to be closely associated with health. He draws attention to the strong inverse relationships between measures of social inequality and measures of the quality of social relations in numerous different data sets. Social status and social affiliations are, in terms of population-attributable risks, among the most powerful influences on population health in the developed world. Wilkinson suggests that an antipathy between hierarchical relations across inequalities of power, income, and status on the one hand, and supportive social relations between equals on the other, is likely to exert a powerful influence on health.

In their rebuttal (Chapter 16), Professors Muntaner and Lynch argue that Wilkinson's model omits important variables (social class), making it vulnerable to biases due to model misspecification. Furthermore, they argue, the "culture of inequality" hypothesis unnecessarily "psychopathologizes" the relatively deprived while omitting social determinants of disease related to production (environmental and occupational hazards) and the capacity of the relatively deprived for collective action. And while shying away from social mechanisms such as exploitation, workplace domination, or classist ideology might avoid conflict, it reduces the income inequality model to a set of useful but simple and wanting associations. Using a nonrecursive structural equation model that tests for reciprocal effects, Muntaner, Lynch, and their coauthor, Gary L. Oates, show that working-class position is negatively associated with social cohesion but positively associated with union membership, and therefore current indicators of social cohesion use middle-class standards for collective action that working-class communities are unlikely to meet. An erroneous characterization of working-class communities as noncohesive could be used to justify paternalistic or punitive social policies.

Finally, Part VI contains analyses of some proposed solutions to the health effects of social inequalities. In Chapter 17, Leiyu Shi and I show how political context and political factors are critical to understanding the growth of inequalities. We analyze the way in which the major political traditions in developed capitalistic countries from 1960 to 1990—the social democratic, Christian democratic and/or conservative, fascist, and liberal traditions—have perpetuated or corrected these inequalities. We show that social democratic governments rooted in large labor movements have been the most successful in reducing social inequalities and improving populations' health and quality of life.

The topic of Chapter 18 is the Third Way, a political position that arose in the United Kingdom (with the Blair government) and the United States (with the Clinton administration) in the early 1990s, supposedly an intermediate position between neoliberalism and social democracy. I select for analysis the most detailed account of the Third Way in the English-speaking world, a book by Anthony Giddens. Giddens stereotypes both the neoliberal and the social democratic positions to an unrecognizable degree, failing to portray the varieties of social democratic policies now in existence in the developed capitalist countries. The Third Way is merely a recycling of liberal positions in some social policy areas and Christian democratic positions in others. Where the Third Way intends to be innovative—as in the U.K. New Deal program—the programs are pale copies of successful labor market policies carried out by northern European social democratic parties. The Third Way, with its questioning of the universalistic welfare state and its preference for assistential and means-tested programs, signifies a break with the social democratic tradition, transforming it into a hybrid between Christian democracy and neoliberalism.

In Chapter 19, Richard Levins and Cynthia Lopez present an ecosocial view of health. Despite declining mortality rates, increased life expectancy, and improvements in diagnostic and therapeutic technologies, the United States has seen the return of infectious disease, a growing gap in health outcomes between rich and poor and between whites and blacks; and a growing discrepancy between what is technically possible and actual health status. And despite its greater expenditures on health, the United States lags behind other developed countries in health outcomes. Professors Levins and Lopez examine four reasons for this: we do not buy more health care, only pay more for it; we receive more health care, but much of it is inappropriate, ineffective, or harmful; only some of us get more health care; and we have created a way of life that makes us sick, then spend more to repair the damage. Levins and Lopez use a broad, ecosocial perspective that rejects the dichotomies social/biological, physical/psychological, genetic/environmental, lifestyle/environment and examines their interrelations rather than assigning them relative weights.

Chapter 20 is a review of the very important work of Amartya Sen, well summarized in his book *Development As Freedom.* In this critique I indicate that although Sen's work represents an enormous advance in redefining the nature and objectives of economic development—making democracy and freedom the major objectives and instruments of economic development—his explanations and project are insufficient. Sen's lack of attention to how economic and political power are reproduced in today's world, and how the political context of economic development actually occurs, limits the understanding of the relationship between economic and political development and how both affect human development. I conclude the chapter and the volume by underlining the critical role of property relations (among others) within and among countries in reproducing the power relations in our societies, stressing the need to understand the role played by such power categories as class, gender, and race and their relations of exploitation and domination in human development and quality of life. An analysis of how these relations are reproduced is of central importance in comprehending and changing those inequalities that constrain the full development of the great potential of every human being.

In the final chapter, I question the position widely held in financial and economic circles that economic globalization has considerably diminished states' power to follow the full-employment and redistributive policies usually identified with the labor and social democratic movements. The chapter provides empirical information that documents how specific governments in developed capitalist countries have been able to pursue such policies during these years of economic globalization, and even monetary integration. It aso documents the fallacy of the supposed exhaustion of the welfare states.

These, then, are the contents of the volume. The reader will notice that the positions presented here differ from and are often in conflict with mainstream explanations of the way in which social inequalities affect health and well-being and the social, political, and economic causes for the production and reproduction of social inequalities. We hope this book will broaden the much-needed debate on the social, political, and economic determinants of populations' quality of life.

Baltimore, May 2000

PART I
Review of the Research

CHAPTER 1

A HISTORICAL REVIEW (1965–1997) OF STUDIES ON CLASS, HEALTH, AND QUALITY OF LIFE: A PERSONAL ACCOUNT

Vicente Navarro

The invitation I received from the organizers of the session expressed their wish that I speak about my life's work on the relationships between class and health within the continuously evolving political context of the past 35 years. I also notice that in the promotion of the session, "An Evening with . . . ," the organizers referred to the growing interest within the academic community in studying the relationship between class and health. This interest seems to have motivated the invitation for a person who has been working on this topic for 35 years to share his experience with the younger generations—those who may like to discover a sense of history and experience—helping to correct the omission of a historical perspective for which U.S. scholarship has frequently been criticized. I will try to establish a linkage and continuity between the past, the present, and the future, sharing with you my experiences, thoughts, and impressions of where we have been, where we are, and where we might like to be.

But first, let me start—as you requested—with a brief biographical note which explains my commitment to the subject. That commitment is not merely academic. It is rooted in a strong experience in my very early youth, when I fought in the Catalan and Spanish antifascist underground, a fight—a good fight—which millions fought for freedom, democracy, solidarity, and social justice, all pointers toward the political objective of achieving, someday, a classless society. Millions—including some of my family and close friends—have fought and died or been killed in the 20th century to achieve this goal. Those years of struggle had an enormous impact on my life and motivated a life-long commitment to the study of class relations in order to transcend them, to allow the development of human society's potential for achieving the level of health and quality of life desired by all people.

I had to leave Spain in 1962 for political reasons; this political exile led me first to Sweden then to the United Kingdom. In those parts of Europe I met many interesting people, but two in particular were to have a huge importance in my life. One was Karl Evang, the Chief Health Officer of Norway at that time, and the other was John Brotherston, a professor at the Usher Institute of Edinburgh University and later the Chief Health Officer of Scotland. While my intellectual life was clearly shaped by studying in Spain under Manuel Sacristan—the Gramsci of Spain—my professional life in the health area was most influenced at that time by Evang and Brotherston. It was they who, with Stampar from Yugoslavia, wrote the famous definition of health in the 1948 World Health Organization Constitution. This, as you will recall, defined health as more than the absence of disease, and declared as the objective of our public health project not just the somatic and psychological but also the social well-being of the individual and of the collectivity. It saw health, therefore, as rooted not only in biological but in social conditions. This was an enormous break with the traditional understanding of health and medicine, putting both in their proper context: the social structure and social relations in our societies.

Very few people have realized that this definition of health—now one of the most frequently cited definitions in medical texts—grew directly out of the pact achieved by the victorious antifascist forces after World War II (and let's not forget that this war was primarily an antifascist war). It was a pact made in response to the high level of expectations created by the end of the war. The enormous sacrifices made by the popular classes during that war had been made with the hope of achieving a better future. The three major forces behind the pact were the New Dealers in the United States, the social democratic governments in Western Europe, and the Soviet Union in Eastern Europe. The political instruments of the working classes and their labor movements in alliance with the middle classes were the main forces behind that pact, establishing the bases for setting out the public's responsibilities for providing social transfers and services that greatly improved the health and quality of life of the majority of people. In Europe, both East and West, the labor movement was rooted in Marxism as the theoretical frame for understanding and changing class relations in those societies. On this side of the Atlantic the Weberian tradition was stronger, although forces rooted in Marxism played an important role in the establishment of the New Deal—also a result of an alliance of the working class with the middle class and southern farmers.

From 1948 to 1965, however, many changes occurred. In the United States, a rapid growth in families' disposable income (at a rate of 2.5 percent per year) and a growing perception of well-being helped to establish the "American dream"—a perception responding to the reality that parents would see their children become better off than they had been. This produced a new understanding—an understanding reproduced by the mainstream media always ready to propagate the views of the dominant forces—that the United States was a middle-class society, with the majority of Americans in the middle.

This was the scene when I landed in the United States in 1965, joining the two million immigrants arriving in the country that year. (I soon realized, incidentally, that having a heavy Spanish accent and a Spanish surname could be a source of negative distinction and suspicion.) I arrived in August of that year, invited by Professor Kerr White to join him at The Johns Hopkins University.

Professor Odin Anderson from Michigan was then the major theoretical voice in the analysis of medicine. In his major opus (*Health Care: Can There Be Equity? The United States, Sweden, and England*, 1972), he concluded his analysis of the United States with a homage to the middle class and to the American dream:

> The middle class was and still is the source of entrepreneurial, technical, and managerial skills, which exploited natural resources, developed the economy, and thus . . . created a social surplus that spilled over into other endeavors such as the arts, education, health services and warring for national honor and expansion.

In this theoretical scenario there were no dominant or dominated classes, or even dominant groups or elites. Terms such as working class were printed in quotation marks to signal the reader that they were suspect terms, used by ideologues who should be excluded from the forum of serious scholarship. It may be difficult for current researchers to believe that, in those times, terms such as class, working class (not to mention class struggle), and just plain capitalism were dismissed as ideological. No serious scholar, aware of the penalty that it would carry, would dare to use these terms. I have in my files several letters from editors of academic journals requesting that I should not use the term working class because it was excessively ideological, and encouraging me to replace it with the less value-laden term socioeconomic status. (They did not seem to realize that such a change was more than a mere semantic modification.) One particularly interesting note, from the then editor of *Social Science and Medicine* (the major journal of medical sociology at that time), recommended "dismissing such inelegant and ideological expressions as working class." I know of another scholar, Professor Ray Elling, who received a similar note from the same editor. (The same journal, incidentally, later published a leading article that was an extremely abrasive review of my work.) Nor did the dissenting voices speak of classes, but rather of interest groups. They interpreted the situation in medicine as resulting from the medical profession's dominance in the practice and institutions of medicine. Their major intellectual reference was Professor Eliot Freidson, the foremost theoretician in the professional dominance school. The radical version of that interpretation of the house of medicine appeared in Health PAC's *American Health Empire*, written by Barbara and John Ehrenreich, who saw the medical establishment as primarily responsible for the sorry state of affairs in medicine.

There was, however, a group of scholars who did not share this vision of the United States. They were the disciples of Henry Sigerist—a figure whose fame and official recognition, incidentally, have always intrigued me. My experience in the United States—particularly in the 60s and 70s—was that, in an intellectual environment that was profoundly ideological, the use of a class discourse was cause for abuse and discrimination. Because of that experience, I have always been perplexed—and, indeed, envious—that an intellectual whose discourse was a class discourse, with frequent references to class power relations affecting the nature of medicine, was actively and enthusiastically supported by the Rockefeller Foundation (a major voice of the U.S. establishment), had his picture on the cover of *Time* magazine, and had a regular radio show on CBS. Sigerist's America was indeed very different from the America I had experienced! The difference between his America and mine was McCarthyism, a class response to the popular expectations raised by the end of World War II. Its objective was to purge from society those voices that supported and wanted to expand these expectations, the realization of which would have reduced the privileges of the U.S. establishment. This explains why, by the mid-60s, the nature of what is "acceptable" and "supportable" in the United States had changed quite dramatically. And it explains why Henry Sigerist left the United States and why his disciples, repressed most brutally by McCarthyism, had to hide their language and discourse. Actually, I will always remember that, shortly after my arrival in the United States, I received a visit from two disciples of Sigerist, Professors Milton Roemer and Leslie Falk (later to become dear friends of mine), who cautioned me about being so open and transparent in my analysis of U.S. society and its medicine; they warned me that such openness would attract rejection and even hostility. Having suffered fascism directly (under a dictatorship in Franco's Spain) I did not pay much attention to their warning. I soon learned, however, that intellectual fascism, McCarthyism, was alive and well in the United States and that its destructive powers could be even worse than the fascism I had experienced in Spain. Many times in my 32 years in the United States I have thought of Milton and Leslie's warning. It proved remarkably accurate.

This dominant anticlass scenario, then, was the theoretical terrain on which I landed in 1965. Repression, however, generates resistance, and this is the history of the study of class and health from 1965 to 1997. Such intellectual and academic resistance in the 60s and 70s was made possible by changes in the political context of the times. The conservatism of the 50s and early 60s was shaken up by the tumult of the 60s, a decade that became known for its social agitation. Intellectual creativity does not occur in moments of conformity but in moments of questioning.

While the historiography of the 60s has focused on the students' protests (which indeed were central in the United States and elsewhere in launching many of the key movements of that decade, such as the anti–Vietnam War movement and the May events in France), the reality is that many forces and classes, including the working classes, played a major role in many countries, including our own. During the May events in France and the hot autumn in Italy, working-class mobilizations paralyzed those countries. Even Sweden saw its mines closed down. And in the United States, besides the impressive anti–Vietnam War mobilization and the splendid civil rights movements, we also saw labor strikes that affected the energy and transport sectors, forcing President Nixon to call out federal troops to put down miners' strikes in North Carolina and Virginia. A common denominator in all of these working-class movements in western nations was their concern for health and quality of life issues rather than just wage or compensatory demands. As the Italian workers who took over the Fiat factories put it so eloquently in a slogan held in front of a factory: "We want to work in factories in which we can sing while working." Thus work itself should be a source of joy and creativity, not just a means to achieving creativity through the world of consumption. Similarly in the United States, the most class-conscious workers, the coal miners, started a strike—one of the largest in U.S. history—about the nature of work, health, and well-being. They were questioning the power relations in the world of production, challenging the class relations dominant in the United States. These power relations were also being threatened by elements of the civil rights movement, which soon realized that the dividing line in the United States is not only race but class. None other than Martin Luther King, one of the most admired persons in the United States, stated that many of the issues in which the civil rights movement was involved were actually class issues. And a few weeks before he was killed, he indicated that "we are engaged in the class struggle, the critical struggle in the U.S." (quoted in D. J. Garrow, *The FBI and Martin Luther King*, pp. 213–215, Penguin Books, 1981).

The Development of Resistance: The Class Approach in the Analysis of Health and Medicine

In that environment of resistance, several events occurred that greatly affected the area of studies on class and health. One was the establishment of the *International Journal of Health Services (IJHS)*. Three individuals played a critical role in this event. Professors Karl Evang and John Brotherston (both very critical of the extreme conservatism of U.S. academic life at that time) had encouraged me to establish a forum for the presentation of critical views suppressed in the mainstream academic journals. Professor Kerr White, however, played the most crucial role. A Canadian liberal in the Bertrand Russell tradition, and a man of maverick convictions who detested conventional wisdom and practices, he gave his full support to the establishment of a journal committed to opening up academia to all positions, provided they were presented with the rigor required in a scholarly journal. Without Kerr, John, and Karl, such a journal could not have been established. They asked me, a junior, nontenured assistant professor, to create such a forum.

Most analytical and critical works that would later have major impacts in the areas covered by the journal—health and social policy, political economy and sociology, history and philosophy, and ethics and law—started in the pages of the *IJHS*, including the research findings and theoretical discussions on the relationship between class and health. Many well-known scholars started their intellectual work in the pages of the *IJHS*, and I am pleased to note that the works of two other speakers celebrated this evening—Professors Elizabeth Fee and Nancy Krieger—were first published in the *IJHS*. Even today, well-established authors send some of their contributions to the *IJHS* knowing that other journals would not dare to publish them. Not uncharacteristically (as happens with most forums in the United States that are critical of mainstream thought), the journal is better known outside than inside the United States.

The East Coast Discussion Group, Later HMO

Contrary to the prevalent individualistic understanding of life, I believe that all intellectual (as well as manual) work is the result of a collective rather than individual endeavor. The enormous intellectual creativity of the 60s and 70s in the studies of class and health was the result of a highly productive exchange among a group of researchers who met regularly (every three weeks), rotating the place of gathering (between Baltimore, Washington, and New York), to discuss theoretical, conceptual, and methodological issues in the study of class, health, and quality of life. Several of us, frustrated with the profound conservatism of U.S. academic life, started the intellectual network that we called the East Coast Discussion Group (ECDG). Howard Berliner, Rob Burlage, Barbara Burney, John Crawford, Robert Crawford, Joe Eyer, Elizabeth Fee, Sally Guttmacher, Jane Halpern, Kim Hopper, Sander Kelman, David and Rhonda Kotelchuck, Joane Lukomnik, Vicente Navarro, Hila Richardson, Len Rodberg, Jack Salmon, Evan Stark, Meredith Turshen, and Grace Ziem were the founders of that group, which later expanded to the west coast with Howard Waitzkin, Thomas Bodenheimer, Richard Brown, and others, many present in the audience today. Our intellectual roots lay in many critical traditions and our concern was the study of exploitation and domination, in their different dimensions—although the group's ever-developing theoretical frame evolved toward viewing the forces of exploitation and their effects on health primarily through the lens of class analysis. This is why we later renamed the group the Health Marxist Organization, or HMO—witnessing ten years later the takeover of these initials by the business establishment to mean health maintenance organization. I regret we did not copyright these initials!

The intellectual productivity of this group was extraordinary. Started by just a few of us, the ECDG (later HMO) soon became a fairly large network. We were creatures of the 60s, and as such we were intense, anarchic in our focus, constraintless (abrasive on occasion) in our positions and practices, and unrestrained in the expression of our emotions and commitments. Many articles and books came out of that intellectual project, products that, for the most part, first appeared in the *International Journal of Health Services*, one of the very few academic journals in the United States that was receptive to this type of critical scholarship. Another such journal was the *American Journal of Public Health*, which also published works by several members of the HMO, including my article "The Underdevelopment of Health of Working America" (Vol. 66, 1976).

It may be of interest to explain the response triggered by the HMO in the United States in the 60s and 70s. The mainstream academic media ignored the group's critical intellectual production. Even by as late as 1982, neither the American Sociological Association nor the U.S.-dominated International Sociological Association had acknowledged the existence of the group's production. The periodical *State of the Art in Medical Sociology* in 1974, 1978, and even in 1982, for example, did not cite any of our works.

More frequently, however, the response was one of overt hostility. *Social Science and Medicine* (whose editor had advised me to avoid the term working class as too ideological) published, as I mentioned earlier, a leading article that was an abusive and abrasive insult to one of us (Vicente Navarro). That article defined Navarro's Marxism as a "disease," concluding that human liberation called for the elimination of that disease (*Social Science and Medicine*, Vol. 19, 1984. For a reply to that attack, see Vol. 20, 1985). I have to assume that the author meant intellectual rather than physical elimination. This abusive article precipitated the resignation from that journal's executive board of Professor Howard Waitzkin, at that time of the University of California. Unfortunately, some of our colleagues from other countries were ready to fill that vacancy, mindless of the need for a cross-border solidarity among critical scholars.

Many of the works produced by the HMO were distributed in a type of underground culture. Students' demands for these works became a stimulus for our production. Slowly but surely the position that we espoused became accepted (as I will soon show), showing once again that to be radical is to have the courage and creativity to think and act 10 or 15 years ahead of one's time.

The establishment of the network created two other responses. One was from Health PAC, whose theoretical framework was primarily in the professional dominance school. Health PAC's response was initially one of hostility, but was soon replaced by one of collaboration within a mutually productive tension. Actually, some of the HMO members who became most productive had started their work as contributors to Health PAC. The other group that viewed us with suspicion was the old left—the disciples of Henry Sigerist—who felt uncomfortable with our transparency, openness, and (sometimes) abrasiveness, and what they perceived, sometimes accurately, as our arrogance. In our defense I must stress that minorities (including intellectual minorities) have to speak louder in order to be heard. And our struggle was not an easy one. Some of Sigerist's disciples chose to ignore us, others attempted to marginalize us, but the majority—and very much in particular Milton Roemer, George Silver, and Leslie Falk—actively supported us. Their supportive letters of reference for us, untenured faculty members at that time, became of crucial importance in our long journey through the academic institutions.

Areas of Work in the Study of Class and Health: 1965–1985

There were four major areas of work in our analyses of health and class during that period. The first was the analysis of class relations in the United States and its house of medicine. We predicted that, given the dynamics of the U.S. capitalist system with its pattern of class relations in which financial capital (the major component of which was the insurance industry) was so dominant and the working class so weak, financial capital (at that time a minority sector within the funding of medicine) would become the major force in the house of medicine, forcing providers to lose their autonomy. A big debate occurred within the HMO on whether or not the medical profession would become proletarianized. I want to emphasize that this prediction—that the logic of capital accumulation (i.e., the logic of optimizing profits as the main motive for organizing the house of medicine) would invade the institutions of medicine and that providers, including the medical profession, would lose their autonomy—was made at a time when nonprofit institutions were the major force in medicine and the medical profession seemed almost omnipotent. It demonstrates the potency and value of our method of class analysis of the reality in the United States that, 20 years ago, we were already able to predict what would happen. Today, what we had called the corporatization of medicine is a reality in the United States. Supermarket medicine, led by insurance companies, with physicians becoming mere agents in a for-profit machine, is the tone of medicine in our times. So much for those of our academic critics who accused us then of being irrelevant, paranoid, or too ideological. No other theoretical frame has proven so powerful in understanding U.S. medicine as that which places class relations at the center of its analysis.

The second area of work focused on the relationship between science and ideology in health and medicine. Our inquiry was aimed at analyzing how class dominance—classism—appeared in scientific medical knowledge, medical institutions, and medical practices. This project—an understanding of classism in medicine—was important for many reasons. One was to oppose the hegemonic understanding of medicine that saw the knowledge, institutions, and practices of medicine as classless. We did not agree with that. The struggle for a classless medicine could not be reduced to improving the distribution of a (supposedly) otherwise neutral-classless product or knowledge. For us, the struggle for a classless society (socialism) was a struggle to change the nature of medicine—the production as well as the distribution of medicine. In that sense we were critical of both the social-democratic and the communist traditions, whose battle for socialist medicine had been limited to better distribution of medicine through state intervention. Although applauding and supporting these endeavors, some of us saw this approach as insufficient and on occasions wrong. I wrote *Class Struggle, State and Medicine: A Historical Review of the British National Health Service* with the intent of critically analyzing the United Kingdom's National Health Service (defined by Churchill as the jewel in the crown of the British welfare state) from a class perspective, showing that this achievement of the British labor movement, splendid though it was, had not changed the pattern of power relations (and the hierarchical order they determined) within the institutions of medicine. I also wrote a critical review of Soviet medicine, *Social Security and Medicine in the USSR: A Marxist Critique*, in which I criticized the reproduction of class relations within Soviet medicine, showing that a new class had developed in the Soviet Union that had become an exploitative force—as shown later by the events of 1989. The writing of that book created considerable hostility in various quarters, including among some disciples of Sigerist. One of them, who will remain unnamed, stopped speaking to me, which caused me great pain and sadness.

A Third Area of Study in the Relationship between Class and Health: Materialist Epidemiology

While many of the HMO's studies centered on the relationship between class and medicine and between class and scientific knowledge, a third, very important dimension was the analysis of the relationship between class relations and health. These studies focused on the analysis of the social context that shapes the nature and level of health of our populations. The HMO rooted that social context in the social relations of production and distribution of resources in our societies. We wanted to focus on these relations as the matrix within which other relations could be understood and interrelated. This is why we chose to refer to these studies as materialist epidemiology rather than the more widely used term social epidemiology, which we considered too unspecific and too unscientific. Society is not a mere set of variables randomly related among themselves. There is a societal hierarchy of relations in which class relations do not determine but do condition most potently how other variables affect the population's health. We called these relations materialist because they are rooted in the society's material relations of production and distribution. We also studied how race, gender, and ethnicity affect health and well-being in our societies. But we analyzed the effects of these variables on health as part of a matrix of relations in which class relations were of great importance in understanding how such variables relate among themselves and with health. We were not class reductionists. But we wanted to stress the enormous importance of class in explaining the level of health and the nature of medicine.

In our investigation of these relationships, we found linear positivist thinking (in which reality is divided into either/or types of categories—either class or race, for example) to be insufficient or erroneous. Reality is not linear: it is dialectical. A 35-year-old black, female, blue-collar worker in the South is black, a woman, a manual worker, and a southerner *all* at the same time; one characteristic is embedded in the other. She is not 30 percent black, 30 percent woman, 30 percent worker, and 10 percent from the South—there is not a linear but a dialectical relationship among these variables. And under capitalism, class relations are relations that structurally define the matrix in which other relations relate. Needless to say, other variables such as race and gender could be conjuncturally more important than class in specific contexts and conjunctions; but class is always there and on many occasions organizes the frame in which other variables relate. This explains why under capitalism, class differentials in mortality are in general larger than race differentials in mortality. As I have shown in an article published in *The Lancet* (Vol. 336, 1990), cardiovascular disease mortality rates are 1.8 times higher among black males than among white males, but are 2.4 times higher among blue-collar workers than among corporate lawyers. Class is the most potent variable to explain mortality and morbidity differentials (for most causes) in the United States.

It was our project not only to demonstrate how this reality was hidden in a society where the language of class was forbidden (and where the federal government mortality statistics were (and still are) published by race and gender but not by class), but also to inquire and conduct research on what it is in class that explains these mortality and morbidity differentials. To answer that question we had to focus more on society than on the individual. In other words, our focus was more on how and where individuals were placed in our societies, how they related to each other and among themselves, than just on the individual. Our criticism of epidemiological research, for example, was that it focused on individual characteristics—called individual risk factors—as the causes of death and disease. Even social epidemiology focused on the impact of specific variables such as income, education, housing, occupation, and other individual characteristics on the health of the individual. We were aware of the excellent work that had been done on that front, since many of us had also contributed to such research. But we considered the individual focus to be insufficient because society is more than the aggregate of its individuals. We therefore wanted to focus on society rather than on the individual so as to understand and explain the level of health of our populations. We needed to understand society in order to explain health and disease. And in that quest we analyzed how relations of exploitation and/or domination (class, race, and gender) were related, were reproduced, and were materialized in everyday life and in death. Some of us, for example, studied how class relations appear in the workplace and in the community and how they affect the level of well-being of workers and residents; others looked at the family, trying to understand the class and gender relations reproduced by and in the family and their effects on the welfare of its members; still others analyzed the causes of economic cycles and their impact on the mortality and morbidity of our citizens.

Looking back, I believe that in spite of our great insufficiencies, the main thrust of our intellectual and professional project—materialist epidemiology—was correct. Recently we have seen the recognition that individual risk factors are not sufficient to explain the variations in mortality and morbidity in our societies. Studies now show that these individual factors explain only a small part of these variations. We have also recently witnessed the call by scholars from Great Britain, such as Professor Richard Wilkinson, to look at social cohesion—we used to call it solidarity—as the most promising avenue for exploring the causes of mortality differentials within and among countries. And we have also seen a growing recognition of the excellent work by scholars in the current generation, such as Professors Robert Karasek, Jeff Johnson, and Ellen Hall, who are the inheritors of our research on the relationship between production and health.

A Fourth Dimension of the Relationship between Class and Health: Imperialism and Health

The most important theoretical frame used in critical analysis to explain international relations in the 60s and 70s was that which considered the world to be divided into North and South, with the South (the developing countries) exploited by the North (the developed countries). The HMO questioned this analysis; we thought the reality was more complex than that. Both the North and the South have classes, and the analysis of those class relations was of paramount importance for understanding the reproduction of poverty in the world. Some of us had first-hand experience in this area. As advisor to the Unidad Popular in Chile, I could clearly see that the forces that deposed Allende's government were the capitalist oligarchy and upper middle classes in Chile. It was these groups that authored Pinochet's fascist coup. Needless to say, the U.S. government also supported the coup. But it was not the United States versus Chile. It was the Chilean capitalist and agricultural-based oligarchies and upper middle classes that carried out the coup, with the support of U.S. corporate interests, very influential in the U.S. government at that time.

Class and class relations were, therefore, also of primary importance to understanding worldwide relations and their impact on health. That understanding was the basis for the establishment by several of us, in conjunction with many colleagues from Europe and Latin America (and later Africa and Asia), of the International Association of Health Policy, which started in Amsterdam in 1974 as an informal group of researchers and scholars from all over the world working in these areas. This worldwide professional association, more than any other, has consistently documented and denounced the alarming growth of inequalities in today's world and its impact on health. And it has been one of the few professional organizations to criticize the technocratic discourse reproduced by WHO and other international agencies, whose financial dependency on the governments of the United States and other developed nations hinders their focusing on the actual causes of inequalities in today's world: the class relations within and among countries, reproduced by international agencies such as the World Bank and the International Monetary Fund, that are seriously damaging the health of the world's population. The advocacy by these agencies of policies of social austerity and structural adjustment that benefit the few at the top at the cost of the welfare of the many is one of the main causes of suffering in today's world. As many articles in the *IJHS* have shown, the proposals for further privatization of health services funding and of pension programs advocated by the World Bank and the International Monetary Fund (about which WHO remains silent) are hurting the popular classes quite remarkably. Such programs, along with the aggressive fiscal policies they advocate, are the major causes of growing income and wealth inequalities, the root of the world's current health problems.

Studies of Class and Health in the 80s and 90s

The studies of class and health in the late 80s and the 90s have focused primarily on several major areas. One area is the consequences of the corporatization of medicine, the phenomenon predicted by the HMO's class analyses in the 60s and 70s. The invasion of the profit-making motive into the house of medicine and business entrepreneurial behavior as the guiding force in medical institutions have become the major threat to the health and well-being of our populations. Very good scholarship has been published, not only by critical authors such as Jack Salmon, David Himmelstein, Steffie Woolhandler, and other inheritors of our tradition, but by mainstream researchers, documenting and denouncing the perverse effects of this invasion. For those of us who had predicted such an invasion (at a time when no one else was talking about it), this event was intellectually satisfying (we were proven right) but humanly excruciating. We would have much preferred to be wrong! Almost powerlessly, we had to witness this corporate invasion of medicine—a consequence of the enormous power of the corporate class and equally enormous weakness of labor in the United States, unparalleled in any other developed capitalist country. Power is indeed a relational concept. One is powerful because one's opponent is powerless. And that was indeed the case in the United States.

Another area in which our predictions proved correct was the collapse of the Soviet Union. We foresaw, when no one else did, that the social relations in that country would change. We criticized the Soviet Union because, as I indicated earlier, a new class had control over the state and over the means of production, control that was obviously being used to optimize its own interests. We showed that class analysis was also valid for analyzing the postcapitalist societies. In our analysis, socialist medicine was not simply medicine better distributed. Unless the hierarchical relations (and the priorities they establish) within medicine changed (establishing different types of priorities), they simply reproduced the class relations that originally shaped them.

The collapse of the Soviet Union has been deliberately and maliciously interpreted as the collapse of socialism in the 20th century. Yet, the empirical data contradict such a conclusion. Political projects whose objectives have been to achieve classless societies by reducing class as well as other forms of inequalities—such as social democracy in developed capitalist societies and revolutionary socialism in developing capitalist countries—have for the most part been more successful than their opponents (committed to maintaining class relations by maintaining inequalities) in improving the level of health and well-being of their populations in the 20th century. I have shown, for example, that an analysis of these experiences during the 20th century, continent by continent, leads to an opposite conclusion from that trumpeted today. In the developed countries, social democracy in Scandinavia and in western continental Europe, for example, has done a much better job since the 1950s in improving the health and quality of life of its citizens than the U.S. government has done for its citizens—a government whose primary consideration has been not the reduction of class inequalities but the reproduction of prevalent class relations. This improvement in the Scandinavian and western continental European countries took place even though, in the 40s and 50s, the well-being indicators (including health indicators) of those countries had been worse than those of the United States. Among the developing countries, prior to its socialist revolution China had much worse indicators of population well-being than did India; by the mid-70s, it had much better indicators. If India had had the same infant mortality rate as China during the 70s, India would have saved the lives of 4 million of its children each year. And in India itself, the state with the best health indicators, Kerala, has been governed by political forces committed to a classless society. In Latin America, Cuba has achieved better health indicators than other Latin American countries at a similar level of economic development. It is in Eastern Europe that the socialist project has had less to show in the way of success. But even there, let's not forget the remarkable achievements of the Soviet Union both within and outside the health sector during the extremely difficult periods of the 40s, 50s, and 60s. Besides playing a critical role in defeating Nazism during World War II, the Soviet Union improved the distribution of resources at a spectacular rate during the 50s and 60s. It is paradoxical, to say the least, that the same forces that celebrate the collapse of the Soviet Union as an indication of the superiority of capitalism remain silent about the collapse of the health situation in the former Soviet countries, a collapse that has been caused by the introduction of the capitalist model these forces promote. A similar process is now underway in China.

I was declared persona non grata in the Soviet Union because of my criticism (from the left) of that society. It is interesting to note, incidentally, that criticism from the right was permitted in that country, but not from the left. My dislike and distaste for the form into which the Soviet system had evolved (clearly predicted by Gramsci, incidentally, and also by Rosa Luxemburg) are well known. But it is revolting to see how much the collapse of the Soviet system is celebrated by those whose capitalist alternative has made the lives of the peoples of the former Soviet Union even worse. Life expectancy has declined spectacularly in these countries. And the Mafia (including the health Mafia), the inheritors of the Nomenclature who ran the Soviet state, are now running these countries. As noted by Professor Daniel Todes, a Johns Hopkins historian and one of the scholars in the United States who is most knowledgeable about Russia, "The Mafia is not a deformation of that system. The Mafia is the dominant force in that system."

In toto, the experience in the 20th century demonstrates not the superiority of capitalism over socialism but rather the need to see the struggles for democracy and for justice as one and the same. However well-intentioned political forces committed to classless societies may be, they must be equally committed to establishing democratic processes to achieve such societies. Meanwhile, and in the absence of any form of restraint, we are witnessing the worldwide spread of neoliberalism, the major cause of growing inequalities and deterioration of health conditions worldwide. Not surprisingly, neoliberalism—the main ideological and political project of the dominant classes today—denies the existence of classes. Instead it sees the individual as the motor of change, with each individual related to others through primarily mercantile relations.

But other positions have recently also denied the importance of class relations in the 80s and 90s. One is the post-modernism project which denies the totalizing nature of capitalism (or of any other social system for that matter) and the centrality of class relations under capitalism; class dilutes itself and finally disappears, replaced by the variety of different social movements that call for separate liberations. This theoretical frame has become particularly powerful in the politics of identities in the United States, within the critical traditions in which class has taken a second row, and many times has disappeared altogether. The appearance of this position, however, is not innocent: it is favored by an official discourse in which the discourse and practice of class are strongly repressed.

I saw the evidence of such an interpretation in the events surrounding the publication in *The Lancet* (Vol. 336, 1990) of my article on the relationship between class, race, and health. In the article I showed that (*a*) class mortality differentials are higher than race mortality differentials, and (*b*) not race but racism explains a large part of the race mortality differentials in the United States; racism puts the majority of blacks in the lower echelons of the class structure. Race mortality differentials therefore are socially not genetically caused.

I must stress here that prior to its publication in *The Lancet*, I had submitted the article to *JAMA* and the *New England Journal of Medicine*, both of which rejected it on the grounds that while I had shown that the working class had higher mortality and morbidity rates than the upper class, I had not disproved the possibility that people were in the working class *because* they had higher rates of disease. In other words, these journals were suggesting that, rather than the social determining the biological, the biological determined the social. Quite remarkable! Nazism was based on such a doctrine, which is now reproduced by Charles Murray and others who see the current social order as determined by biology.

The Lancet, however, accepted my article right away and, without my asking it to do so, published it along with an editorial under the title "U.S. Is Not a Classless Society."

It is important to describe also what happened after the publication of this article. As I have already indicated, the United States is one of the very few developed countries that does not publish mortality statistics by class. The federal government publishes mortality statistics by race, gender, age, region, and ethnicity, but not by class. When my article appeared, the then U.S. Secretary of Health, Dr. Sullivan (the only black in President Bush's cabinet), liked it. He instructed the Centers for Disease Control to explore the possibility of publishing mortality statistics by race and by class as I had suggested in the article: publication of statistics by race alone is misleading since race is not the issue—racism is—and this is why (among other reasons) it was important to add class. Shortly afterwards, however, the Centers for Disease Control received a communication from the Domestic Council of the White House instructing them to discontinue the project. President Bush was on record claiming in a speech he gave at Georgetown University in 1990 that classes did not exist in the United States.

I invite you to ask: Why is the U.S. establishment so strongly opposed to class analysis and class discourse in our society? Why do we see the reproduction of such an ideological and unscientific perception of the United States as a middle-class society, despite the overwhelming evidence that it is indeed a class society? In a September 1997 Gallup poll, incidentally, 62 percent of Americans identified themselves as working class.

The answer to these questions became very clear to me during the 1988 Presidential campaign, when I was the senior health advisor to Reverend Jesse Jackson. I had been his advisor in 1984, when he chose to run as the voice of the minorities, of those excluded from the American dream. He ran as the conscience of America, as the voice of the marginalized. I saw considerable sympathy toward his 1984 campaign from the major instruments of the U.S. establishment. *The New York Times*, for example, wrote an editorial very supportive of Reverend Jackson's campaign.

In 1988, however, Reverend Jackson returned as a class candidate. He openly appealed to a working-class mobilization, trying to make white blue-collar workers aware that they have more in common with black blue-collar workers because they are all workers than with the bosses because they are all white. And indeed, the mortality and morbidity figures showed Reverend Jackson to be absolutely right. This time, in 1988, the U.S. establishment responded with enormous hostility. *The New York Times* published an extremely hostile editorial, accusing Reverend Jackson of trying to destroy the country with that type of discourse. His advisors became concerned about his safety. We remembered what happened to Martin Luther King, shortly after defining class as the central conflict in the United States. I could see the U.S. establishment was in a panic about the mobilization of the working class around a class project that undoubtedly could curtail that establishment's class privileges. It is precisely the absence of a class discourse in the United States that is the best indicator of the enormous class dominance in this country.

I have seen evidence of this also in the way the U.S. establishment has responded to me and my work. If I had wanted to play by its rules and be a Latino (as I proudly am), I probably could have received all the honors that the U.S. establishment can bestow, as many of my colleagues have. I did not choose to play that role. Rather, in all my work I have emphasized class and have tried to serve the working people of this country in the best way I know. Actually, the hostility I have faced may be the best proof of my thesis.

Finally, let me try to answer the question of why we are seeing the renaissance of an interest in class today. The material reality of our people shows why. In spite of the triumphalist discourse of the U.S. establishment, the heartbreaking reality is that the majority of working people in this country (and in the world) are hurting. Disposable income has been declining for the majority of the working class. And, for the first time since the end of World War II, more Americans think that their children will be worse off rather than better off than their parents. We are witnessing the end of the American dream.

Along with this situation we are witnessing a marked polarization of U.S. society. In 1974 the average income of a chief executive officer was 34 times greater than that of a worker, but by 1994 it was 179 times greater! In the health sector we have seen a decline in the numbers of people with health benefits coverage. According to a recent Commonwealth Fund report, 52 million people are without health insurance at some time during each year! This polarization, incidentally, is also taking place among minorities. We have seen a considerable increase in the size of the black and (to a lesser degree) Hispanic middle classes, a result of the breaking down of the barriers of discrimination with the help of race-oriented affirmative action programs. Such antidiscriminatory projects must be continued since we should oppose all forms of race and gender discrimination. But let's not confuse these programs with the much needed programs that would better the lives of the vast majority of blacks, Hispanics, and other minorities, who are members of the working class. As the size of the black middle class has been increasing, for example, the disposable income of the majority of the black working class has been declining. Actually, in the United States today, as Professor William Julius Wilson has shown, social polarization among blacks is even wider than among whites: while the top 20 percent of whites consume 44 percent of all white income, the top 20 percent of blacks consume 49 percent of all black income.

The best way of improving the life and well-being of working-class blacks, Hispanics, Asians, and whites is to follow class-oriented programs that benefit the working and middle classes—that is, universal programs such as full employment policies and a national health program (among others) that would benefit all workers, and very much in particular those in the lower echelons such as the minorities. Public policies therefore should be class (as well as race and gender) oriented. In the health sector these class policies mean:

1. Continuing to pressure our government to publish information on class (as do most European countries) as well as race and gender—and I don't mean socioeconomic status or other Weberian gradient categories, but relational class categories. This can be done with the information that the government already collects.
2. Establishing a U.S. Presidential commission that (like the Black commission in the United Kingdom and countless other commissions in other countries) documents and monitors the state of class inequalities in the nation. An excellent doctoral thesis by one of my students, Lisa Miller Schalick, has shown how class mortality differentials are increasing in the United States.
3. Implementing the recommendations of the Annapolis NIH conference on the development of an infrastructure for collecting data—as published in the *IJHS*—that can help our government relate the changes in class structure to the health and well-being of our population.
4. Establishing as one of the top priorities for our national government's health policy the reduction of class mortality and morbidity differentials, as well as race and gender differentials.
5. Continuing the civil rights project through affirmative action programs, but stressing the need to:
    a. establish, also, universal social-rights—race-neutral—programs that benefit the majority of our working and middle classes, such as a full employment program with living wages and a national health program;
    b. discontinue the neoliberal policies, at home and abroad, that are stimulating the growth of inequalities in today's world; and
    c. evaluate the impact of foreign policy, including trade, on the social and civil rights of the world's populations.

This is a practical and realistic proposal that would undoubtedly improve the health and well-being of our populations. It is feasible in today's United States, but will require our government to become far more responsive than it now is to the wishes and needs of our working people—the working class and the popular classes, which are far too removed from our political institutions. Pointers of change seem to be appearing, such as the growing interest in class themes in the United States and the excellent changes now occurring in the U.S. labor movement, the great hope for reform in this country. I invite you, scholars and researchers, workers in the production of knowledge, to assist and support this movement.

Finally, allow me to finish with some remarks to the younger generation. You are fortunate to be working at a time when the political and academic institutions have become somewhat more sensitive to class issues (although not yet to class discourse). In a country like ours, without much sense of history, you need to remember that we have reached this point only because others have labored in the fields in which you are now harvesting. Many others, including my own generation, paid a high personal price for our commitment to asking forbidden questions. Lives were lost (we all miss Eric Holtzman), jobs were denied, professorships and chairs were withdrawn after offers had been made because of political pressure; tenures were never granted or greatly delayed because of our commitment. As the new generation, you need to be aware of this reality—silenced for too long—and you should not allow it to be forgotten. You need to know this history, to establish a continuity between the past, the present, and the future. I hope I have contributed to that.

PART II
Causes for the Growth of Inequalities and Their Impact on Health and Quality of Life

CHAPTER 2

NEOLIBERALISM, "GLOBALIZATION," UNEMPLOYMENT, INEQUALITIES, AND THE WELFARE STATE

Vicente Navarro

I. THE NEOLIBERAL "ORTHODOXY" AND ITS ECONOMIC AND SOCIAL CONSEQUENCES

Since the early 1980s, a new orthodoxy has appeared in western economic thought that considers the state and its interventions as obstacles to the economic and social development of western populations. This new orthodoxy was facilitated by the electoral victories during that period of many conservative and liberal parties in the majority of the OECD countries, and very much in particular by the elections of President Reagan in the United States in 1980 and Prime Minister Margaret Thatcher in the United Kingdom in 1979. Since then, this orthodoxy has become hegemonic in national and international centers of economic and political power, and it has dominated in academia and in the mainstream media on both sides of the Atlantic. Initially referred to as "Reaganomics" in the United States and "Thatcherism" in the United Kingdom, this new orthodoxy is more frequently known as neoliberalism—although this term is less used in the United States, where the term "liberalism" is usually applied to public policies that in Europe would be called social democratic. This neoliberal "orthodoxy" is characterized by the following positions:

1. *Public deficits are intrinsically negative.* They absorb national savings, increase interest rates, and reduce investments. Consequently, neoliberalism calls for reducing and even eliminating public deficits, freeing up resources needed for private investment, reducing interest rates, and shifting resources from the public to the private sectors.

2. *State regulation of the labor market is also intrinsically negative.* It adds rigidities to the labor market, hindering both economic growth and job production. Labor should be considered like any other commodity and thus should be unregulated, with wages determined by the forces of the international and national markets.

3. *Social protection guaranteed by the welfare state and its redistributive policies hinders economic growth.* It does so by increasing collective consumption and reducing private savings, in particular, by reducing the savings ability of the wealthiest sectors of the population. The latter groups are the most negatively affected by the redistributive policies of the welfare state—and are also those that have the greatest propensity for saving. Based on this assumption of an inverse relationship between redistributive policies and savings and investments, the neoliberal position calls for the reduction and even, in the most extreme cases, the complete elimination of the welfare state. Newt Gingrich, the leader of the Republican Party in the U.S. Congress, has called for the virtual elimination of the U.S. welfare state (1).

4. *The state should not intervene in regulating foreign trade or international financial markets.* The free flow of goods, services, and financial capital is the best way of guaranteeing an efficient and equitable worldwide distribution of resources.

Due to the worldwide influence of the governments of the United States and the E.U. countries (the majority of which were governed, during the 1980s and early 1990s, by conservative and liberal parties), these neoliberal positions became dominant among the OECD countries and among the international agencies that those governments controlled or heavily influenced. It is important to clarify that the degree of application of these neoliberal policies has varied considerably among the OECD countries; some countries have resisted the implementation of at least some of the more extreme neoliberal positions. But it also must be stressed that important elements of neoliberal public policies became key components of the public policies of many governments, and have continued to be reproduced in the mid and late 1990s, even though the political orientations of many of these governments have changed. As of spring 1998, most developed OECD countries have left-of-center governments, yet many of the neoliberal policies remain in place. One reason for this is the widely held belief that these neoliberal public policies have been more successful than the public policies they replaced (usually referred to, erroneously, as Keynesian public policies) in improving the efficiency of these economies. The post–World War II public policies, however, went farther than the typical Keynesian policies. Indeed, the dominant public polices in the major developed OECD countries were characterized not only by a considerable expansion of public and social expenditures, but also by an active intervention in the sphere of production through state interventions that had a most significant influence in orienting the economic development of these countries. The three most important capitalist economies at that time—the United States, Western Germany, and Japan—had state policies that went farther than Keynesianism (expansion of demand); they were heavily interventionist in the realm of production. For this reason I will use the term "state interventionist public policies" rather than the more widely used term "Keynesian policies." (I will expand on this point in a later section.) These policies were supplanted in the late 1970s and early 1980s by neoliberal policies that claimed to be superior to those they were replacing. Since then, not only conservative and neoliberal but also some left and left-of-center governments have shared that perception of the superiority of neoliberal policies over state interventionist policies in improving the efficiency of their economies.

In the first section of this chapter I analyze the evidence presented in support of the assumed superiority of neoliberal policies. The data presented here are part of a long-term research project in which I am currently engaged, analyzing the economic and social consequences of neoliberalism. Living and working in both the United States and Europe provide the advantage of not only easy access to international and national data, but also the ability to observe firsthand the impact and consequences of neoliberal policies. No other OECD country, for example, has followed these policies as closely and extensively as the United States. Since the election of President Reagan in 1980, other countries have also adopted such policies; consequently, there is now sufficient empirical information in the United States and elsewhere to allow scholars to study the evidence put forward by advocates of the neoliberal thesis in support of their position. Needless to say, many years ago, when neoliberalism began its successful journey to implementation, its scientific validity could be sustained only by its internal coherence in its critique of what was then defined as Keynesianism—the then-dominant theoretical frame in economic and social policies. Today, however, 20 years later, we have enough empirical evidence to determine whether its scientific credibility can be sustained. The evaluation of this empirical evidence is the purpose of the first section of this chapter.[1]

IMPACT OF NEOLIBERAL POLICIES ON ECONOMIC PERFORMANCE

Economic Growth, Inflation, and Profits

One claim made by neoliberal authors in support of the superiority of neoliberal policies is the increased rate of economic growth experienced in the 1980s, which is assumed to have resulted from the implementation of important elements of neoliberal policies in the OECD countries. This superiority of neoliberal policies seems to be confirmed by Table 1, for example, which shows that the rate of economic growth was higher in the 1980s than in the 1970s. However, this table shows two other equally important realities that question the

[1] In this section, I am profoundly indebted to the work of several colleagues, including the late David Gordon, Professor of Economics at the New School for Social Research in New York (whose death was an enormous loss for the international academic community), and John Schmitt of the Economic Policy Institute in Washington, D.C. Also, a debt is owed to Professor John Eatwell of Cambridge University. Their assistance is greatly appreciated.

Table 1

Annual growth rate of total output (GDP) for the period 1960–1993, in percent[a]

	1960–73	1973–79	1979–82	1982–90	1990–93
United States	4.0	2.4	–0.1	3.6	1.2
Europe (OECD)	4.8	2.6	0.9	2.7	0.6
Japan	9.6	3.6	3.7	4.5	2.1
OECD	4.9	2.7	0.8	3.5	1.1

[a]Sources: OECD, *Historical Statistics* and *Economic Outlook.* Figures for 1993 from OECD, July 1993, Table 2.1.

superiority of such policies. First, the rate of economic growth in the 1980s was lower than in the 1960s, when state interventionist economic policies were in full swing. Second, in the 1990s, when neoliberal policies were still in operation, the rate of economic growth declined quite substantially, to even lower levels than in the 1970s. If, rather than looking at the annual growth of GDP, we look at the GDP per capita and for longer periods in the 1990s (Table 2), we find that, for most of the developed OECD countries, the rate of growth was lower in the 1990s than in the 1980s, and lower in the 1980s than in the 1970s. Only in Germany, Denmark, Ireland, and Norway were rates of economic growth per capita greater in the period 1979–1997 than in the period 1979–1989. All these countries—all with highly regulated labor markets and extensive social protection—had greater economic growth than the United States. *From the data in Tables 1 and 2 one cannot conclude that neoliberal policies were more successful in stimulating economic growth than the state interventionist policies they replaced. Quite to the contrary: they were less successful.*

Needless to say, there was not a linear relationship between the rate of economic growth and the application of neoliberal public policies. But the point that merits stressing is that during the periods in which neoliberal public policies were applied, economic growth was slower in general than during the periods in which the public policies were state interventionist. Moreover, the United States and the United Kingdom, the countries where neoliberal policies were most strongly implemented, did not have better rates of economic growth per capita than other countries with more regulated labor markets and more extensive social protection.

The neoliberal policies, however, do seem to have been successful in controlling inflation. As is evident in Table 3, the rate of inflation was lower (except in Japan) in the 1990s than in the 1980s, and lower in the 1980s than in the 1970s. The table shows how the reduction of inflation was particularly accentuated in OECD-Europe. This reduced inflation was primarily the result of (*a*) the development of monetary and fiscal policies aimed at reducing inflation; (*b*) the growth

Table 2

Annual growth rate of total output (GDP) per capita for the periods 1973–1979, 1979–1989, and 1989–1997, in percent[a]

	1973–79	1979–89	1989–97
United States	2.5	1.8	1.1
Japan	3.5	3.2	1.7
Germany	3.1	1.7	1.8
France	3.0	1.8	1.0
Italy	3.1	2.3	1.0
United Kingdom	2.4	2.2	1.2
Canada	3.7	1.9	0.2
Australia	2.3	1.8	1.5
Austria	3.8	2.0	1.2
Belgium	3.0	1.8	1.2
Denmark	2.2	1.8	2.0
Finland	2.9	3.3	0.1
Ireland	3.4	2.7	5.7
Netherlands	2.4	1.3	1.9
New Zealand	0.8	1.8	0.8
Norway	4.3	2.2	3.2
Portugal	2.9	2.6	2.3
Spain	2.7	2.3	1.8
Sweden	1.7	1.8	0.2
Switzerland	1.3	1.6	–0.5

[a]Source: Schmitt, J., and Mishel, L. *An Evaluation of the G-7 Economies of the 1990s,* Table 1B. Economic Policy Institute, Washington, D.C., January 30, 1998.

Table 3

Average annual growth of inflation for the period 1973–1990, in percent[a]

	1973–79	1979–90	1990
OECD	8.8	5.2	4.4
Europe (OECD)	9.7	5.7	3.8
United States	8.0	4.6	4.1
Japan	8.1	1.9	2.1

[a]Source: OECD, Inflation, *Historical Statistics,* 1960–1990.

of unemployment, which had a moderating impact on the rate of wage increases; and (*c*) a decline in the price of raw materials in the international market, especially in the price of oil.

Another area where neoliberal policies have been successful is in increasing profit shares and profit rates, an increase that is particularly evident in the manufacturing sector. Table 4 shows how net profit share increased in manufacturing in the OECD countries (except Japan). This increase was especially evident in Europe, particularly in Great Britain, The Netherlands, Belgium, and Sweden, countries whose profit share increased by 10 percent (2). This profit increase was primarily the result of a decline in wages rather than an increase in investment, which did not occur. In some countries, such as Great Britain, the profit share increased substantially (even though wages also increased) because high unemployment led to an increase in productivity, primarily in sectors such as the coal and steel industry where unemployment increased markedly, producing the so-called "Thatcher productivity miracle." That miracle was based on an employment rate in 1989 that was one-third of that in 1945 (3). In most OECD countries, profit share increased at the cost of reduction in salary share and decline in the rate of wage increases (4). This situation has been particularly accentuated in the United States, where Lawrence Mishel (5) has shown that if the rate of profits of both manufacturing and financial capital had been the same in the 1980s as in the 1970s (rather than growing at an unprecedented speed), the rate of wage growth would have doubled from 1980 to 1990.

Business Investments

The impressive growth in profit rates and net profit shares that did occur in the 1980s did not produce an increase in the rate of investment. Quite the contrary. Table 5 shows how the rate of business investments declined both in business in general and in manufacturing in particular (with the exception of Japan). This decline challenges a basic tenet of the neoliberal position: the claim that there is a *direct relationship between profit rates and rate of business investment*. Actually, the entire neoliberal justification for calling for preferential treatment of business, facilitating the growth of profits, is to increase investments. But the remarkable

Table 4

Manufacturing profit shares, rate of annual change, in percent[a]

	OECD	E.U.	U.S.	Japan
1973–1979	–4	–6	–2	–13
1979–1989	+6	+8	+2	–0.8

[a]Source: reference 2, Figure 2.1

Table 5

Average annual growth rate of capital stock, in percent[a]

	1960–73	1973–79	1979–89
Business			
United States	3.7	3.7	3.5
Europe (OECD)	5.2	3.8	2.9
Japan	12.4	6.6	7.3
Manufacturing			
United States	4.0	3.9	2.3
Europe (OECD)	5.1	2.4	1.3
Japan	12.4	5.4	6.3

[a]Source: reference 2.

increase in profit rates and share during the 1980s did not translate into higher investment rates. Investment rates continued to decline, confirming Armstrong, Glyn, and Harrison's (2) thesis that growth of profits is not a necessary or sufficient condition for growth in the rate of investments.

Nor do we see any evidence for another basic thesis of the neoliberal position that justifies the preferential fiscal treatment of upper income groups: the claim that there is a positive relationship between growth of savings and increase in investments. As indicated above, this position assumes that the upper income groups are the social groups most able to save, and thus policies aimed at favoring these groups stimulate savings and investments. As is evident in Table 6, however, in the United States—which has some of the better statistics on savings and where neoliberal policies have been most fully developed—there was no relationship between net investments and personal savings or net private savings during the entire 1955–1989 period. The table shows that the rate of increase in savings was highest (8.2 percent) in the period 1973–1978, when state interventionist policies were still in effect, and declined considerably during the 1980s when neoliberal policies were operating at full steam. In the 1980s, savings declined along with the decline in fixed nonresidential investment. As Table 6 shows, there is no relationship between savings and investment: periods of high savings have been periods of low investment, and vice versa. Moreover, savings and investment declined at a time when neoliberal policies were most highly developed (6).

Side-by-side with the decrease in private investment was a decrease in public investment in most OECD countries, with major declines in Great Britain, Germany, Sweden, Belgium, Denmark, Australia, and New Zealand. And this brief summary of investments should conclude with yet another finding: the

Table 6

Net fixed non-residential investment and personal savings in the United States, as percent of potential output[a]

	Fixed investments	Personal savings	Net private savings
1955–59	2.8	4.6	7.6
1959–66	2.8	4.0	7.0
1966–73	3.8	5.0	7.4
1973–78	3.0	5.5	8.2
1978–89	2.6	3.7	5.0

[a]Source: Adapted from Gordon, D. The macro relationship between investment and saving. In *Macro-economic Policy after the Conservative Era,* edited by G. D. Epstein and H. M. Gintis, Table 3.2, p. 63. Cambridge University Press, Cambridge, England, 1995.

decline in private and public investments was accompanied by increased investment in services and finance, with a financial flow from the production of goods to the production of services and, most importantly, to financial transactions. All OECD countries underwent a notable increase in financial investment and a decline in productive investment (4, pp. 38, 39).

Productivity

The decline in the rate of increase in productive investment in Europe during the neoliberal period was accompanied by a decline in the rate of increase in productivity (both in general and in manufacturing) (Table 7). In some countries, however, productivity increased even though the rate of increase in investments declined; this was due to the large increase in unemployment, such as occurred in Thatcher's Britain, as mentioned above. In the United States and Japan productivity barely changed, although it increased in the manufacturing sector in the United States.[2] A similar picture appears when we look at the disaggregated data, the annual growth rates of labor productivity in the business sector during several periods: 1960–1973, 1973–1979, and 1979–1996 (Table 8). We can see that the rate of growth in productivity has been declining in most countries, including the United States, although it increased somewhat in the 1980s and 1990s.

Unemployment and Social Inequalities

Increased unemployment has been a trademark of the 1980s and 1990s (Table 9). In the OECD countries, only Australia, Sweden, and the United States had

[2] Overall productivity increased but productivity per employed person declined (see Table 14).

Table 7

Productivity growth, average annual percentage rate[a]

	U.S.	Japan	Europe
Business			
1960–73	2.2	8.6	4.8
1973–79	0.0	2.9	2.6
1979–90	0.5	3.0	2.2
Manufacturing			
1960–73	3.3	10.2	6.0
1973–79	1.2	4.5	4.0
1979–90	2.6	4.8	3.0

[a]Sources: OECD, *Economic Outlook,* June 1992, Table 48; and U.S. Bureau of Labor Statistics, *Monthly Labor Rev.,* April 1993, Table 50.

lower unemployment rates in 1990 than in 1980; in all other OECD countries, unemployment was higher. The growth in unemployment in all OECD countries was accompanied by an increase in wage inequalities, facilitated by deregulation of the labor markets (7, 8). This growth of wage inequality has not been uniform, however. Although highly accentuated in the case of the United States and the United Kingdom among men, it has not occurred in other OECD countries, such as Japan, Germany, and France (Table 10). This increase in salary differentials was accompanied in most European countries by a lessening of progressive fiscal policies, with an increase in indirect taxes and reduction of the top tax rates (Table 11). In Belgium, France, Germany, Luxembourg, and Great Britain direct taxation declined (9, Table A.8.2), and the United States and Great Britain saw the largest reduction in top tax brackets, with a 40 percent decrease in their tax rates. All these countries experienced *an increase in social inequalities, with an increase in capital and a decline in labor's share* (4, p. 50).

Social Expenditures

Another factor contributing to the growth of social inequalities was the reduced rate of increase in social expenditures stimulated by neoliberal policies. The average annual rate of increase in these expenditures for the OECD countries during the 1970s had been 8.2 percent; this declined to 1.6 percent during the 1980s (see 10, Tables 5–10, for an analysis of the evolution of the different components of the social expenditures during these periods in the E.U. countries). The decline was particularly accentuated in Germany, Great Britain, The

Table 8

Labor productivity in the business sector, annual average growth rate, 1960–1996, in percent[a]

	1960–73	1973–79	1979–96
United States	2.6	0.6	0.8
Japan	8.4	2.8	2.2
Germany	4.5	3.1	1.1
France	5.3	2.9	2.2
Italy	6.4	2.8	2.1
United Kingdom	4.1	1.6	1.8
Canada	2.9	1.5	1.0
Australia	3.2	2.4	1.3
Austria	5.7	3.1	2.3
Belgium	5.2	2.7	2.0
Denmark	3.9	2.3	2.1
Finland	5.0	3.2	3.6
Ireland	4.8	4.3	3.9
Netherlands	4.9	2.6	1.6
New Zealand	2.1	–1.1	1.3
Norway	3.8	2.7	1.8
Portugal	7.5	0.5	2.4
Spain	6.0	2.8	2.8
Sweden	3.7	1.4	2.0
Switzerland	3.3	0.8	0.4

[a]Source: Schmitt, J., and Mishel, L. *An Evaluation of the G-7 Economies of the 1990s,* Table 2A. Economic Policy Institute, Washington, D.C., January 30, 1998.

Netherlands, and, to a lesser degree, in Belgium, Sweden, New Zealand, and Australia. In some countries, however, these expenditures increased, as was the case for Spain, France, Italy, Norway, Finland, and Greece (4, p. 28). (See section IV of this chapter for an analysis of the consequences of neoliberalism for the welfare state.)

Poverty and Family Debt

One consequence of the growth in social inequalities has been the growth in poverty in five of the 11 E.U. countries (particularly in Great Britain) and in the United States, as well as a decline in the internal demand by the popular

Table 9

Unemployment in the OECD, European Union, United States, and Japan[a]

	Unemployment, %	
	1974–79	1980–90
OECD	4.2	7.4
European Union	4.4	7.9
United States	6.7	7.2
Japan	1.9	2.5

[a]Source: Adapted from reference 4, Table 2.4, p. 26.

Table 10

Trends in male earnings dispersion ratio of 90th to 10th percentile earnings[a]

	1979	1989	1995
United States	3.18	4.04	4.35
Japan	2.59	2.85	2.77
Germany	2.38	2.29	2.25
France	3.39	3.49	3.43
Italy	2.29	2.17	2.64
United Kingdom	2.45	3.08	3.31
Canada	3.46	3.81	3.77
Australia	2.74	2.81	2.94
Austria	2.64	2.72	—
Belgium	—	2.26	—
Denmark	—	—	—
Finland	2.44	2.61	2.53
Ireland	—	—	—
Netherlands	—	—	—
New Zealand	—	2.85	3.17
Norway	—	—	—
Portugal	—	3.85	4.13
Spain	—	—	—
Sweden	2.11	2.16	2.20
Switzerland	—	2.44	2.54

[a]Source: Schmitt, J., and Mishel, L. *An Evaluation of the G-7 Economies of the 1990s,* Table 8A. Economic Policy Institute, Washington, D.C., January 30, 1998.

Table 11

Expenditures and revenues, as percent of GNP[a]

	Public expenses		Direct taxes		Indirect taxes		Social security contributions	
	1985	1994	1985	1994	1985	1994	1985	1994
Belgium	61	56	19	16	11.8	11.6	15.8	16.4
Denmark	58	62	27	29	16.8	16	1.9	1.5
France	52	55	7.7	7.6	13	11.7	19.3	19.5
Germany	47	49	13.3	12.2	9.8	10.6	13.9	15.2
Luxembourg	50	53	22	17	12	13.7	12.6	13.7
Netherlands	58	55	11.6	14.7	11.3	12.1	19.5	18.2
Great Britain	44	42	15	12	11.7	12.1	6.8	6.3
Italy	50	55	12	16	8.8	11.4	12	13.3
Portugal	43	42	8	9	13.5	14.2	8.2	8.4
Spain	52	48	7.5	11.7	8.3	10.7	11.9	14.6
Greece	48	57	6.1	7.4	15	18	12.5	12.4
Ireland	51	42	12.6	14.2	16	14	5.4	5.5

[a]Source: reference 9, Figure A.8.2, p. 296.

classes (11). Wages declined as a percentage of national income in most OECD countries, and during the 1980s family savings declined by 7 percent in Norway, Italy, Sweden, Great Britain, Finland, and France, forcing families to borrow and thus (because of the high interest rate) increasing family debt. Only Germany and Italy were able to avoid this situation. Great Britain, on the other hand, experienced the largest increase in family debt ever, doubling it in ten years. Interest payment increased from 4.1 percent of family income in 1978 to 8.6 percent in 1989. The large number of family bankruptcies is an indicator of the damaging consequences of such an increase for a very large number of families.

Business Credit

It was the marked increase in the rate of profit and profit shares during the 1980s that allowed many large enterprises to self-finance their investments. Small businesses, however, had severe problems in getting credit because of the very high interest rates, especially in Europe. This situation was particularly accentuated in Spain, with one of the highest interest rates in Europe. Besides difficulty in obtaining credit, small businesses faced yet another problem: the enormous instability of capital markets (national and international) with volatile currency exchanges. This volatility explains the extreme mobility of the financial markets, which together with the deregulation of these markets was a major cause of economic instability.

As we can see from this brief summary of economic and social indicators during 1979–1996, a period dominated by neoliberal public policies, *the "success" of these policies is highly questionable.* Except for control of inflation and growth of profits, most other indicators (such as economic growth, unemployment rate, rate of investment, productivity, growth of social inequalities, and poverty rate) are less than impressive, particularly when compared with the economic and social performance of the 1960s and 1970s when state interventionist policies were dominant. Table 12 shows how, along with control of inflation and growth in the rate and share of profits (the success stories), there has been an increase in unemployment and poverty in most OECD and E.U. countries. We have also seen the growth in wage differentials that these policies have facilitated, along with a spectacular growth in inequalities (to be discussed later), due to economic and fiscal policies that favor large employers and the best-off in the OECD and E.U. countries. The social costs of these policies have been quite high, and these costs include massive unemployment, one of the largest social problems in these countries.

II. CAUSES OF UNEMPLOYMENT

In this era of high unemployment, it is sometimes difficult to remember that in the post World War II period, up to the early 1970s, the majority of OECD countries had full employment. International trade increased substantially during this same period, with a rate of growth unseen before or since. The world experienced huge economic growth and productivity increases, with the largest-ever surge of internal and international demand (including in the developing countries) due to a much increased demand for products from the developed world. This was, after all, as aptly defined by Marglin and Schor (12), the "golden age of capitalism."

It was during this time that state interventionism became dominant in public policy circles. According to these policies (partially influenced by Keynes), wage increases, along with the expansive social expenditures and redistributive policies of the welfare state (favoring consumption by the popular classes), stimulated the internal aggregate demand. Moreover, social expenditures were perceived as an investment in human capital, responsible for the increases in labor productivity. The welfare state, according to state interventionist thought, also fostered social cohesiveness and the establishment of a social pact between labor and capital that facilitated economic growth and increased productivity. The state played a critical role in this theoretical framework (*a*) by expanding social consumption as a way of increasing internal demand to reach full employment and as a way of

Table 12

Economic and social indicators, 1973–1990[a]

	Average annual rate of inflation, %		Profit shares in manufacturing, % variation		Unemployment, %		Poverty, as % of population below 50% of median income	
	1973–79	1979–89	1973–79	1979–89	1974–79	1979–89	1980	1979–85, change
OECD	8.8	5.2	−3.7	5.6	4.2	7.4	—	—
United States	8.0	4.6	−3.0	1.8	6.7	7.2	—	—
Japan	8.1	1.9	−13.0	−0.5	1.9	2.5	—	—
Sweden	10.6	8.1	−7.3	11.1	1.9	2.4	5	—
Finland	12.6	7.4	5.2	3.9	4.4	4.9	—	—
Norway	8.2	6.9	−0.3	−0.5	1.8	2.8	5	—
Austria	6.1	3.9	—	—	1.5	3.3	—	—
Denmark	10.2	5.9	−2.8	6.9	5.5	8	13	2.3
Belgium	8.1	4.3	−11	14	6.3	10.8	8	−0.7
Netherlands	7.4	2.6	0.0	15	4.9	9.7	9	0.8
Germany	4.7	3.1	−3.1	2.5	3.2	5.9	5	1.7
France	10.9	6.8	−4.6	2.1	4.5	9	18	−0.2
Italy	17.1	11.3	2.7	3.1	6.6	9.5	9	2.3
United Kingdom	16	7	−7	10.8	5	10	8	2.8
Ireland	14	7.6	−1.5	—	7.6	15.6	17	5.1
Spain	18	9	—	—	5.2	17.5	20	−0.5
Greece	15	18	—	—	1.9	6.6	24	−0.2
Portugal	19	18	—	—	6	7.3	28	0.2

[a]Sources: Inflation: OECD, *Historical Studies,* 1960–1990; and OECD, *Economic Outlook,* 1993. Profit shares: OECD, *Historical Studies,* 1960–1990; and reference 2. Unemployment: OECD, *Historical Statistics* and *Economic Outlook.* Poverty: Bundrman, B., et al. Equivalence scales, wellbeing, inequalities and poverty. *Rev. Income and Welfare* 34(2): 115–142, 1988; and O'Higgins, M., and Jenkins, S. Poverty in the EEC. In *Analysing Poverty in the European Community,* edited by R. Teekens and Van Prage, 1990.

stabilizing economic cycles, and (*b*) by regulating capital markets to prevent a financial crisis, guiding investments toward productive sectors and halting the flow of capital, thus enabling the country to reassert its sovereignty (12). The low unemployment or full employment during this period resulted from the implementation of state interventionist policies, carried out by governments of very different political hues—let's not forget that even U.S. President Richard Nixon, a Republican, defined himself as a Keynesian. It was none other than President Nixon's Secretary of Defense, Caspar Weinberger, who described the U.S.

Defense Department as directing the largest industrial policy in the West. He was right. But these policies, as indicated in the previous section, went farther than Keynesianism. They included the active, direct intervention of the state in the spheres of production through active industrial policies largely responsible for the remarkable growth of productivity after World War II (13; see especially the chapter by Hooks (14)). It was these policies, together with the Keynesian policies of stimulation and manipulation of demand, that became the dominant state interventionist policies finally adopted by the social democratic parties and the labor movement in the European Union and by the New Dealers in the United States, later to be reproduced by other political movements as well. These were the social democratic decades, regardless of who was in power.

After the 1970s, however, unemployment increased in all OECD countries, and in particular in the OECD-Europe countries. As Table 13 shows, West Germany had the largest increases in unemployment rate in OECD-Europe (although its starting point was quite low). In some countries, such as Italy, the growth in the unemployment rate was not so marked, but the starting point was much higher than in Germany. Other countries such as the United States, Canada, and Japan also experienced increased unemployment.

This increase in unemployment was first interpreted as a consequence of the oil crisis and increased oil prices, which forced many governments to slow their rate of economic growth. Such an explanation is now difficult to accept, however, given the continuing growth in the unemployment rate in the 1980s and 1990s. Moreover, the price increases of some critical raw materials that occurred during the Korean War and the sudden increase in the price of oil in 1986 did *not* trigger a growth in unemployment such as that seen in the 1970s. It seems that variations in the price of oil or other raw materials cannot explain the massive increase in unemployment.

Table 13

Unemployment in G-7 countries, 1964–1973 and 1983–1992: Average unemployment rate for each decade, percent[a]

	1964–73 (*A*)	1983–92 (*B*)	Ratio (*B/A*)
West Germany	0.79	6.03	7.63
France	2.23	9.70	4.35
Italy	5.48	10.13	1.85
Great Britain	2.94	9.79	3.33
United States	4.46	6.69	1.50
Canada	4.23	9.64	2.28
Japan	1.22	2.71	2.22

[a]Source: OECD, *Main Economic Indicators,* 1964–1992.

Another consideration merits attention here: the limited response of the unemployment rate to variations in the economic cycle. Until recently, periods of economic expansion were accompanied by creation of employment, even though in each successive expansionary period the rate of job production was slower than in the last. Also, for each period of recession, the unemployment rate was higher than in the previous recession. And to further complicate matters, recent periods of economic expansion have not produced any increases in employment (15). The relationship between employment/unemployment and the economic cycle has been substantially weakened. A most worrisome development. Why has this happened? Some other theories for the rise in unemployment are considered below.

New Technologies?

Besides the oil crisis of the early 1970s, another common theory about the cause of growing unemployment attributes the increase to the introduction of new labor-saving technologies, such as information and electronic technologies, that permit enhanced rationalization of the production, distribution, and administrative processes by eliminating jobs. Yet, if these new technologies were truly labor-saving, we would have expected an increase in productivity since they would allow the production of goods and services with less labor time. But we have not seen such a productivity increase. Quite the opposite; in the 1980s the rate of growth in productivity per employed person (including in the manufacturing sector) declined in the majority of OECD countries, and this decline has continued into the 1990s (Table 14). As Eatwell (16) has indicated, because the rate of productivity growth during the 1980s and 1990s declined at a lower rate than the reduction in aggregate demand, employment has been maintained at levels that would not have been sustainable if the rate of productivity growth had remained the same as in the 1960s. The level of aggregate demand in the 1980s and 1990s was lower than in the 1960s (even in the manufacturing sector) due to a decline in the disposable income of the overall population, rather than a nonexistent market saturation. Large sectors of the OECD populations (not to mention populations in underdeveloped countries) lacked an adequate level of consumption. Further decline in this aggregate demand, nationally and internationally, due to the decline in disposable incomes and public expenditures (rather than the introduction of new technologies), has contributed to the slow economic growth and limited job production (17).

The thesis that new technologies are causing mass unemployment has been promoted by Jeremy Rifkin in his famous book, *The End of Work: The Decline of the Global Labor Force and the Dawn of the Post-Market Era* (18). He predicts in his book that the introduction of labor-saving technology will create a future without work. This thesis seems to be reinforced by the widely held perception that employers are constantly "downsizing" their labor force, assisted by the

Table 14

Productivity growth rate, GDP per employed person[a]

	1961–70 (*A*)	1981–90 (*B*)	Ratio (*B/A*)
West Germany	4.3	1.9	0.45
France	5.0	2.0	0.40
Italy	6.2	1.9	0.31
Great Britain	3.3	2.0	0.60
United States	1.9	1.1	0.58
Japan	9.1	3.0	0.33
	Manufacturing		
	1964–73 (*A*)	1983–92 (*B*)	Ratio (*B/A*)
West Germany	4.0	2.4	0.60
France	5.3	2.6	0.49
Italy	5.1	2.6	0.51
Great Britain	4.2	3.6	0.85
United States	3.1	2.8	0.90
Canada	4.0	2.6	0.65
Japan	9.6	5.7	0.59

[a]Source: OECD, *Main Economic Indicators*, 1961–1992.

introduction of new technologies. The mainstream press, such as the *New York Times* and the *Washington Post*, constantly refer to the spectacular downsizing of General Motors (a quarter of a million jobs lost in 1978–1993), General Electric (170,000 jobs lost in 1981–1993), U.S. Steel (100,000 job lost in 1980–1990), and many other companies as indicators of a future of mass unemployment created by the introduction of technologies.

And yet, the reality is different. *There is no evidence that the introduction of new technologies is behind the increase in unemployment. Nor is there evidence that the amount of work is declining*. Quite the contrary: the overall number of working hours per week has been increasing (during 1960–1990) in all the G-7 countries, precisely those countries at the forefront of technological innovation. And it has been in the United States and Japan (the countries with the greatest technological innovation) that the working hours per week have been increasing most rapidly (19, Fig. 2).

Another reality that refutes the "end of work" thesis is the constancy in the average rate of job production in the major capitalist societies over long periods. In the United States, for example, the rate of job production during the period

1974–1995 was 1.8 percent, slightly below the 2 percent rate during 1960–1973. A similar situation occurred (on average) for the 12 E.U. countries, whose average rate of job production during the period 1974–1995 (0.2 percent) was only slightly lower than the rate during 1960–1973 (0.3 percent). Thus no major decline in the rate of job production has occurred in the United States or in the European Union, despite a major increase in the rate of technological innovation on both continents. Moreover, the almost constant rate of job growth on both continents occurred within a context of a dramatic decline in the rate of economic growth in both the United States and the European Union. The annual rate of economic growth for the United States declined quite significantly, from 4.3 percent in 1960–1973 to 2.5 percent in 1974–1995. Similarly for the European Union, the rate declined from 4.8 percent in the first period to 2.2 percent in the second period. Given this large decline in the annual rate of economic growth on the two continents while the rate of job production remained practically the same, we must conclude that *the ability of the economy to produce jobs increased rather than declined* during these 30 years. If the "end of work" theories were correct, the ability of these economies to produce jobs would have declined rather than increased with the increasing introduction of technology! The reasons for increased unemployment, therefore, are to be found somewhere other than in the introduction of new technologies.

Finally, another reality that contradicts the "end of work" thesis is that in the last 20 years we have seen significant variations in the rate of job production within the E.U. countries, variations that cannot be explained by the different rates of technological introduction in those countries.

Thus we have not seen a decline in the ability of these countries to produce jobs. What we have witnessed, instead, is a significant change in the types of jobs that are being produced. Table 15 shows the changes in self-employment, part-time work, and temporary work as percentages of overall employment from 1973 to 1993 in all major OECD countries. But even here we cannot detect an overall pattern of change. Self-employment and temporary work have increased in some countries and declined in others. The only change that may represent a real trend is the growth of part-time work. In most of the countries shown in Table 15, there has been an increase in the percentage of all work that is part-time. But these changes are unlikely to be related to the introduction of technologies.

Another point worth clarifying is that, contrary to Rifkin's claims, there has not been a general trend toward job insecurity. As the International Labor Organization survey of employment for 1996–1997 shows, job security (measured as the number of years that a worker stays in the same job) has remained fairly steady, or has increased—even after standardizing by demographic structure, a standardization that is required since a more mature population has more stable employment than a younger one (19, p. 35). The only two exceptions are the United States and Spain, where job security has declined for both women and men. As the ILO report indicates, only these two countries have seen declines

Table 15

Type of work (work modalities) other than full-time work[a]

	Self-employment (in non-agricultural sector), % of all employment		Part-time work				Temporary work, % of all employment	
			% of all employment		Women, %	Involuntary, %		
	1973	1993	1973	1993	1993	1993	1989	1993
United States	6.7	7.7	15.6	17.5	66.2	30.7	—	—
Canada	6.2	8.6	9.7	17.2	68.9	36.0	—	—
United Kingdom	7.3	11.9	16.0	23.3	84.5	15.3	5.5	5.7
Japan	14.0	10.3	13.9	21.1	67.7	9.2	10.3	10.8
Germany	9.1	7.9	10.1	15.1	88.6	10.9	9.9	10.32
France	11.4	8.8	2.9	13.7	83.3	39.7	3.3	10.0
Italy	23.1	24.2	6.4	5.4	70.5	47.7	6.6	5.8
Spain	16.3	18.7	—	6.6	75.6	19.6	15.6	32.0
Portugal	12.7	18.2	—	7.4	66.3	25.8	13.1	8.6
Greece	31.0	28.2	—	4.3	61.6	—	16.2	9.3
Ireland	10.1	13.0	—	5.1	71.6	36.3	6.1	9.0
Belgium	11.2	13.3	3.8	12.8	89.3	33.7	5.4	4.7
Netherlands	9.2	8.7	—	33.4	75.7	17.9	5.8	10.0
Sweden	4.8	8.7	—	24.9	81.3	27.1	—	—
Austria	11.7	6.3	6.4	10.1	89.7	—	—	—
Norway	7.8	6.2	23.0	27.1	80.5	—	—	—
Finland	6.5	9.5	—	8.6	63.1	41.1	—	—
Denmark	9.3	7.0	—	23.3	74.9	23.5	12.5	10.7
Australia	9.5	12.9	11.9	23.9	75.3	32.4	—	—

[a]Source: reference 19, p. 26.

in security for those who have jobs, even when jobs are standardized by demographic factors.

International Trade?

Another frequently cited reason for mass unemployment in most OECD countries is the "invasion" of OECD markets by commodities produced in low-wage countries, particularly those of the Pacific Rim—an invasion that has destroyed jobs in employment sectors affected by this competition. An abundant pool of cheap labor in such countries and an increased mobility of manufacturing are replacing labor and destroying jobs in the developed countries (20; for a critique of this argument, see 21). To support this thesis, its proponents refer to the vast growth in imported goods in the developed countries during the 1980s and 1990s. In the G-7 countries, for example, imports represented only 1 percent of all manufactured products consumed in 1968; this number had jumped to 10 percent by 1995 (16, p. 7). There is no question that these imports are destroying jobs (predominantly unskilled labor) in the affected employment sectors, but this has been accompanied by an *increase* in employment in the exporting sectors of the developed economies, whose exports have increased significantly. These exporting sectors tend to employ skilled labor. Thus it is not clear that international trade is causing a growth in unemployment in the developed countries. International trade destroys and produces jobs at the same time. There is a large body of literature produced by labor and trade economists that details the impact of foreign trade on unemployment. I will try to summarize this bibliography in a later section dealing with globalization. Suffice it to say here that despite considerable disagreement on the impact of foreign trade on employment, there is fairly widespread agreement that the growth of international trade is causing a change in the labor force, particularly in the manufacturing sector (the largest sector, by far, that produces tradable commodities). This change is shifting the labor force toward more skilled workers in developed capitalist countries, adding impetus to the process of educating the labor force, a point to be discussed later.

Another important consequence of international trade is its impact on wage levels in those sectors affected by increased international competition, and therefore its impact on inequalities. Indeed, the fear of jobs being moved to low-wage countries forces labor to accept reductions in wages and benefits that it would not otherwise tolerate. As David Gordon (22) has indicated, however, the lowering of wages is a general phenomenon that is also affecting sectors not subject to this international competition. There is no clear evidence, then, that trade is responsible for the growth of wage inequalities, at least to the degree that could explain the enormous growth of these inequalities (23).

Decline of Internal Demand and Liberalization of Financial Markets

While not denying the possible role of the forces discussed above in increasing unemployment, I believe the most important cause is the reduction in aggregate demand that has been responsible for the decline in economic growth during the 1980s and 1990s—a period in which the rate of economic growth in Europe, for example, was half that in the 1960s (24). This decline in economic growth occurred in most OECD countries, in the E.U. countries, and in the majority of the developing world, except for China and the countries of Southeast Asia, until recently.

A main reason for this decline in demand was the implementation of neoliberal policies, begun in the 1970s and fully developed in the 1980s and 1990s. Of the neoliberal policies that dramatically increased social inequalities, both within and among countries, a very important one was the liberalization of international financial markets. The collapse of the Bretton Woods agreements and the liberalization of currency exchanges that took place at the beginning of the 1970s created a much increased mobility of financial capital and equally impressive fluctuations in the value of foreign currencies. In the semiperipheral countries (such as Spain), with low internal demand, governments responded with a constant devaluation of the currency and establishment of monetarist policies that further reduced the internal demand, creating higher unemployment.

Another consequence of the liberalization of financial markets was the growth in financial mobility in search of higher and quicker profits (25). It is interesting to note, for example, that before the collapse of the Bretton Woods agreements, 90 percent of all currency exchanges corresponded to commercial transactions and long-term investments. After the collapse of Bretton Woods, however, an impressive 88 percent of all these transactions were of a speculative nature. The daily financial flows that respond to speculative activities are larger than the monetary reserves of all G-7 governments put together (16, p. 10). It is easy to see that the liberalization of financial markets and currency exchanges has created an extremely unstable economic climate in which speculative transactions can overpower any state. This power of the financial markets is based on their ability to penalize any government that they deem "irresponsible." Governments, aware of this reality, then formulate economic policies with the primary objective of being perceived by the financial markets as "respectable," "credible," and "acceptable." A key element of "respectability" is the implementation of monetary policies acceptable to the financial markets. It is interesting to note that because financial markets respond to information and perceptions rather than to the reality behind them, these markets operate according to perceptions framed within a financial culture having little scientific value but enormous ideological content. As Eatwell notes (16, p. 38):

> Money markets and foreign exchange markets become dominated by simple slogans—larger fiscal deficits lead to higher interest rates, an increased money supply results in higher inflation, public expenditures bad, private expenditures good—even when those slogans are persistently refuted by events.

This heavily ideological culture, full of slogans and empty of scientific credibility, becomes the guide for governments' monetary and fiscal policies. Their primary objective, then, is to be seen as "credible" by the financial markets. And part of that "credibility" and "maturity" is keeping interest rates high, public deficits low, and public expenditures low. The high interest rates together with the instability of international markets affect production most substantially, slowing down economic growth and increasing unemployment. The high interest rates, and the fluctuations, variability, and instability of the currency and monetary markets, affect primarily the small enterprises responsible for most new job production.

A final point about the financial markets. Given the great instability and variability of money and currency markets, it is extremely difficult or practically impossible to coordinate the fiscal policies of the E.U. countries or of the G-7 countries—a cooperation that is essential for a collective response to the enormous problem of unemployment. Such a response requires (*a*) coordination of the rate of currency exchange to eliminate currency fluctuations, one of the primary reasons for the international flows of speculative money, and (*b*) regulation of the financial markets.The current lack of coordination and regulation is due to the absence, in Europe and elsewhere, of institutions that could realize such coordination; there is a huge resistance by the financial markets to the establishment of such institutions. Yet, as Lester Thurow (26) has indicated, it is this political unwillingness and inability to regulate the international financial markets that explains the high interest rates, one of the most important causes of high unemployment. And it is precisely this, rather than the supposed rigidity of the labor markets, that is, in part, contributing to the unemployment in Europe. The European labor markets have been much less rigid in the 1980s and 1990s than they were in the 1970s when unemployment was much lower. Actually, the liberalization of labor markets in the 1980s and 1990s occurred along with the growth in unemployment.

Based on this brief survey of the evidence supporting or questioning the various theories put forward to explain unemployment (to be expanded on later in this chapter), we can conclude that neoliberal policies—which increase social inequalities, decrease aggregate demand, stimulate speculative financial flows, create economic, financial, and monetarist instability, and produce high interest rates—are major causes of unemployment in Europe. The dominant economic culture continues to support these neoliberal positions, despite the evidence for their failure to create jobs and improve the standard of living for the majority of our populations, because these policies have created a dramatic increase in the standard of living for the wealthiest sectors (27). These sectors have increased their power and influence in western societies, shaping the contours of the economic and political discourse, which claims that the interests of the bourgeoisie and allied classes are indeed universal—the interests of everyone. The popular classes, the majority of people in our societies, have not benefited from these policies.

III. EUROSCLEROSIS VERSUS U.S. DYNAMISM

One of the most persistent arguments put forth in support of neoliberal policies is their success in the United States, the country in which such policies have been most highly developed. In this argument, the United States is presented as a dynamic and vibrant economy, in contrast to the stale, sclerotic European economies. As expressed in an editorial in *The Economist*, one of the most influential neoliberal periodicals, "Reality speaks for itself. America's phenomenal success in creating new jobs contrasts with Europe's abject failure to do so" (28). The same editorial attributes the U.S. success to its greater labor flexibility and lesser social protection. The OECD secretariat, another neoliberal international think-tank, has until recently adopted a similar position. The OECD has presented the United States as an example for Europe, advising its member countries to implement policies that have already proved so successful in the United States: that is, to make their labor markets more flexible, to cheapen the price of labor, and to decrease social protection and unemployment insurance coverage (29).

In support of their thesis, *The Economist*, the OECD, and other neoliberal agents cite (*a*) the creation of 18 million jobs in the United States during the 1980s (when the neoliberal policies were fully implemented), a much larger number of new jobs than in any other OECD country; (*b*) the creation of 10 million jobs during the period 1993–1997; and (*c*) the low unemployment rate (5.4 percent) in the United States in 1997, lower than in most OECD countries.

The citing of 18 million new jobs as proof of the potency of the U.S. economy is highly misleading, however. It is incorrect to use the absolute number of jobs produced by an economy as an indicator of its job-producing ability. A large country, after all, is likely to produce more jobs than a small one. A much better indicator of job-producing ability is the *rate of job creation*: the new jobs created in a certain time period as a percentage increase over the number of jobs existing at the start of that period. For example, the second column in Table 16 (new jobs as percentage of total employment in 1979) shows that from 1979 to 1989, employment in the United States increased by 18.7 percent, compared with a 26.5 percent increase in Austria and 20.1 percent increase in Canada. These latter countries were more successful than the United States in producing employment, even though they have less labor flexibility and more social protection. Moreover, the fourth column of Table 16 shows that, from 1989 to 1992 (when neoliberal policies were in effect), the rate of job creation in the United States was 0.2 percent, *the lowest among all OECD countries with growth in employment, including The Netherlands (6.6 percent), Japan (5.2 percent), Italy (1.9 percent), Western Germany (5.3 percent), and France (0.8 percent). The table shows that, contrary to the claims of* The Economist *and the OECD, the United States was not more successful than other countries (with more extensive welfare states and more regulated labor markets) in producing employment during the period 1979–1992.*

A similar situation has occurred since 1992. Here again, the 10 million new jobs created from 1993 to 1997 are presented as further proof of the job-producing miracle of the U.S. economy, but 10 million new jobs in a labor force

Table 16

Jobs produced in 10 countries (G-7 plus Austria, Sweden, and The Netherlands), 1979–1992[a]

	Jobs created in 1979–89, thousands	New jobs, as % of employment in 1979	Jobs created in 1989–92, thousands	New jobs, as % of employment in 1989
Austria	1,617	26.5	–34	–0.4
Canada	2,091	20.1	–246	–2.0
France	550	2.6	180	0.8
Germany	1,730	6.8	1,450	5.3
Italy	840	4.2	400	1.9
Japan	6,460	12.0	3,120	5.2
Netherlands	730	13.7	400	6.6
Sweden	364	8.7	–218	–4.8
Great Britain	1,410	5.7	–890	–3.4
United States	18,518	18.7	256	0.2

[a]Source: reference 53, p. 223.

of 120 million represent an annual growth of about 1 percent, which is a lower rate of job production than in the period 1979–1989 (1.7 percent), and much lower than in the pre-neoliberal decade, 1969–1979 (2.4 percent). During this period the rate of job production has been lower in the United States than in several European countries. In 1996, for example, Spain, the European country with the highest unemployment (20 percent), had a higher job production rate (1.8 percent) than the United States. Other Western European countries—Ireland, The Netherlands, and Norway—also had higher job production rates than the United States.

These figures show that in any given year, some countries with more generous welfare states and more regulated labor markets have higher rates of job production than the supposedly miraculous United States.

Moreover, if we analyze the gross rates of job production rather than the net rates, we find even more compelling evidence that the image of sclerosis in the E.U. countries and dynamism in the United States is a great simplification. Table 17 shows that during the 1980s and 1990s and for similar economic cycles, Denmark, France, and Sweden (all with more regulated labor markets and more comprehensive welfare states than the United States) had *higher* gross rates of job production than the United States. Moreover, a more detailed look (Table 17) also shows that while the United States was more successful than France, Denmark, and Sweden in producing jobs through the opening of new establishments, these

Table 17

Job creation and job destruction in the United States and selected E.U. countries, average annual rates as percent of total employment[a]

	Denmark 1983–89	Finland 1986–91	France 1984–92	Germany 1983–90	Italy 1984–92	Sweden 1985–92	U.K. 1985–92	U.S. 1984–91
1. Gross job gains	16.0	10.4	13.9	9.0	12.4	14.5	8.7	13.0
Openings	6.1	3.9	7.2	2.5	3.9	6.5	2.7	8.4
Expansions	9.9	6.5	6.7	6.5	8.4	8.0	6.0	4.6
2. Gross job losses	13.8	12.0	13.2	7.5	11.1	14.6	6.6	10.4
Closures	5.0	3.4	7.0	1.9	3.8	5.0	3.9	7.3
Contractions	8.8	8.7	6.3	5.6	7.3	9.6	2.7	3.1
3. Net employment change	2.2	–1.6	0.6	1.5	1.3	–0.1	2.1	2.6
4. Job turnover	29.8	22.4	27.1	16.5	23.4	29.1	15.3	23.4

[a]Source: OECD, *Employment Outlook*, 1995.

three countries, as well as Italy, Germany, Finland, and the United Kingdom, were more successful than the United States in producing new jobs through the expansion of existing establishments. Why, then, did these European countries not have a higher net rate of job production than the United States? The answer becomes clear when we look at the second row of Table 17: the rate of job destruction was higher in this group of European countries (except Germany and the United Kingdom) than in the United States. Most of these job losses in Europe were due to firms reducing employment (contractions) rather than closing down (closures)—precisely the opposite of the situation in the United States. Notice, incidentally, that by summing the jobs created and jobs destroyed we find a higher turnover rate (a major indicator of labor flexibility) in these European countries (except Germany and the United Kingdom) than in the United States.

A critical difference, therefore, between the European Union and the United States in this period was the higher rate of job loss in the E.U. countries. Why did this occur? One explanation put forward by conservative and neoliberal authors alike is that labor market rigidities and excessive social protection in Europe have been (and remain) responsible for the higher rate of job loss. But if that were the case, how would these authors explain the higher gross rate of job production in three of the most regulated labor markets—Sweden, Denmark, and France—than in the United States? And how would they explain the higher rate of job expansion in *all* major European countries than in the United States? Those who support the arguments about "excessive" rigidity and social protection cannot have it both ways.

A more plausible answer is rooted in the different evolution of the economic and employment structures on each side of the Atlantic. The European countries have (on average, for the entire continent) an economic and employment structure that resembles that of the United States of 30 years ago. This 30-year delay explains why, in the European Union, 12 percent of the total employment is in agriculture (versus 1.2 percent in the United States) and 14 percent in industry (versus 11 percent in the United States). Consequently, the pool of jobs to be destroyed is larger in Europe than in the United States. And these jobs are indeed being destroyed faster in Europe (Table 18), because the rate of productivity growth is higher (in both employment sectors) in Europe. This is occurring within a worldwide context of demand stagnation. Services, however, are growing at a rather similar rate on both sides of the Atlantic. As Table 19 shows, the composition of the services sector is different in Europe and the United States. For example, more people are employed in commerce, business, and social and personal services in the United States than in Europe. But Table 19 also shows that the rate of employment growth in social and personal services (the largest employment component of the services sector on both continents) is larger in the European Union, but not large enough to absorb the flow of job seekers displaced from agriculture and industry. This, incidentally, is why the French government wants to expand the rate of growth in community and social service employment

Table 18

Annual growth of employment per capita[a] in different economic sectors during the period 1973–1990 for the United States and OECD-Europe, in percent[b]

	Agriculture	Industry	Services
United States	−1.6	−0.7	1.5
OECD-Europe	−3.9	−1.6	1.3

[a]The annual growth of employment (per capita) is the annual growth of employment minus the annual growth of the active population.
[b]Source: OECD, *Historical Studies*.

Table 19

Employment in services, United States versus OECD-Europe[a]

	Commerce	Transport and communications	Business and finance	Social services	
Employment, as % of all employed population, 1992				Private and community	
OECD-Europe	18.4	6.0	8.5	29.1	
United States	22.2	5.6	13.2	31.5	
Annual growth of employment per capita, average for 1979–1990				Private	Public
OECD-Europe	0.6	−0.4	3.3	2.7	0.6
United States	0.9	0.2	3.3	2.2	0.2

[a]Source: OECD, *Historical Studies*, 1979–1992.

through public funding and subsidy of that sector. It also shows that *the welfare state, rather than being a drag on the economy, contributes to the creation of employment.*

The historical delay in the European economic and employment structure has another consequence that further complicates the employment situation in Europe: the lower percentage of women and young people in the European labor force than in the U.S. labor force. To the degree that this situation is changing (and it is changing very rapidly), we are seeing an enormous growth in demand for jobs from women and young people in Europe—higher for both groups than in the United States. Actually, in the United States (with a percentage of women in the labor force that is one of the highest in the OECD, lagging only the Scandinavian countries) we have witnessed a decline in the number of young people looking for jobs. For example, 4.6 million fewer young people (aged 16–24 years) were looking for jobs in 1995 than in 1979. This is precisely the opposite of what is occurring in Europe, where more women and young persons are looking for jobs now than ten years ago.

Higher Unemployment in Europe than in the United States?

A detailed comparison of the rates of unemployment in the United States and the E.U. countries (Table 20) also fails to demonstrate the supposed sclerosis of the E.U. economies. This table shows the rates of unemployment for the period 1983–1996 (following the major recession of the early 1980s) and during the subperiods 1983–1988 and 1989–1994 that roughly coincide with the economic cycles of that period. As is evident from the table: (*a*) variability in unemployment rates was greater among the E.U. countries than between the United States and the European Union; (*b*) for the period 1983–1996, the United States had higher annual unemployment (6.5 percent) than Sweden (4.3 percent), Portugal (6.4 percent), Norway (4.2 percent), Western Germany (6.2 percent), and Austria (3.8 percent); (*c*) for the period 1983–1988, the United States had higher unemployment (7.1 percent) than Sweden (2.6 percent), Norway (2.7 percent), Italy (6.9 percent), Western Germany (6.8 percent), Finland (5.1 percent), and Austria (3.6 percent); and (*d*) for the period 1989–1994, the United States had higher unemployment (6.2 percent) than Sweden (4.4 percent), Portugal (5.0 percent), Norway (5.5 percent), Western Germany (5.4 percent), and Austria (3.7 percent). Actually, for the *entire period 1983–1996, about 30 percent of the OECD-European population lived in countries with average unemployment rates lower than the U.S. rate* (30).

Recently, however, the U.S. unemployment rate has been lower (5.4 percent) than the E.U. average (11.5 percent). But people can drown in a river that is—on average—only two feet deep! Averages do not reveal the enormous variability of unemployment rates within Europe. According to the OECD *Employment Outlook* report of 1997 (31, Table B, p. 163), the U.S. unemployment rate in 1996 was higher than in Switzerland (3.8 percent), Norway (4.9 percent), Luxembourg (3.3 percent), Ireland (3.7 percent), and Austria (5.3 percent), and only one percentage point lower than in Denmark and The Netherlands. The United Kingdom, with the least regulated labor market in the European Union, had one of the largest unemployment rates (8.2 percent), higher than in Sweden (8.0 percent), Portugal (7.5 percent), and the other countries listed above.

Is the relatively low unemployment in the United States due to its more flexible markets and lower social protection? Not necessarily. As I have shown, other countries with more regulated labor markets and greater social protection maintain lower unemployment rates than the United States. Moreover, young,

Table 20

Unemployment rates in the United States and OECD-Europe, in percent[a]

	1983–96 Total	1983–88 Total	1989–94 Total
Austria	3.8	3.6	3.7
Belgium	9.7	11.3	8.1
Denmark	9.9	9.0	10.8
Finland	9.1	5.1	10.5
France	10.4	9.8	10.4
Germany (Western)	6.2	6.8	5.4
Ireland	15.1	16.1	14.8
Italy	7.6	6.9	8.2
Netherlands	8.4	10.5	7.0
Norway	4.2	2.7	5.5
Portugal	6.4	7.6	5.0
Spain	19.7	19.6	18.9
Sweden	4.3	2.6	4.4
Switzerland	1.8	0.8	2.3
United Kingdom	9.7	10.9	8.9
United States	6.5	7.1	6.2

[a]Source: reference 30, Table 1.

unskilled workers (the most vulnerable group in the labor market) have higher unemployment rates in the United States and Great Britain than in several E.U. countries. The answer is rooted in the data provided above on job production, job destruction, and rates of growth of job demand and job supply on both continents. In the United States the rate of job destruction is lower than the rate of job production, while the rate of growth in the demand for jobs has been declining faster than the rate of growth in the supply of jobs. Almost the reverse is the case for the European Union. The decline in the rate of growth in the demand for jobs in the United States is due to several factors, including (*a*) a greater number of people who have given up looking for work because of the poor quality of available jobs, (*b*) a larger dependency on part-time jobs by people who would prefer but cannot find full-time work, and (*c*) a larger number of people incarcerated. When these groups of people are included in the unemployment figures, the data on unemployment change quite significantly. Table 21 shows that, with the exception of Great Britain, unemployment rates for men (although not for women) are lower in the E.U. countries than in the United States. This table also shows that—contrary to the findings of the recent OECD report *Implementing the OECD Strategy* (32, p. 29)—the unemployment figures change quite

Table 21

Alternative measures of unemployment rates, as prepared by the U.S. Bureau of Labor Statistics, 1993, in percent[a]

	Women	Men[b]
France	17.7	11.2
Germany	16.5	7.3
Italy	21.9	8.8
Great Britain	10.5	14.3
United States	10.4	11.7
E-4	15.2	10.4

[a]The U.S. Bureau of Labor Statistics, in its estimates of unemployment among men, includes (for all cited countries) the number of people who are looking for a job, plus those who have given up looking for a job because they cannot find one, plus half of part-time job holders who would like to work full-time. Source: U.S. Bureau of Labor Statistics, 1993.

[b]The number of adult men (aged 16–64) incarcerated in each country has been added, from Maner, M. The international use of incarceration. *The Prison Journal,* March 1995, pp. 113–123; and *Statistical Abstract of the United States 1996,* Table 350. See reference 37.

considerably when these three groups of unemployed people are added to those counted in the official unemployment figures.

Another piece of information I should stress here is that unemployment rates for young people (15–24 years old) in some countries, for example Germany, are lower than in the United States, for both young men and women. For the period 1988–1995 the average rate of unemployment in Germany was 6.4 percent among young men, about half that in the United States (13 percent), and 7.1 percent among young women, much lower than in the United States (11.6 percent) (33). As these facts show, the supposed "rigidities" of the German market do not seem to hinder a major integration of new entrants into the labor force. Moreover, during the period 1984–1990 the unemployment rate in Germany among young male unskilled workers (making up 12 percent of all male workers) was 31.6 percent, almost identical to the rate, 32 percent, in the United States (where such workers represented 15 percent of all male workers) (34). These figures reveal almost identical possibilities for integration of young male unskilled workers into the labor market in both countries, even though jobs for these workers are better paid, have better benefits and social protection, and are less temporary in Germany than in the United States. A similar situation exists in Austria and Denmark, where jobs are also better paid, have better benefits and social protection, and are more long-term than in the United States. Actually, it is principally Great Britain—with the least regulated labor market of the OECD—that has a higher rate of unemployment among young male unskilled workers (35).

This reality refutes the widely held position among neoliberal and conservative authors that a good way of facilitating the integration of young male unskilled workers into the labor force is by lowering the wages, social protection, and security for these entry-level jobs. This position, which has become almost a dogma in neoliberal and conservative circles, is being reproduced despite the current evidence that clearly challenges it. As Nickell and Bell (36) have indicated in their detailed study of the impact of wages and insecurity on the employability of young unskilled workers, there is no evidence that the major unemployment in the European Union is a result of greater difficulty in finding jobs for unskilled workers in the European Union, or of higher wages, more social protection, and more secure jobs in the European Union than in the United States.

The same authors also show, incidentally, that the growth of unemployment in the United States and the E.U. countries (with the exception of Italy) is not concentrated only among the unskilled but also affects skilled workers. The OECD itself has indicated that one characteristic of the most recent recession was the destruction of jobs for both unskilled and skilled workers, including white-collar workers who had previously been considered to be unaffected by recessions. Moreover, the OECD has indicated that in the last economic recovery, the workers that saw the most rapid growth of employment were the unskilled workers (32, p. 38).

Social Protection in the Workplace: Comparisons between the United States and the European Union

The U.S. situation, as described in section II of this chapter, challenges a widely held neoliberal position that attributes the large unemployment in the E.U. countries to the overly generous social protection of European workers and, in particular, "excessive" unemployment insurance. Actually, unemployment insurance is much lower in Italy than in the United States, while unemployment is much higher in Italy. Moreover, unemployment has been increasing in the European Union while the comprehensiveness of unemployment benefits and the percentage of unemployed who receive them have declined quite considerably (32, p. 38).

The neoliberal position that attributes the higher unemployment in the European Union to more generous unemployment benefits and coverage also ignores the marked variability in such benefits and coverage within the European Union. In France, for example, 44 percent of the unemployed received unemployment benefits in 1991, compared with 64 percent in Germany, a meager 19 percent in Italy, 62 percent in the United Kingdom, and 34 percent in the United States. As to the degree of comprehensiveness of unemployment benefits, in France they represented 57 percent of salary for a 40-year-old worker with a spouse (without children) during the first three months of benefits coverage, compared with 40 percent in Germany, 15 percent in Italy, 24 percent in Great Britain, and 31 percent in the United States (37, Table 13). This degree of variability in the comprehensiveness and coverage of unemployment benefits does not have a direct and clear relationship with the rate of unemployment, either acute or chronic, the latter being the more problematic in the European Union. As noted above, Italy, with a very low coverage and comprehensiveness of benefits, has very high chronic unemployment (5.8 percent of the active population), while Germany, with some of the most generous unemployment benefits in the European Union, has a very low chronic unemployment (2.4 percent) (37, Table 6). All the available evidence seems to indicate that the comprehensiveness and duration of unemployment benefits help the unemployed to find a more attractive job, rather than fostering a situation of chronic unemployment. Indeed, studies of social psychology in the United States and in Sweden show that work is much wanted and much needed by the majority of the adult population, since work gives people a sense of purpose and identification with society—thus destroying the neoliberal's perception of the unemployed as lazy individuals who do not want to work.

In the light of all this evidence (in particular, the absence of a direct relationship between the "generosity" of unemployment benefits and rate of unemployment),[3] it is remarkable that the OECD, in one of its reports on unemployment, wrote of a wide consensus that the variability in the rate of unemployment in the OECD countries is related to the generosity of unemployment benefits coverage (32, p. 52). Contrary to the OECD's claims, no such consensus exists. Far from it. Not only is there plenty of evidence that questions such a direct relationship, but even the sources cited by the OECD in support of that consensus, such as the well-known studies by Atkinson and Micklewright (39), come to an opposite conclusion: there is no direct or clear relationship between unemployment insurance and the rate of unemployment. In recognition of this evidence, the OECD has finally had to accept that "there is not an immediate link between unemployment rates and unemployment benefit entitlements" (40, p. 17). It cannot be concluded, therefore, that higher unemployment in the European Union than in the United States is the result of Europe's higher unemployment benefits.

All these data show that the United States—the model for neoliberal authors—has not *necessarily* been more successful than other countries, with larger welfare states and more regulated markets, in producing jobs or reducing unemployment.

[3] There is an extensive literature reviewing the evidence (or lack of it) for a relationship between the level of comprehensiveness and coverage of unemployment benefits and the rate of unemployment. See the recent review questioning this relationship by Esping-Andersen (38).

The Causes of the Growing Inequalities: Wage and Benefits Inequalities in the United States versus the European Union

A similar situation appears when we analyze wages and fringe benefits. As is evident from Table 22, which compares the annual rates of growth of the top, median, and bottom deciles of salaries for men and women in several countries during the periods 1973–1979 and 1979–1990:

1. European salaries for men and for women have increased more rapidly than U.S. salaries (with the exception of the top decile of women in Italy, who had a lower salary growth than the top decile of women in the United States).
2. This larger growth in European than in U.S. salaries occurred for all deciles (with the exception noted above).
3. In the United States there was a decline in wages for men below the median wage and for the bottom decile of women.

This decline in wages in the United States has continued since 1990 (except for women in the top decile). Moreover, if we consider all workers, not just full-time workers, the hourly wages during the period 1979–1995 fell 6.9 percent, a decline that also affected the top decile, whose hourly wages fell 4.8 percent (41; 42, p. 7).

A similar decline has occurred in workers' fringe benefits (health and pension benefits). The percentage of workers with employer-provided health insurance coverage declined in the United States from 71 percent in 1979 to 69 percent in 1993, and employer-provided pension coverage declined from 48 to 45 percent during the same period (43). In the United States, one million persons lose their health benefits coverage every year.

One explanation of the decline in U.S. wages and benefits that is usually given by neoliberal authors is the growing percentage of the labor force that works in the services sector, which has a lower productivity and therefore lower salaries than manufacturing. But this argument is unsustainable, since the decline in wages and benefits has also occurred among manufacturing workers. Table 23 shows how hourly wages in manufacturing have been declining in the United States, while they have been increasing for the majority of OECD countries (with the exception of Denmark for the period 1979–1989).

The decline in wages and benefits affects skilled as well as unskilled workers, including professionals. The hourly income for professionals with an academic degree (with 1 to 5 years of experience) underwent an annual rate of decline of 1.59 percent for men and 1.28 percent for women from 1989 to 1995, showing that education is no protection against declines in income.

Nevertheless, this decline in the rate of growth of salaries has been more accentuated for the unskilled than the skilled sectors, and for the lower than for the higher echelons of the labor force. Only the top 8 percent has undergone a significant increase in the rate of wage growth. This situation has led to a very

Table 22

Rate of annual growth of wages in the top (90%), median (50%), and bottom (10%) deciles, in percent[a]

	Men		Women	
	1973–79	1979–90	1973–79	1979–90
France				
Top decile	2.4	1.1	3.2	1.8
Median decile	1.8	0.6	3.4	1.1
Bottom decile	2.0	0.6	3.0	0.7
Germany				
Top decile	—	3.7	—	4.7
Median decile	—	3.5	—	4.6
Bottom decile	—	4.2	—	4.4
Italy				
Top decile	—	2.2	—	1.6
Median decile	—	0.5	—	1.7
Bottom decile	—	2.0	—	3.9
Great Britain				
Top decile	—	3.4	—	4.2
Median decile	—	2.2	—	3.0
Bottom decile	—	1.2	—	2.0
United States				
Top decile	0.5	0.4	1.0	1.7
Median decile	0.5	–0.6	1.3	0.7
Bottom decile	0.5	–1.4	2.7	–0.4

[a]Source: OECD, *Employment Outlook,* 1993, Table 5.3.

fast and dramatic polarization of earnings for men and women in the United States. Tables 24 and 25 show how the United States has the largest wage polarization among those OECD countries where such information is available. It is interesting to note, incidentally, that similar, although less marked earnings inequalities have also occurred in other OECD countries, but this growth of earnings inequalities has not occurred in all countries. For example, a decline of earnings inequalities among men has occurred in Germany since 1979, and in Japan, France, Canada, and Finland since 1989. For women, a decline of earnings inequalities has occurred in Germany and Italy since 1979, and in Australia, Finland, and Switzerland since 1989.

Table 23

Hourly wages in manufacturing:
Average annual growth rate, 1979–1992[a]

	1979–89	1989–92
Canada	0.2	1.5
Denmark	–0.2	2.0
France	1.9	0.7
Germany	1.9	3.1
Italy	1.5	0.5
Japan	1.3	3.1
Netherlands	0.5	1.1
Sweden	0.9	0.3
Great Britain	1.7	2.4
United States	–0.6	–0.1

[a]Source: Bernstein, J., and Mishel, L. A comparison of income, wage and employment. In reference 53, p. 202.

Table 24

Trends in male earning dispersion ratio of 90th to 10th percentile earnings[a]

	1979	1989	1995
United States	3.18	4.04	4.35
Japan	2.59	2.85	2.77
Germany	2.38	2.29	2.25
France	3.39	3.49	3.43
Italy	2.29	2.17	2.64
United Kingdom	2.45	3.08	3.31
Canada	3.46	3.81	3.77
Australia	2.74	2.81	2.94
Austria	2.64	2.72	—
Finland	2.44	2.61	2.53
New Zealand	—	2.85	3.17
Sweden	2.11	2.16	2.20

[a]Source: Schmitt, J., and Mishel, L. *An Evaluation of the G-7 Economies of the 1990s,* Table 8A. Economic Policy Institute, Washington, D.C., January 30, 1998.

Table 25

Trends in female earning dispersion ratio of 90th to 10th percentile earnings[a]

	1979	1989	1995
United States	3.06	3.65	3.96
Japan	2.19	2.34	2.24
Germany	2.65	2.42	2.26
France	2.60	2.82	2.94
Italy	2.99	2.17	2.80
United Kingdom	2.26	2.86	3.06
Canada	3.73	4.17	4.01
Australia	2.40	2.61	2.53
Austria	3.36	3.45	3.69
Belgium	—	2.18	2.22
Finland	2.06	2.17	1.98
New Zealand	—	2.51	2.62
Portugal	—	2.79	3.25
Sweden	1.65	1.78	1.82
Switzerland	—	2.70	2.54

[a]Source: Schmitt, J., and Mishel, L. *An Evaluation of the G-7 Economies of the 1990s,* Table 8B. Economic Policy Institute, Washington, D.C., January 30, 1998.

Wage polarization increased quite substantially in the United States during the 1980s and 1990s, contributing to the country's growing income polarization. The most important cause of income polarization, however, is not the wage or earning dispersion but rather the unprecedented growth of income derived from capital—this explains the spectacular growth in the income of the top 5 percent of the population. Profits, for example, have increased at unprecedented levels. Given the lack of a similar growth in productivity, one has to conclude that the increased profits are due to the decline in wages (i.e., a transfer of income from labor to capital). As Blanchard has indicated, "the high profits of financial capital and the decline of wages and labor costs explains a transfer of income from labor to capital" (quoted in 5). Lawrence Mishel (5) notes that if the rate of profits of financial and entrepreneurial capital had remained constant (instead of growing at an unprecedented rate) from 1980 to 1990, the rate of growth in wages would have doubled during that period.

This transfer of income from labor to capital has been one of the explicit purposes (and consequences) of neoliberal public policies, and has been responsible for the unprecedented growth in social inequalities. Indeed, one of the primary purposes of neoliberals' calls for labor's wage moderation has been to facilitate the growth of profits that—in theory—will be converted into investment and economic growth. But, as indicated in section I of this chapter, the rate of profits has increased at unheard-of levels since the early 1980s in most OECD countries without any significant increase in employment or investment. During this entire period, wages have increased at lower rates than productivity (reversing the situation in the 1970s, when wages increased faster than productivity), while unemployment has not declined (32, p. 42).

The outcome of neoliberal policies, with their reduction in social expenses, their deregulation of labor markets, and their public policies favorable to capital, has been an enormous impact on the income and wealth distribution of the countries in which these policies have been implemented. Consequently, it is in the countries where neoliberal policies have been most thoroughly implemented—the United States and the United Kingdom—that social polarization has been most accentuated.

IV. THE SOCIAL CONSEQUENCES OF NEOLIBERALISM: THE GROWTH OF SOCIAL INEQUALITIES AND POVERTY

Atkinson, Rainwater, and Smeeding (44) have documented the growth of income inequalities in the majority of OECD countries, showing that the United States and the United Kingdom have had the largest increases in inequalities—as measured by the ratio of the median income of the top decile to the median income of the bottom decile (Table 26).

As indicated in section III, important causes for the growth of such inequalities have been (*a*) the enormous and unprecedented transfer of income from wages (income from work) to profit and rent (income from ownership of capital), and (*b*) the growing dispersion among wage earners—both situations being largely attributable to the neoliberal policies detailed in this chapter.

Other factors that have also been considered as causes of the growing inequalities are the introduction of new technologies (which seemingly eliminated or cheapened unskilled labor) and the globalization of the world economy (with imports from low-wage countries destroying jobs or lowering wages for unskilled workers). I have already criticized the increased technology argument. Section V will question the globalization thesis as an explanation for the wage polarization and growth of unemployment in developed capitalist countries. Suffice it to say here that (*a*) rather than globalization, what we are witnessing today is an economic (and political) regionalization of production and commerce among countries at similar levels of economic development (North America, Europe, and Southeast Asia) and with similarly qualified labor forces; (*b*) imports from less developed capitalist countries into developed capitalist countries (as a percentage of all imports) have diminished rather than increased during the last 30 years; and (*c*) imports from less developed countries have been increasingly high value-added commodities rather than labor-intensive products.

Table 26

Income inequalities, measured by the ratio between the income of the top decile (90th) and the income of the bottom decile (10th), incomes as percentages of overall median income[a]

	Bottom decile (10th) *(P10)*	Top decile (90th) *(P90)*	Ratio *(P90/P10)*
Finland (1991)	57	158	2.75
Sweden (1992)	57	159	2.78
Belgium (1992)	58	163	2.79
Norway (1991)	56	158	2.80
Denmark (1992)	54	155	2.86
Luxembourg (1985)	58	172	2.95
Netherlands (1991)	57	183	3.05
Italy (1991)	56	186	3.14
Germany (1988)	54	172	3.21
Austria (1987)	56	187	3.34
Switzerland (1982)	54	185	3.43
France (1984)	55	193	3.48
Spain (1990)	49	198	4.04
Japan (1992)	46	192	4.17
Ireland (1987)	50	209	4.18
United Kingdom (1990)	44	206	4.67
United States (1991)	36	208	5.78

[a]Source: Smeeding, T. M. *American Inequality in a Cross National Perspective: Why Are We So Different?* Working Paper No. 157. Luxembourg Income Study, 1997.

Maher, Jesuit, and Roscoe (45) have studied the impact of commerce and investment on the growth of social inequalities in the OECD countries, and have concluded that neither commerce nor investments are the cause of the growth in such inequalities. It is worth repeating that *the most important causes of the growth in inequalities are political, such as the implementation of neoliberal public policies by neoliberal and conservative (and on occasion, social democratic) governments and the consequent weakening of the labor movement and the trade unions; the fiscal policies implemented by these governments; the decentralization of collective bargaining agreements; the dismantling of social pacts governed by tripartite arrangements (government, employers, unions); and the weakening of universal social policies.* Gottschalk and Joyce (46) have shown, for example, that countries with a strong labor movement (with strong unions), strong social pacts (between government, employers, and unions), and highly centralized collective bargaining agreements have lower income inequalities than countries such as the United States and the United Kingdom, where trade unions are very weak and governments have followed neoliberal policies favoring the well-to-do.

Sweden, The Netherlands, Germany, Italy, and France, for example, all of which have centralized bargaining systems, have lower income inequalities than the United States and the United Kingdom. The strong labor movements and unions, strong social pacts between employers and unions, strong public commitment to welfare states, centralized bargaining agreements, and highly regulated labor markets are indicators of the class power relations in existence in these European countries. *It is therefore a political relation rather than economic determinism (which is behind the globalization position) that underlies the level of inequalities in any country.*

The countries that have been successful in reducing income inequalities have done so through redistributive public policies and through the reduction of wage differentials and dispersion. As the OECD *Employment Outlook 1997* recognizes, countries with social pacts (and centralized bargaining systems), with high trade union density and extensive coverage of the working population by centralized collective bargaining agreements, were able to achieve lesser wage and income inequalities than those without these agreements (31). The report concludes that income differentials have grown more rapidly in countries without such arrangements.

It is also important to indicate that while many countries have experienced a growth in income differentials, others have been able to reduce them. Spain, governed by a social democratic government, reduced its income differentials during the 1980s through its fiscal policies and expansion of its welfare state (in particular, pensions, health services, and education), although its economic policies—contributing to the creation of high unemployment—were responsible for slowing the redistributive effects of these social policies.

In summary, the growth of inequalities in most OECD countries was due to *(a) the economic and fiscal policies favorable to property and to the best-off in these societies, including a weakening of the progressivity of the tax code and tax changes that benefit capital over labor; (b) the growth in wage inequalities among and within economic sectors as a result of weakening of the trade unions and decentralization of the collective bargaining process; (c) reduction of the welfare state, with declines in the rate of growth of social expenditures (despite a larger growth in social needs) and weakening of the indexation of benefits that adapts benefits to levels of inflation; and (d) economic policies that gave priority to the reduction of inflation via monetarist policies that reduced the rate of economic growth and increased unemployment.* This reduction of economic growth and the changes in progressivity of the tax code were responsible for the decline in public revenues, with a consequent decline in social expenditures.

Needless to say, the intensity and direction of these interventions and events have varied quite considerably among the OECD countries, and several of them have taken corrective measures to reduce their negative impact on income distribution. But the great majority of countries, by following such policies, did not succeed in reversing the trend toward higher inequalities (47).

Poverty and Public Policy

A consequence of the growth in inequalities has been the increased poverty in large numbers of OECD countries. Table 27 shows that, of the 14 countries in the OECD, ten had increased poverty during the 1980s. The United States and the United Kingdom, the two countries that went farthest in implementing neoliberal policies, had the greatest increases in poverty, remaining at the end of the 1980s and into the 1990s the countries with the highest percentages of the population living in poverty. As Table 28 shows, that poverty was extended to all groups of the population—elderly, adults, and children. In the United States, one of every four children live in poverty, while in Great Britain almost one in four of the elderly live in poverty. The table also shows that, regarding poverty, there are three groups of countries. In the first group, the United States and Great Britain, poverty is a mass phenomenon, affecting large percentages of the population, adults, elderly, and children. These are the countries that neoliberals present as models for their policies. In the second group of countries, Ireland and Spain, poverty is an important although not massive phenomenon. Both countries are recent democracies after long periods under conservative regimes (40 years of fascist dictatorship in the case of Spain). Spain, with the largest income inequalities in the European Union, was able to reduce its inequalities and poverty during the period 1982–1994 (under a socialist government), although at the end of the period high levels of inequalities remained, with a still considerable level of poverty among the elderly, adults, and children. The third group of countries consists of those where poverty affects a small percentage of the population, but the percentage is growing in some of these countries as well.

The data in Tables 27 and 28 also permit some other observations. One is that poverty is an expansion of income inequalities, maintaining a direct relationship between the two: the larger the social inequalities, the larger the percentage of the population living in poverty. In the Scandinavian countries (where the social democratic model has been dominant), inequalities are low and poverty is low. The United States and the United Kingdom (where the neoliberal model is dominant) have high levels of both inequalities and poverty.

A second observation is that the differences in the rates of poverty between the social democratic and neoliberal models are quite extensive. The child poverty level is almost 25 percent of all children in the United States and 18.5 percent in Great Britain, but only 2.7 percent in Finland, 3 percent in Sweden, and 4.9 percent in Norway. These differences cannot be explained by differences in the degree of globalization of the economies or in the degree of technological innovation, or by any other economicist arguments prevalent today. These

Table 27

Changes in poverty levels[a]

	Year	Poverty ratio, %
United States	1979	16.6
	1994	19.1
United Kingdom	1979	9.2
	1994	14.6
Australia	1981	12.5
	1989	12.9
Canada	1981	12.6
	1991	11.7
Spain	1980	12.2
	1990	10.4
Denmark	1987	10.4
	1992	7.5
Belgium	1985	4.6
	1992	5.5
Sweden	1981	5.4
	1992	6.7
Norway	1979	5.0
	1991	6.6
Finland	1987	5.7
	1991	6.2
France	1979	8.2
	1989	7.6
Germany	1986	4.9
	1991	6.7
Netherlands	1986	4.9
	1991	6.7
Italy	1986	10.6
	1991	6.5

[a]Source: reference 48, p. 14.

Table 28

Poverty rates (defined as 50 percent of median disposable income) among age groups in several OECD countries, in percent[a]

	Total	Elderly	Adults	Children
United States (1994)	19.1	19.6	16.4	24.9
United Kingdom (1991)	14.6	23.9	10.7	18.5
Ireland (1987)	11.1	7.6	9.6	13.8
Spain (1990)	10.4	11.4	9.2	12.8
Germany (1989)	7.6	7.5	7.3	8.6
Denmark (1992)	7.5	11.3	7.3	5.1
France (1984)	7.5	4.8	8.1	7.4
Netherlands (1991)	6.7	4.1	6.6	8.3
Sweden (1992)	6.7	6.4	8.1	3.0
Norway (1991)	6.6	13.5	5.4	4.9
Italy (1991)	6.5	4.4	6.1	10.5
Finland (1991)	6.2	14.4	5.8	2.7
Belgium (1992)	5.5	11.9	4.6	4.4
Luxembourg (1985)	5.4	12.9	4.1	5.2

[a]Source: reference 48, p. 14.

differences are due to the different public policies followed by governments, of which the public social policies are of key importance. For example, the very low percentage of poverty among children in Scandinavian countries is a result of the wide availability of family-oriented social services (such as child care centers and domiciliary home care services). These services have facilitated the integration of women into the labor market, helping to maintain family income, including that of single-parent families. Another reason for the family income maintenance in these countries is the equal wage policies followed by the labor movements and implemented by the social democratic governments. These two policies—women receiving the same wages as men, and the welfare state helping families care for children and elders—are responsible for the very low levels of poverty, including for single-parent families, in the Scandinavian countries. The level of poverty among single-parent families is 59 percent in the United States, 49 percent in Great Britain, and 37.1 percent in Spain, compared with only 5 percent in Sweden, 19 percent in Norway, 7.7 percent in Finland, and 13.8 percent in Denmark (48, Table 4).

It is important to emphasize that although Spain, Ireland, and Italy are countries of Catholic culture, a culture that rhetorically emphasizes the importance of family, they in fact follow public policies that clearly handicap the development of the family. For example, the absence of family-oriented social services such as child care and home care services overburdens families (especially women), and is responsible for the very low fertility in these countries (among the lowest in the world today) and the high level of child poverty (13.8 percent in Ireland, 12.8 percent in Spain, and 10.5 percent in Italy). The practical insensibility of public policies toward the family (and toward women) is also the reason why infant mortality in these countries (7 per 1,000 live births in Spain and Italy) is larger than in Sweden (4 per 1,000 live births) (49).

Table 28 also shows that the United States and the United Kingdom have very high poverty rates among the elderly (19.6 percent in the United States and 23.9 percent in the United Kingdom). Spain and Ireland also have large percentages (although lower than the United States and the United Kingdom) of elderly in poverty (11.4 percent in Spain and 7.6 percent in Ireland). France (4.8 percent), The Netherlands (4.1 percent), Sweden (6.4 percent), and Italy (4.4 percent) have low percentages of elderly persons in poverty. It is surprising, however, that Luxembourg, Belgium, Finland, Norway, and Denmark, all of which have low levels of overall poverty, have high levels of poverty among the elderly, comparable to or even higher than the levels in Spain and Ireland. A plausible explanation is the limited emphasis on social transfers, with a focus instead on social services. This situation should be a warning to those countries that are advocating a transfer of funds from the elderly to the young and/or from social transfers to services. The much needed expansion of the pro-family social services described above should not be paid for by reducing transfers of funds to the elderly via pensions and other means.

Table 29 shows how those countries with higher poverty rates are also, in general, those with public policies that are less redistributive of funds. The United States and the United Kingdom, for example, have higher overall poverty rates and less redistributive public policies. A similar situation occurs for poverty among the elderly, adults, and children.

In all these comparisons, the clearest contrast is between the United States and the majority of E.U. countries. While Belgium's public policies, for example, reduce its overall rate of poverty from 28.4 to 5.5 percent of the population (a reduction of 80.6 percent), the United States reduces its poverty from 26.7 to 19.1 percent (a reduction of only 28 percent). This is a marked contrast between the poverty reduction rates of the United States and Belgium. Similarly, while Belgium's public policies reduce poverty among the elderly by 86.6 percent, among adults by 77.5 percent, and among children by 74.4 percent, U.S. public policies reduce poverty only by 66.5 percent for the elderly, 15.9 percent for adults, and a mere 13.2 percent for children.

Another observation we can make from data in Table 29 is that the level of poverty among adults is not directly related to the level of unemployment. The United States, for example, has a low unemployment rate but the highest poverty rate among the countries considered. Poverty is related as much to the level of

Table 29

The rate of effectiveness of redistributive public policies in different OECD countries[a,b]

	Total poverty			Poverty in elderly			Poverty in adults			Poverty in children		
	B	*A*	*% R*	*B*	*A*	*% R*	*B*	*A*	*% R*	*B*	*A*	*% R*
Belgium (1989)	28.4	5.5	80.6	88.9	11.9	86.6	20.4	4.6	77.6	17.2	4.4	74.4
Sweden (1992)	34.1	6.7	80.4	91.6	6.4	93	23	8.1	64.8	18.4	3.0	83.7
Denmark (1992)	26.9	7.5	72.1	69.9	11.3	83.8	19.5	7.3	62.6	11.6	2.7	76.7
Netherlands (1991)	22.8	6.7	70.6	65.5	4.1	93.4	17.6	6.6	61.8	15.2	8.3	45.4
Norway (1991)	21.8	6.6	69.7	68	13.5	80.1	12.9	5.4	58.1	12.7	4.9	61.4
Germany (1989)	22.0	7.6	65.5	65.8	7.5	88.6	12.5	7.3	41.6	11.7	8.6	26.5
France (1984)	21.6	7.5	65.3	79.9	4.8	94.0	23.5	8.1	65.6	27.4	7.4	73.0
Italy (1991)	18.4	6.5	69.7	55.7	4.4	92.1	13.6	6.1	55.1	11	10.5	4.5
Ireland (1987)	30.3	11.1	63.4	54.9	7.6	86.2	30.4	9.6	68.4	30.3	13.8	54.5
Spain (1990)	28.2	10.4	63.1	68.2	11.4	83.5	23.3	9.2	58.7	20.7	12.8	38.2
United Kingdom (1991)	29.2	14.6	50.0	68.5	23.9	65.1	19.5	10.7	45.1	28.7	18.5	35.5
United States (1991)	26.7	19.1	28.5	58.7	19.7	66.6	19.5	16.4	15.9	28.7	24.9	13.2

[a]*B* = poverty level *before* the intervention of redistributive public policies (i.e., before *subtracting* taxes and fees and *adding* social transfers benefits to the individual disposable income).

A = poverty level *after* the intervention of redistributive public policies (i.e., after *subtracting* taxes and fees and *adding* social transfers benefits to the individual disposable income).

% R = percentage of poverty reduction as a result of redistributive public policies.

[b]Source: Adapted from reference 48, p. 34.

wages and salaries as to the rate of unemployment. Actually, the level of salaries and wages is more important than the rate of unemployment in explaining the high level of U.S. poverty. In the United States, 82 percent of adult men who are poor are employed (50). This is why one of the most effective ways of reducing poverty is to increase the minimum wage and the wages of the most poorly paid jobs, which are concentrated among unskilled workers. The most successful antipoverty programs are not the welfare antipoverty programs (usually means tested), but rather public policies that intervene directly in the labor market, increasing employment and wages, as well as universal programs (such as pensions) and family-oriented social programs that facilitate the integration of women into the labor market.

Another conclusion from Table 29 is that the poverty rate among adults and children is also clearly affected by the redistributive effects of public policies. Countries with highly redistributive policies have lower levels of poverty.

Furthermore, Table 29 shows that it is the elderly who benefit most from these redistributive public policies. In all countries listed, the large majority of elders would be living in poverty if they had not benefited from the redistributive public policies of the welfare state. It is among this group that the redistributive effect is most accentuated. This situation has led some authors to claim that the welfare state is too oriented toward the elderly, that it is an unfair arrangement in which the elderly are absorbing resources that should be focused on younger age groups. According to some of these authors, conflicts between the generations have replaced the conflicts among classes. This argument, however, assumes that (*a*) the elderly are living in relative abundance, wasting resources that could better be used in other groups, but Table 29 shows that most elders would be poor without the welfare state; (*b*) the welfare state has reached its limit in terms of expansion, an assumption that is difficult to sustain given the enormous growth of national income in most countries; and (*c*) the transfer of funds to the elderly benefits only the elderly, whereas in fact, children of the elderly benefit greatly from their elders' security, which explains the enormous popularity of these programs.

The Reasons for the Growth in Inequalities: The Forgotten Political Variables

I have shown that, contrary to the claims of conservative and neoliberal positions, the United States is not more successful than other countries with more regulated labor markets and more developed welfare states. Actually, we find more labor instability, more labor insecurity, more unemployment (among men), and more low-wage jobs in the United States than in many E.U. countries. Why this situation? What are the reasons for these differences? As shown earlier, when comparing the labor market behaviors of the United States and the E.U. countries, the labor market differences cannot be explained by different degrees of technological innovation or by different degrees of integration in the supposedly globalized world economy. Indeed, the actual causes of these differences are not economic but political, including the power of the political and social forces that shape the nature of the labor markets, the strength of the different political and social instruments used by these forces, and the type of institutional arrangements that configure the labor market relations. Among the political and social instruments, the strength (or weakness) of the trade unions and of the social democratic parties and their political adversaries is of key importance in explaining the existence (or lack) of full-employment policies, the existence and level of the minimum wage, and the degree and type of development of the welfare state (51).

A critical element, therefore, for understanding the behavior of the labor markets, the existence of inequalities, and the nature of public social policies is to analyze the power of social and political instruments, such as the trade unions. How powerful are the unions in a country? A major indicator of union power has been the percentage of the labor force that is unionized. This way of measuring the power of the unions (e.g., 52), however, is a mistake. In the United States, for example, 16 percent of the labor force was unionized in 1994, a higher percentage than in France (9 percent). In the United States, however, the arrangements achieved by collective bargaining agreements covered only 18 percent of the whole labor force, more or less the same percentage of workers who were unionized since, in general, U.S. unions represent only those workers who are unionized. Moreover, the collective bargaining powers in the United States are highly decentralized, affecting only small sectors of the labor force. In France, however, collective bargaining agreements covered 95 percent of all workers—unionized and non-unionized. Collective bargaining agreements, negotiated by the unions and by the employees' associations, are highly centralized in France, covering the overwhelming majority of the labor force. French unions, therefore, have far more power than U.S. unions, despite the lower percentage of unionized workers in France.

Because of this point, frequently ignored in many analyses of the labor movement, it is important to differentiate between the percentage of the labor force that is unionized and the percentage that is covered by collective bargaining arrangements. From Table 30 and from the information provided in previous sections of this article, we can reach several conclusions.

First, unions in particular, and the labor movement in general, are weaker in the United States than in the European Union, which is one of the major reasons why labor market conditions are worse, why social inequalities are greater, and why public policies are less redistributive in the United States than in the European Union. Similarly, the weakening of labor under the conservative governments in the United Kingdom was a primary reason for the growth of inequalities, for the decline in the redistributive effects of public policies, and for the deterioration of labor market conditions in that country.

Table 30

Union density and coverage of the labor force by collective bargaining agreements, in percent[a]

	Union density			Collective bargaining agreements		
	1980	1990	1994	1980	1990	1994
Australia	48	41	35	88	80	80
Austria	56	46	42	98	98	98
Belgium	56	51	54	90	90	90
Canada	36	36	38	37	38	36
Denmark	76	71	76	69	69	69
Finland	70	72	81	95	95	95
France	18	10	9	85	92	95
Germany	36	33	29	91	90	92
Italy	49	39	39	85	83	82
Japan	31	25	24	28	23	21
Netherlands	35	26	26	76	71	81
New Zealand	56	45	30	67	67	31
Norway	57	56	58	75	75	74
Portugal	61	32	32	70	79	71
Spain	9	13	19	76	76	78
Switzerland	31	27	27	53	53	50
United Kingdom	50	39	34	70	47	47
United States	22	16	16	26	18	18

[a]Source: reference 42, Table 3.3, p. 71.

A second conclusion is that Germany, one of the largest economies, witnessed a lesser erosion of union power and also had lower unemployment rates (among the top four E.U. countries), greater increases in the level of wages (particularly among low-wage workers), and lower growth in inequalities.

The power differentials between the E.U. and U.S. labor movements explain why all E.U. countries have larger labor and social rights, such as longer vacations, greater worker participation in the workplace, better and more extensive occupational health and hygiene rights and services, more comprehensive medical care, more active professional training, larger unemployment insurance (except in Italy), and a higher minimum wage than the United States (53). Actually, the minimum wage in the United States is not only lower than in the majority of E.U. countries but has been declining faster. For example, the E.U. minimum wage, which represents 60 percent of the median wage, has remained practically constant since the middle 1970s. In the United States, however, the minimum wage declined from 45 percent of the median wage in the 1970s to 35 percent in the 1980s (Table 31).

This weakness of U.S. labor is also evident in the absence of institutional structures that would permit the establishment of tripartite social pact arrangements among government, unions, and employers (as occurs in many E.U. countries), arrangements that would enable the development of full employment and other types of public policies. As Nickell (30) has shown, for example, the countries that have had long periods of low unemployment (lower than the United States) are those—such as Austria, Germany, Norway, Sweden, and Portugal—that have had tripartite central arrangements between unions, employers, and government aimed at achieving full employment. Moreover those countries—such as Sweden—with a recent growth in unemployment have undergone a decentralization of their collective bargaining arrangements, breaking with the social pact between unions, employers, and government, a break that responded more to political than to economic causes (38).

Alternatives to Current Neoliberal Policies

The reduction of inequalities requires two types of interventions: in the labor market and in the state. For the first, a critical element is the reduction of unemployment and the creation of well-paid employment. We have already seen that neoliberal policies to reduce unemployment (via the deregulation of labor markets and reduction of social protection) have failed. Most European countries have deregulated their labor markets and reduced their social protection, yet unemployment has continued to increase. Actually, all the evidence shows that

Table 31

Minimum wage:
International comparisons[a]

	% of median salary 1988–91
Belgium	66
France	61
Greece	67
Netherlands	72
Portugal	73
Spain	54
United States	35

[a]Source: *Unemployment: Choices for Europe*. CEPR, 1995.

those measures have contributed to the increase in unemployment, job instability, and insecurity in the labor force in these countries.

An alternative way of reducing inequalities is to expand the welfare state to increase social cohesion and invest heavily in human and physical capital. Both policies would require an active state intervention. Even prominent voices within the business establishment—such as William Woleman, business correspondent of *Business Week* (quoted in 54)—have recently called for a more active state intervention to resolve the unemployment problem and the growth of social inequalities in the United States. These expansionist policies are usually dismissed by conservative and neoliberal political forces (and increasingly by some social democratic forces) as unfeasible, as well as unwise, due to the globalization of the world economy. It is assumed that economic globalization has considerably reduced or even eliminated the possibility for states to intervene—via economic and fiscal policies—in the resolution of their social and economic problems, including the reduction of inequalities. In this new scenario, globalization is the justification for public policies—reduction in public social and physical expenses, deregulation of labor markets, and elimination of social protection—that are increasing inequalities. And, again, in this scenario, the primary role of the state is to facilitate the integration of the national economy into the globalized economy, following policies favorable to capital. As I have shown, these pro-capital policies are increasing unemployment and inequalities by reducing the welfare state and making the fiscal policies more regressive. The E.U. country that has followed these policies most extensively has been Great Britain, where, during the period 1979–1994: (*a*) the rate of unemployment among unskilled workers increased by 33 percent; (*b*) the income gap between the top and bottom deciles increased enormously, creating levels of inequality equal to those in the United States, with the largest income inequalities in the OECD (44); and (*c*) there was a 28 percent decline in the level of pensions (taking the median wage as the point of reference).

These policies, however, respond to political rather than economic necessities (such as the needs created by the process of globalization). Indeed, the expansion of the welfare state as a way of reinforcing social cohesiveness and solidarity, as well as a way of creating employment through full-employment policies, is opposed by capital because such policies strengthen labor and increase the level of labor's demands, thus reducing capital's prerogatives. During the 1960s and 1970s, for example, the expansion of the welfare state strengthened the working class considerably, escalating its level of demands for participation in and/or control over decision-making in the world of production. It was the escalation of these demands that triggered capital's response through neoliberalism. Neoliberalism is indeed the capitalist's response to the escalation of demands by the working classes of the western world (55), which explains why the opposition to full-employment policies is rooted in political rather than economic reasoning.

V. ECONOMIC GLOBALIZATION?

One of the most powerful positions in political and economic circles in the West is that the world now has a globalized economy, with a worldwide globalization of trade and commerce, of investments, and of finance (for a good definition of what has become known as globalization, see 19, Chapt. 1; 56, Chapt. 1). This phenomenon, presented as new and unprecedented, is assumed to be responsible for the decline of the world's states and of their ability to intervene in economic and political affairs within their own borders. The forces behind globalization determine the economic and political policies of the governments, greatly reducing the options from which these governments can choose. Thus we are witnessing the appearance of a discourse that promotes a certain economic determinism, diminishing quite considerably the importance of the political sphere. In this discourse, governments appear as prisoners of international economic forces that determine what they can do. This economic determinism is now guiding many public policies that, despite their clear unpopularity, are being imposed on the world's western, eastern, northern, and southern populations. It is constantly being said, for example, that global competitiveness is forcing governments to institute unpopular policies, such as deregulating labor markets and reducing social protections. These public policies are thus presented as unavoidable: there is no other way. The working classes and popular masses of the developed capitalist countries are being asked to reduce their standard of living, to accept lower wages and social benefits, because (using a quasi-military language) they are "threatened" by an "invasion" of imported products from low-wage underdeveloped countries. This "invasion" will destroy people's existence, jobs included, unless they follow these unpopular austerity policies. As a recent report of the European Commission concluded (57, p. 45):

> The most important phenomena that the countries of the European Union are facing is the globalization of the economy, in which all countries compete in an open worldwide market. They are seeing their markets invaded by products imported from less developed countries whose production costs we cannot match.

More recently, the United Nations distributed a draft paper in which it discusses the impact of structural changes in the world economy on the lives and well-being of the populations living and working in developed capitalist countries, concluding that (58, pp. 14–15):

> until recently, the world was divided into rich countries, characterized by high productivity and high wages, and countries with low productivity and low wages. This situation, however, has changed. From the 1970s and from the 1980s we are seeing a very dramatic change with the appearance of undeveloped countries with high productivity and low wages.

The U.N. report further expands on the implications of this new situation, indicating that it will also force lower wages in high-productivity countries because in today's worldwide labor market we have full accessibility of capital and labor across countries. What this report does is add strength to the widely held position that governments must respond to globalization by reducing the costs of production (in particular, wages and social benefits) to enable the developed capitalist countries to compete with the less developed countries.

Before analyzing the empirical evidence for or against this globalization position, I should clarify what is meant by globalization. Many different realities are grouped under this rubric, and because of this confusion we need to disaggregate the concept of globalization, both conceptually and empirically, into its different categories: the globalization of commerce, the globalization of productive investments, and the globalization of financial capital. I believe it is very important to make this separation since each category requires a different approach to analyzing its historical novelty and its extension. In other words, it is important to ask to what degree globalization (in its three main dimensions—globalization of commerce, of productive capital, and of financial capital) corresponds to reality and, when it does, whether or not it is a new phenomenon. It is in the responses to these questions that much confusion has arisen.

Another subject that merits our attention is an analysis of the mechanisms through which globalization affects the levels of wages, social protection, and employment in the countries involved. In this regard, the globalization of commerce is assumed (*a*) to destroy jobs or lower wage levels in developed countries that are being "invaded" by products from low-wage developing countries, and (*b*) to produce jobs in the newly industrialized countries that export such products to developed capitalist countries. To the degree that markets for products in developed countries are being taken over by products made in less developed countries, unemployment is increasing. Moreover, the newly displaced workers are forced to look for new jobs, increasing the pool of job seekers and lowering wages in the entire labor force. Employers also use the international competitiveness argument as a way of forcing employees to accept cuts in wages and benefits (for an excellent presentation of this argument, see 59).

The globalization of productive investment, with the majority of investment going from developed to less developed countries, also destroys jobs in those industries that move from developed to developing countries, while increasing employment in the developing countries. Moreover, governments compete with each other to create conditions that attract investments, such as lowering the tax burden on capital, making fiscal policies more regressive, and pressuring for decreases in wages. Employers also use the threat of moving to low-wage countries to gain concessions from their own labor force.

The globalization of financial capital also forces governments to reduce their deficits and follow austerity policies that reassure the financial markets of their "credibility." These austerity policies reduce the stimulating effect of welfare state policies, lowering the rate of economic growth and the production of employment.

Besides these negative impacts of globalization, other, positive effects have been argued for. The globalization of commerce, for example, while destroying unskilled jobs with imports from low-wage countries, is also creating new high-wage skilled occupations in export-oriented industries. Also, the globalization of productive investments to other countries is perceived as stimulating the production of jobs in the country where investments originate, since satellite production units continue to rely on the parts and components produced by the headquarters of the industry in its home country. (For a summary of the pros and cons of globalization, see 19, Chapt. 1, p. 4.)

As the reader will already have grasped, it is not easy to estimate the number of jobs that are being produced and destroyed, or the impact of globalization on wages and social protection, in the countries involved. There is an extensive bibliography on each of these points, partially summarized in other sections of this article. What I will try to do here is to analyze not so much the detailed impact of the globalization process, but rather the empirical data that sustain or question the major positions of the globalization theorists.

Globalization of Commerce

A simple perusal of the products sold in any large shopping mall in the United States or in the European Union would seem to confirm that a very large number of goods are made in less developed countries. Moreover, many families on both continents know of some enterprise that has closed and moved to another country. And many workers (particularly in manufacturing) in developed capitalist countries have heard from their employers that they had better scale back the levels of their demands, or else (the "else" being the move of the industry to other countries where labor is cheaper and/or more docile). All these experiences are extremely powerful and constitute the material bases on which the ideology of globalization is reproduced.

It is important, however, not to reach conclusions based only on individual experiences. We must look at the data to learn about the extent of this phenomenon, and here is where the evidence of globalization is less clear and convincing than the globalization theorists assume. Table 32 shows the evolution from 1913 to 1993 of the percentage of national consumption in manufacturing that is met by imports for the United States, Japan, the four largest E.U. economies, and the four smallest E.U. economies. The data seem to confirm the thesis of globalization for the United States (whose import penetration increased quite rapidly, from 3 percent in 1963 to 16 percent in 1993) and for the European economies (whose important penetration increased, for the largest economies, from 11 percent in 1963 to 29 percent in 1993, and for the smallest economies,

Table 32

Import penetration of domestic markets for manufacturing, 1913–1993, in percent[a,b]

	1913	1950	1963	1971	1980	1993
United States	3	2	3	8	9	16
Japan	34	3	4	5	5	6
Four largest E.U. countries	13	6	11	17	21	29
Four smallest E.U. countries	24	20	26	33	45	57

[a]Numbers represent imports as percentage of consumption.
[b]Source: reference 66, p. 6.

from 26 percent in 1963 to 57 percent in 1993). A much lower growth of import penetration occurred in Japan (from 4 percent in 1963 to 6 percent in 1993).

But before embracing the globalization thesis one needs to keep several facts in mind: (*a*) the overwhelming majority of these imports are from OECD countries and not from less developed countries—only 5.5 percent of all imports into developed capitalist countries are from the developing countries, and of these, the great majority are from only five countries, the Southeast Asian countries (60, p. 105); (*b*) the rate of growth of all manufacturing imports has declined during the 1990s; and (*c*) manufacturing represented only 18 percent of all employment in the OECD in 1994, and that percentage is declining in all OECD countries (31, Table 4.2, p. 105). Manufacturing employment—even when it includes related, non-manufacturing employment—has been declining. The highest employment is in services, which, except for tourism, is little affected by globalization.

Regarding exports, Table 33 shows the evolution from 1913 to 1994 of the value of exports (measured in current prices) as percentage of GDP for the United States, Europe, Japan, and the OECD. We can see that the value of exports actually declined in Europe from 1984 (29.8 percent) to 1994 (28 percent), when it was at approximately the same level as in 1913. Table 33 also shows that the growth of exports has been increasing quite slowly since World War II, and in the case of Japan has even declined. A similar decline is likely to occur in Europe after establishment of the monetary union, since most export-import activity in Europe occurs within the European Union.

From these figures, it seems questionable whether the lowering of wage levels and social protection can be attributed to the globalization of economies, since exports have been increasing rather slowly and even declining in most developed capitalist countries, and manufacturing imports from low-wage countries represent a very low percentage of overall employment. Despite this evidence, globalization is presented as the reason for continuing the reductions in wages

Table 33

Exports (measured in current prices) as percentage of GDP, 1913–1994[a]

	1913	1950	1960	1973	1984	1994
United States	7	4.6	5.2	6.9	7.9	10.6
Europe	23	16.7	19.7	24.2	29.8	28
Japan	20	11.8	10.2	10.0	15.0	9.5
OECD	16	10.5	12.7	15.3	19.0	18.4

[a]Sources: OECD, *Historical Statistics;* and reference 66, p. 6.

and social protection, reproducing the arguments made in 1911 when Norman Segel wrote that "the world economy has become so interdependent as to make national independence an anachronism" (quoted in 61). He also indicated, incidentally, that the world economy had become so integrated that it made intercountry wars impossible. Two world wars challenge the accuracy of Segel's analyses.

Globalization of Investments

A situation similar to that described above also appears in the case of globalization of investments: the overwhelming majority of investment transfers take place between developed countries. Actually, total investments in less developed countries represent only 3 percent of all the capital stock in existence in developed capitalist countries. Table 34 shows that, during the period 1967–1991: (*a*) the majority of investments continued to take place in developed capitalist countries; (*b*) the European Union attracted more foreign investment than the United States, questioning the image of "eurosclerosis" put forward by neoliberals; (*c*) the percentage of investments going to less developed countries declined rather than increased (from 30.6 percent of all investments in 1967 to 23.4 percent in 1991); and (*d*) there was an important shift of investments from Latin America to the Asian countries.

All these facts challenge the image of a "threat" posed by the developing to the developed countries. The reality shows that the actual drama in the less developed countries is their marginalization and exploitation, given the larger flow of capital from less developed to developed countries (due in large part to payments of foreign debt and interest accrued on that debt) than from developed to developing countries. According to a recent study, the net gain in the capital flow for developed countries was $163 billion for the period 1984–1988 (cited in 62).

Another way of measuring the importance of foreign investments is to calculate these investments as a percentage of all domestic investments. Table 35 shows the

Table 34

Foreign direct investment, 1967–1991, in percent[a,b]

	1967	1980	1991
United States	9.4	16.4	22
European Union	23	37	37
Less-developed countries	30.6	22	23.4
Latin America	17	12	7
Africa	5.3	2.6	2.1
East Asia	4.8	6.2	13

[a]The numbers represent the percentage of all foreign investments taking place in the designated country or region.
[b]Source: reference 56, Table 1.9, p. 33.

Table 35

Foreign direct investment 1984–1994, as percent of gross domestic investment[a]

	OECD	U.S.	Japan	E.U.
Inward	3.8	5.0	0.1	5.1
Outward	5.0	3.4	3.1	7.8

[a]Source: UNCTAD, *World Investment Report,* 1996, Table 5; cited in reference 66, p. 6.

evolution of foreign investment (as a percentage of domestic investment) in the OECD, United States, Japan, and European Union for the period 1984–1994. In Europe, inward flow of foreign investment represented only 5.1 percent, and European investment outside Europe represented only 7.8 percent of all domestic investments. In the United States, the inward flow of foreign investments represented only 5.0 percent, and U.S. investment abroad represented only 3.4 percent of all domestic investments. Here again, the numbers are quite low when seen in perspective. Actually, recent studies carried out by the National Bureau of Economic Research in the United States show that production by multinational corporations (MNCs) represents only 22 percent of all world production, of which only 6 percent of industrial production (including manufacturing, mining, transport, communications, construction, and commerce) and only 0.2 percent of service production took place outside the country of origin of the MNC (63). Because of this situation, the International Labor Organization has concluded that these flows of investments are unlikely to have had a large impact on unemployment or on wage levels (64). Actually, salaries and wages (measured as hourly wages) in the United States, for example, declined in all sectors of the economy from 1974 to 1997, regardless of the degree of import penetration or foreign investment in the sector. Wages in manufacturing, for example, declined by 10 percent, and an almost identical decline occurred, on average, in other sectors. Moreover, the large majority of imports and investments are from other developed capitalist countries with higher wages than the United States. Sixty percent of all imports in the United States are from E.U. countries and Japan, with higher wages than the United States. David Gordon (65, p. 82) has estimated that wages in manufacturing (the sector most affected by imports) are 25 percent higher in Japan and 14 percent higher (on average) in the European Union than in the United States. The claim that the United States needs to lower wages and social protection in order to face competition from countries with lower wages and less protection is therefore untenable. To the contrary, wages and social protection are higher, not lower, in these competing countries than in the United States. The reasons for the declines in U.S. wages and social protection have to be sought elsewhere.

There has been a similar overstatement of the importance of investment flows in less developed countries. From 1979 to 1989, the overall number of jobs created by all foreign investment in manufacturing (from developed capitalist countries) in less developed countries was 60,000 jobs, barely sufficient to explain the destruction of jobs in the more developed countries (the employment created by manufacturing MNCs increased from 1.02 million in 1979 to 1.08 million in 1989) (65, pp. 193–194).

For globalization of finance, it is also important to note that while these financial transactions have increased enormously—as I will be discussing later—their importance has also been exaggerated. Even in the most open financial markets such as that in the United Kingdom, only one-fifth of all pension funds have been invested or deposited outside the country, and only a quarter of all financial assets are non-British owned (66, p. 42).

Globalization or Regionalization? The Importance of the State

As I have shown, most trade and investment flow occurs within developed capitalist countries. Here I will focus on the importance of the state (and thus of the political space) in shaping the nature of those flows. Indeed, contrary to the globalization thesis, the state plays a critical role in establishing trade and investment flows.

Paul Hirst and Graham Thomson (67) have conducted the most detailed studies of the flows of commerce and investments in today's world. They have shown that rather than globalization, what we are witnessing is a regionalization of commerce and investments within a system of production in which the most international entities, the MNCs, are actually transnational rather than international. Most of the production and sales of MNCs take place within the region where the MNCs are based. Regarding sales, for example, 65 to 75 percent of all sales of MNCs (which, as noted earlier, represent approximately 22 percent of all commerce in the world today) occur in the country and region where they are located. MNCs of the United States, the United Kingdom, and The Netherlands are the most transnational, that is, most disperse in their sales. But, even in these countries, sales outside the country and region (North America in the case of the United States; the European Union in the case of the United Kingdom and The Netherlands) represent less than 20 percent of all sales. Table 36 shows the percentage of sales of German, Japanese, British, and U.S.-based MNCs (in manufacturing and in services) that take place in the region where they are based. As the table indicates, the overwhelming majority of their sales occur in their home region, for both manufacturing and services. Table 36 shows a similar picture for investments by the MNCs; the overwhelming majority take place within the region where the MNC is based. Actually, the percentage of investment in the home region increased from 1987 to 1993, and dispersion declined.

A similar situation occurs for employment by MNCs. For U.S. MNCs, for example, 78 percent of all fixed capital, 70 percent of all sales, and 73 percent of all employment take place in the United States (68, 69). These multinationals are basically national corporations with a rather limited degree of dispersion, a dispersion that has not changed much in the last 30 years.

These multinational—or better, transnational—corporations rely heavily on the government of the country in which they are based for creating the national and international conditions favorable to their reproduction and expansion. Actually, a

Table 36

Percentage of sales and assets of MNCs in the country or region of origin, 1987–1993[a]

	Manufacturing		Services	
	1987	1993	1987	1993
Sales				
Germany	72	75	—	—
Japan	64	75	89	77
Great Britain	66	65	74	77
United States	70	67	93	79
Assets				
Japan	—	97	77	92
Great Britain	52	62	—	69
United States	67	73	81	77

[a]Source: reference 67, Tables 4.1 and 4.2.

characteristic of our times has been the mobilization of corporate interests to influence and shape the nature of state interventions, a situation that would not be occurring if the importance of states had diminished. Moreover, regional arrangements such as NAFTA and the European Union are centered about the member states of those arrangements.

Globalization of Finance

I have left globalization of finance to be considered last because it has different dynamics from the globalization of commerce and of investments. Indeed, I have shown that the latter two forms of globalization are not as new and/or extensive as is claimed, and the evidence suggests that they may be declining. The growth of imports plus exports as percentage of GNP—for both developed and less developed countries—was more rapid in the period 1950–1989 than in 1980–1989 (67, p. 28). Moreover, Hirst and Thomson (67) have also shown that in some sectors—such as the energy sector—internationalization (globalization) was far more accentuated at the beginning than at the end of the 20th century.

A process that is newer, however, is the *international flow of financial capital for speculative purposes*. This development is of critical importance for understanding the slowing of economic growth in the OECD countries. The collapse of the Bretton Woods agreements in 1972 and the subsequent deregulation of currency exchanges and, later, of the financial markets created an enormous mobility of financial capital, of a speculative character. This has been responsible for an unprecedented monetary instability, which, together with the associated power of the financial markets, has produced large numbers of economic and social problems that are wrongly attributed to the globalization of commerce and investments. The liberalization of currency exchanges and their great instability—occurring after the termination of Bretton Woods—caused a constant mobility of financial capital, looking to optimize the rate of profit in the shortest term possible. A worldwide international casino society has thus been established, in which mere speculation is the most important characteristic of the financial markets. The markets are constantly moving, seeking the best currency transactions, whose prices are constantly changing. This mobility includes the buying of bonds and securities that are shifting constantly. Table 37 shows the degree of penetration of this financial flow into government bonds, including eurobonds.

Actually, the end of Bretton Woods was supposed to free currency values from dependence on the dollar, allowing the fluctuation of the dollar. But rather than an increased autonomy for these currencies, we have seen them become enormously dependent on the financial markets that, in theory, are constraining the power of governments to intervene in their own economies. A frequently cited example of such constraint is the reversal of policies carried out by

Table 37

Penetration of financial capital in government bond markets, 1983–1989[a]

	1983	1985	1988	1989
Australia	20	33	55	54
Belgium	4	10	13	14
Canada	16	21	31	37
France	4	2	6	15
Italy	3	4	4	6
Japan	6	6	4	4
Netherlands	33	28	35	37
Spain	0	0	2	5
United Kingdom	9	11	15	15
United States	13	14	17	19

[a]Source: reference 67.

President Clinton immediately after his election. Clinton's election in 1992 was partially a result of his call for expansion of welfare state policies and more investment in human and physical capital. Shortly after his election, *Washington Post* reporter Robert Woodward wrote that Mr. Rubin, Secretary of the Treasury (and an ex-president of a major Wall Street financial corporation), warned the President that he could not carry out these programs since the financial markets would not allow such expansionary policies. If Clinton were to go ahead with these policies, the financial markets would withdraw from the government bond market and raise interest rates. The alternative they demanded was abandonment of these policies (on the basis of which Clinton was elected) and reduction of the public deficit; President Clinton complied (resulting in the loss of Democratic control of Congress in 1994). This situation forced the *Washington Post* to report (70):

> The financial markets and the central banks that fix the interest rates are the generals of a war that has been occurring in the last twenty years, and that in theory is justified by the need to control inflation but in practice has emptied governments of their power, impoverishing democracy. Afraid of increasing taxes and terrified of threatening the markets of bonds and securities, politicians have surrendered to financiers in the battle of the budget and fiscal policies.

President Clinton gave in to financial markets because he was afraid that those markets would abandon the bonds and dollar deposits, forcing a financial instability that would slow down the economy—a situation Clinton did not want to face so soon after his election. Abiding by the financial markets' wishes, he made reduction of the federal deficit his top priority. He expected that this would reassure the financial markets, and that interest rates would decline. But they did not. They did decline somewhat in 1993, but rose again soon after, in 1994 (71, p. 136). Why?

It is part of the neoliberal dogma that public deficits are responsible for the rise of inflation, the decline of investment, and the decline in economic growth. These are, incidentally, the assumptions behind the criteria for the establishment of the European monetary union: a condition established (by the Maastricht Treaty) for joining the monetary union is to maintain a public deficit below 3 percent of GNP. Basically, the neoliberal position assumes that (*a*) private investment is the key condition for economic growth; (*b*) private saving is the main source of investment; (*c*) the reason for slow economic growth is lack of private savings; and (*d*) government consumes too much, reducing the pool of savings by borrowing from the market and leaving fewer funds for the private sector. The problem for the neoliberal position, however, is that each one of these assumptions can be tested empirically (as I have done in section I of this chapter), and there is no evidence to support them. Indeed, items (*a*) through (*c*) assume public and private investment are independent of each other—that is, they compete for scarce savings. But the data do not support this proposition. Contrary to neoliberal thinking, this is not a zero sum game. The efficiency of private investment depends to a large degree on the efficiency of public investment. Actually, one reason for the low growth in productivity in the United States is the reduction of public investments. Aschauer (72), of the Economic Policy Institute, has shown that this reduction of public investment in the United States is responsible for half of the decline in the rate of growth in productivity in this country. Rather than competing, public investment may be a condition for the efficiency of private investment.

Another neoliberal assumption that is challenged by the data is that public borrowing produces a shortage of private investments. Robert Eisner, president of the American Economic Association and professor of economics at Northwestern University, has analyzed the evolution of public deficits and private investments from 1959 to 1991 and has observed a situation opposite to that claimed by neoliberals. Professor Eisner (73) has found that periods of large public deficits have been accompanied by large—rather than small, as neoliberals would predict—domestic private investments. The reason for this is that public investments and expenditures stimulate demand in the private sector, which is responsible for the growth of private investment. Moreover, in an economy that operates below full employment (and therefore functions below its capabilities), growth in demand does not have to cause an increase in inflation. Only in a full-employment situation, when the full potential of the economy is realized, could a growth in the public deficit create inflation. Such a condition has not occurred in any OECD country in the last 20 years.

The most important factor in stimulating investment is not the size of the public deficit, nor the level of interest rates, but rather the level of demand. The most detailed study of the behavior of enterprises, conducted in the United States in 1993 by economist Steve Fazzari (74) of Washington University, shows that the most important variable (far above any other variable) in explaining enterprises' investments is the amount of actual and projected sales—that is, the demand for products. As economist Robert Blecker (75) of American University has indicated, "The interest rates can be as low as you want, but unless the business person believes he is going to sell what's produced he or she is not going to invest."

The logic of the economic system is that an increase in demand is what stimulates investments, leading to a growth of sales, income, and savings, a process opposite to that suggested by neoliberals (saving leads to investments). Actually, we are seeing a very dramatic growth in profits and savings (particularly among the top income sector of the population) that is not being translated into investment and economic growth. This is a result of the stagnation of demand in the OECD countries, which is attributable to (*a*) a decline in the relative income of the majority of the population, due to the growth of social inequalities and social polarization; and (*b*) a decline in public deficits that also diminishes demand. This is precisely what is happening in the European Union as a consequence of the monetarist and austerity policies that are being carried out to comply with the criteria established for monetary union. It is these monetarist policies that are responsible for the growth of unemployment in the European Union, rather than "globalization," "rigid" labor markets, "excessive" welfare states, or increased technology in the workplace.

This interpretation of E.U. unemployment was confirmed during the recession of 1991–1993. We can compare the behavior of the E.U. governments with that of the U.S. government during the recession of 1989–1992. The U.S. government (which was, incidentally, Republican) reacted to the recession by substantially increasing demand via a large growth in the federal budget (at an annual rate of 1 percent of GNP) and a lowering of interest rates (which remained low during the entire recession). The E.U. governments, however, responded to their own recessions with opposite policies: they reduced government expenditures (at an annual rate of 0.5 percent of the aggregate E.U. GNP) and maintained very high interest rates (during the entire recessionary period). These policies caused a further slowing down of economic growth and increased unemployment (76, p. 89). It was these anti-expansionary policies of the E.U. governments, rather than the supposed rigidity of labor markets or overly generous welfare states, that increased unemployment.

These anti-expansionary policies of the E.U. governments—still in effect at the time this article is being written—are contributing to the large unemployment in the European Union. They have been implemented, in theory, to reduce inflation; but in practice they are a response to the interests of financial capital. Actually, these policies are unnecessary as anti-inflationary measures since a condition for expansionary policies to become inflationary is that the economies must be running at full speed with full employment—conditions that do not exist in the European Union, and have not existed for some time now. Even if the European economies were in a full-employment situation, inflation could be prevented if a social pact were reached between government, employers, and labor unions to develop anti-inflationary income policies (76, p. 90). But the absence of economic institutions at the E.U. level (except for the European Central Bank) makes it impossible to establish such social pacts at the European level. Thus the European Union becomes the dream of neoliberalism: the disappearance of the state in a market fully governed by financial capital. It is precisely this dominance by financial capital that is contributing most to the largest social problem in Europe: unemployment and slow economic growth, the nightmares of the European populations.

Against Financial Determinism

In view of the situation described thus far, we might ask whether it is impossible to change this dominance by the financial markets. The fact that the U.S. President had to abide by the dictates of these markets would seem to be further proof that nothing can be done to reverse this dominance. The financial markets, however, are not omnipotent, and the perception that they are omnipotent is what makes them so. This perception is based on a political rather than economic reality. Indeed, as we already have seen, the reversal of President Clinton's policies—abandoning expansionary policies immediately after being elected and implementing a federal deficit reduction program, with a marked reduction of the deficit from $255 billion in 1993 to $164 billion in 1994—did not lead to a lowering of interest rates. To the contrary, interest rates almost doubled during the period 1993–1994, a situation that so enraged President Clinton that he wanted to fire the Chairman of the U.S. Federal Reserve Board, Alan Greenspan, and appoint Mr. Felix Rohatyn (who would have reduced interest rates as a way of facilitating economic recovery). The Republican-dominated U.S. Congress, however, did not allow this change of chairmanship—all of which proves that interest rates are politically rather than economically determined; they depend on who controls the U.S. Federal Reserve Board.

The financial markets are immersed in institutions that are of a political character and respond to political decisions. This is the reason why decisions that are basically political are presented as economic or monetary decisions. Even *The Economist*, one of the most influential neoliberal organs, has recognized that many governments are carrying out highly unpopular policies that respond to financial interests, "hiding" (the expression used by *The Economist*) behind the excuse that these changes are needed to respond to the imperative of financial markets.

Meanwhile, the austerity policies, with the unprecedented growth in inequalities, are threatening to create a worldwide recession that could resemble the Great Depression of the 1930s. As President Roosevelt indicated in his second inaugural address (when he introduced the New Deal), "We have known that greed was bad morals, but what we have found is that it is also bad economics" (77).

Today, daily international transactions amount to $1.2 trillion, the majority of which is speculative in nature. In every four days of international bank transactions, the money being manipulated across international borders exceeds the value of all production in the United States during one year! And in Great Britain, a country with marked inequalities and high levels of poverty, the City of London, one of the most important financial centers in the world, manipulates $460 billion every day just in currency exchanges—most of which are speculative and do not enrich the production of goods or services (62, p. 38). This mobility, instability, and speculative nature of international monetary flows is hurting the productive capacity of the OECD economies, slowing economic growth. The unprecedented financial instability hampers economic growth, which causes a rise in public deficits. This reality is increasingly recognized, even by experts close to the financial interests. None other than Mr. Volcker, past Chairman of the U.S. Federal Reserve Board (during Republican administrations), noted in a report on the world economic situation that "since the beginning of the 1970s, economic growth of the most developed countries has been reduced by half (from 5 to 2.5 percent). And a very important cause of that decline has been the financial instability created by the large variability and instability of the price of currencies" (quoted in 62, p. 250). This report also recognized that the growth in unemployment and decline in productive investments, caused by the liberalization of currency exchanges and financial markets, have been responsible for the growth of public deficits. It is quite remarkable that this conclusion is finally reached by individuals representative of the financial interests that have benefited enormously from the liberalization of currencies and markets: the rates of profit of banking currency transactions are the highest of all capitalist enterprises in the world today (62, p. 299). *It is not rigorous, therefore, to accuse the welfare state of being responsible for the slowdown of the economies.* Actually, if the rate of economic growth of the 1950s and 1960s had been maintained during the 1970s, 1980s, and 1990s, today we would have full employment with enough funds to maintain and even expand the rate of growth in social expenditures.

It is very important to question the dogma, applauded by the right and lamented by the left, that the financial markets are the institutions that determine the austerity policies followed by today's governments. These policy decisions are political and as such respond to the class power relations in each state. The European recession of 1991–1993, for example, was politically caused. It was the result of the German government's decision to integrate (some may say absorb) East Germany into West Germany. This integration increased the supply of

German marks to the East, creating the possibility for rising inflation in Germany. To avoid this, the Bundesbank raised the interest rate, forcing other European countries to do the same. Those monetary policies contributed substantially to the European recession. This and many other examples show how political considerations are always the critical ones. There are no omnipotent financial markets that have forced governments to carry out austerity policies. To the contrary, the financial markets are immersed in the political institutions that shape them. The liberalization of the financial markets is political: it was instituted by governments, in particular by the U.S. and U.K. governments, which liberalized those markets as a way of facilitating the expansion of U.S. and U.K. banking interests (78). Similarly, the criteria for establishing European monetary union (with the requirement that public deficits be under 3 percent of GNP, and public debt under 60 percent of GNP) were based on political decisions that responded to financial interests, well represented by the enormously influential Bundesbank.

The liberalization of financial markets can be reversed, however. There is nothing omnipotent or sacred about the liberalization of these markets. They can be controlled and/or regulated and/or slowed down if governments, either cooperatively or individually, so desire. Andrew Glyn (79) has recommended, for example, the reintroduction of tight capital controls. James Tobin (80) has advised taxing speculative currency exchanges. And many governments have unilaterally intervened to avoid short-term transactions that are the most speculative in character (78).

VI. PUBLIC POLICIES AIMED AT RESOLVING THE UNEMPLOYMENT PROBLEM: THE NEOLIBERAL SOLUTION—DEREGULATING LABOR MARKETS

The most important public policy interventions to reduce unemployment in western capitalist developed countries have been the deregulation of labor markets and reduction in social protection, because unemployment is considered to be the result of labor market rigidities and an excessive welfare state. In these interventions, the United States and United Kingdom have been presented as successful models, with very low unemployment. But, as I have indicated earlier in this chapter, unemployment is not the best indicator of the efficiency of a labor market, and the United States and United Kingdom are not good examples of job-producing countries. In this section I will analyze the behavior of labor markets on both sides of the North Atlantic, and will question many of the assumptions of the neoliberal position on these labor markets.

But, first, a brief outline of some elementary positions is called for; indeed, any analysis of labor markets has to start by establishing where adult people are in the labor force. People can be employed (let's call this position *E*), unemployed looking for a job (*U*), or non-participatory (*N*). But just as important as knowing where people are in these three mutually exclusive positions in the labor market, we need to understand the flows among these positions. An important dimension of labor flexibility is the ease with which people go from one position to another, and is measured by the flows among these three positions, *E*, *U*, and *N* (Figure 1).

Thus *EU* defines the flow of people from being employed to being unemployed, either because they get fired or because they leave a job. *NU* defines the flow from being non-participatory (outside the labor market) to looking for a job, although not yet finding one. The sum of *EU* and *NU* defines all the people who join the unemployed (people without a job who are looking for one). As is immediately evident, the number of people who are unemployed depends on the number of people who have left a job (and are looking for one) plus the number of people who were not looking for a job, but now are looking for one. Thus two countries with the same rate of job production can have different rates of unemployment, depending on their level of job destruction and/or termination of contracts and/or the level of job demand from people who previously were not looking for work (such as new entrants into the labor market).

Similarly, the total flow of people from work to non-participation in the labor force is the sum of the flow of people from employed to non-participatory (*EN*) and the flow of people from a position of job seeking to a position of giving up (*UN*). Thus two countries with identical rates of job production could have very different unemployment rates, depending on the nature of the jobs produced; low-paying jobs discourage people from looking for jobs (*UN*) or make it less attractive to hold on to a job (*EN*). The country producing less attractive jobs may have lower unemployment because fewer people are interested in finding a job.

On the other hand, the flow of people leaving unemployment is the sum of the number who have found a job (*UE*) and the number who have given up looking for a job (*UN*).

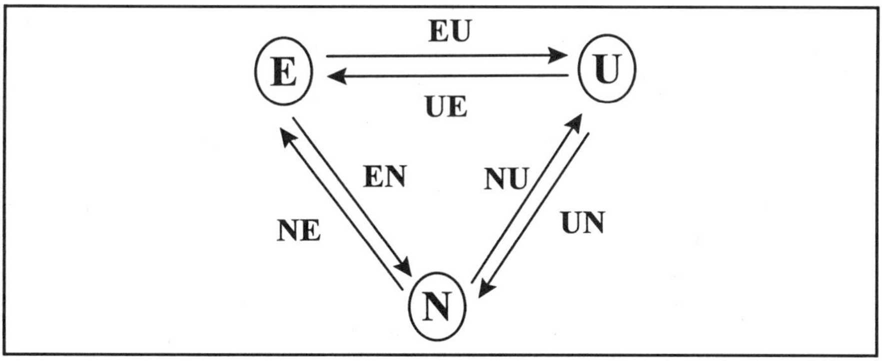

Figure 1. Flows within the labor market between employment (*E*), unemployment (*U*), and non-participation in the labor force (*N*). The flows are described in detail in the text.

Within this flow of people, the number of new contracts, or hirings (*H*), is equal to *UE* + *NE* + *EE;* that is, the number of people who find a job after some time looking for one (*UE*), plus the number who find a job as soon as they begin looking (lucky them!) (*NE*), plus the number who change jobs (*EE*). The number of discontinuations of contracts, or severances (*S*), is equal to *EU* + *EN* + *EE*; that is, the number of people who become unemployed after having had a job (*EU*), plus the number who having had a job no longer have one and are not looking for one (*EN*), plus the number who leave one job for another (*EE*).

The total number of job changes is *S* + *H*; that is, the sum of new contracts plus discontinued contracts. Worker's turnover (*WT*) is a measure of the degree of mobility among contracts:

$$WT = \frac{H+S}{E} = \frac{(UE+NE+EE)+(EU+EN+EE)}{E}$$

$$= \frac{UE+NE+EU+EN+2EE}{E}$$

Table 38 shows the value of these and related indicators for France, Germany, Spain, Great Britain, and the United States. It shows that the worker's turnover of the labor market in the United States (51.80) is lower than that in France (59.55), although larger than in Germany (43.80), Spain (40.72), and Great Britain (13.16). The latter country had the lowest worker's turnover in 1987 (81).

The great difference between the labor markets in the United States and those in the European countries is not so much the overall "worker's turnover" or even the move from one job to another (*EE*),[4] but rather the mobility to unemployment (*EU* + *NU*) and to non-participation (*EN* + *UN*) and vice versa, from unemployment and non-participation to employment (*NU* + *UE* + *NE*) (82).

Actually, in the flow from contract to contract (*EE*) the U.S. labor market *has greater rigidity due to the privatization of its welfare state*. Pension benefits and health care benefits, for example, are funded by employer and employee contributions, paid to private insurance companies according to terms negotiated in highly decentralized collective bargaining agreements. Consequently, the level of pension and health care benefits for workers and their families depends on the type and place of work, and changes with the employment center at which the worker is hired. Thirty percent of adult male workers, for example, would like to change their place of work but do not do so because they are afraid of losing their health benefits coverage, or having it reduced (83, p. 97). The privatization of the welfare state, which gives employers huge power over employees (who lose not only income but also pension and health benefits coverage for themselves and their families when fired), adds enormous rigidities to the U.S. labor market. *In*

[4] OECD (1994) data show that several European countries have the same rate of mobility *EE* as the United States; Italy has an identical rate to the United States.

Table 38

Indicators of labor market flexibility in several OECD countries, 1987, as percent of the population base[a]

	France	Germany	Spain	Great Britain	U.S.
Flow of people who become unemployed (*EU* + *NU*)	3.88	3.0	1.61	7.8	23.88
Flow of people who leave unemployment (*UE* + *UN*)	69.62	93.33	16.80	120.40	545.47
Rate of new hirings (*H/E*)	28.86	22.33	19.80	6.55	25.27
Rate of contract terminations (*S/E*)	30.69	21.47	20.92	6.61	26.53
Worker's turnover (*WT* = (*H* + *S*) /*E*)	59.55	43.80	40.72	13.16	51.80
Average length of unemployment, months	8.2	8.04	6.12	10.67	5.04
Percent of unemployment that is chronic	39.52	36.98	51.48	42.16	12.66

[a]Source: reference 81, Table 2.2, p. 10.

that respect, the universalization of social rights, such as pensions and health care, typical of the E.U. countries, eliminates such rigidities in those countries.

The rigidities of the U.S. labor market are particularly centered in the flows from contract to contract (*EE*), and are due to the privatization of the welfare state, a privatization that is based on employee-employer negotiations. The decentralized nature of these collective bargaining processes, and the absence of collective bargaining agreements for large sections of the labor force, explain the enormous variability and, in general, the poverty of workers' benefits. The vast majority of workers and employees do not have the same type of benefits as their E.U. counterparts. Pensions, unemployment insurance, health care benefits, occupational health and safety, vacation time, parental leave, and other benefits are lower in the United States than in the majority of E.U. countries (53).

Another characteristic of the U.S. labor market is that the flow of people from contract to contract (*EE*) is, for the most part (68 percent for blue-collar workers and 61 percent for white-collar workers), to lower paying jobs (84, p. 47).

Where labor mobility in the United States is much larger than in the European Union is from employment to unemployment (*EU*) or to non-participation (*EN* and *UN*) and vice versa, from non-participation to participation, and from unemployment to employment (*NU, NE*, and *UE*). This type of mobility explains two other characteristics of the labor market in the United States: the overall duration of unemployment is shorter and the proportion that is long-term is lower than in Europe. We can see in Table 38, for example, that the average duration of unemployment in the United States is 5.04 months, compared with 10.67 months in Great Britain, 6.12 months in Spain, 8.04 months in Germany, and 8.2 months in France. And the percentage of unemployment that is chronic is 12.66 percent in the United States, much lower than in Great Britain (42.16 percent), Spain (51.48 percent), Germany (36.98 percent), and France (39.52 percent).

Another characteristic of the U.S. labor market that is a consequence of greater labor mobility (*EU* + *EN* + *NU* + *NE*) than in the European Union is that the active population in the United States experiences unemployment more frequently than the E.U. population; that is, there is a greater probability of being unemployed in the United States than in the European Union. This probability is not randomly distributed among the active population, but rather is concentrated in particular sectors, which explains why, according to the annual Economic Policy Institute report *The State of Working America*, "a third of all the labor force in the United States is in a situation of constant instability" (50, p. 241). Actually, when all the periods of unemployment in the lifetime of a worker are added, the overall time an average worker spends in unemployment is most likely larger in the United States than in the European Union.[5]

Labor instability (largely, flows from employment to unemployment and vice versa) is concentrated in the lower level of the labor force, but the threat of being unemployed is much larger and affects the majority of the active U.S. population. According to Princeton Survey Research Associates, 66 percent of the U.S. labor force has a feeling of labor instability and stress (85).

This fear of being laid off and the associated stress is particularly accentuated among workers who have entered the labor market for the first time, especially women and young people, the majority of whom have first jobs that are temporary. According to an OECD report on employment, 34 percent of low-wage workers in the United States are stuck in low-wage jobs without the possibility of moving to higher-wage positions, compared with only 16 percent of such workers in Germany (32, p. 44). It is because of this that the U.S. labor market is not divided into those who have work (insiders) and those who do not (outsiders), but rather those with a fixed (long-term) contract and those with

[5] The way in which the U.S. Bureau of Labor Statistics collects information about employment and unemployment allows for the calculation of the overall time of unemployment for a worker during his or her lifetime. No such possibility exists with information in the European Union, which means the comparison must be based on national experiences and observations.

a temporary (short-term) contract. In the United States, *the latter group constantly leaves and enters the labor market (EU–UE–EU–UE, etc.). This situation is what gives the impression of greater flexibility in the U.S. than in the E.U. labor market.*

The U.S. experience should challenge the proposition put forward by neoliberal and conservative authors in the United States to facilitate the firing and/or discontinuation of workers in the European Union as a means of creating employment on that continent. Experience in the United States shows that this type of intervention condemns large sectors of the labor force to a constant cycling between unemployment and employment in temporary jobs that are not stepping stones toward better-paying positions. Actually, the unattractiveness of this constant cycling explains another characteristic of the U.S. labor market: *the large number of people that abandon their job search (UN and EN) because of their failure to find a job that is stable and meets their expectations.* The low salaries and low quality of these jobs explain the large number of people who have abandoned the labor market in the United States. They also explain why, contrary to the predictions of neoliberal economics, the increase in the U.S. minimum wage increased rather than decreased the percentage of the population that is employed. The betterment of jobs promoted the demand for jobs and the flow *NE* (86). The percentage of the active population that has abandoned the search for a job, because of being discouraged about finding a job that will meet their expectations, is larger in the United States (0.8 percent of the employed population) than in the E.U. countries where such surveys have been carried out—for example, France, Italy, Great Britain, and Greece (for which the overall aggregate is 0.5 percent) (37). Actually, one reason why there are more people looking for jobs in the European Union than in the United States is that entry-level jobs are better in Europe than in the United States. It has been estimated, for example, that if France now had the same rate of job demand as in 1973, the rate of unemployment among men would be 6.8 percent and among women (who represent 60 percent of the unemployed in France) would be 4 percent.

Consequences of Labor Instability

The great facility that exists in the United States for firing workers, and the large mobility and flow between employment and unemployment (*EU* + *UE*), have not led to a pronounced increase in the number of more stable and better paid jobs. To the contrary, the widely perceived labor instability has resulted in a lowering of wages for the majority of workers, including those for highly paid workers. As Chairman of the U.S. Federal Reserve, Mr. Greenspan, recognized recently, a primary reason for the low pressure to increase wages has been the widespread perception of labor instability (quoted in 87):

> In 1991, in the moment of deep recession, a survey among workers of large enterprises showed that 25 percent were afraid of losing their jobs. In 1996, in spite of lower unemployment, the same survey showed that a larger percentage, 46 percent, were now afraid of losing their jobs.

Labor instability, the actual risk and the fear of losing one's job, is the cause of wage stagnation and even wage declines for most workers in the United States. This situation worsened during the period 1989–1995, with an increased rate of firing and discontinuation of contracts (*EU*), particularly among mature workers (40–55 years old); an increased percentage of the labor force in temporary jobs; and an increase in the percentage of involuntarily part-time work (88).

The Council of Economic Advisors to the U.S. President has questioned this widely held perception in the United States that wages are declining, referring to a larger growth in the high-wage (on average) sectors than in low-wage sectors (89; for a critique see 90). The Council, however, does not refer to the actual wage levels of the newly created jobs; rather it refers to the average wage in each sector where those jobs are produced. But given that the average wages of these sectors are declining (a fact that the Council does not deny), the new occupations are clearly lower paid than the existing ones. Moreover, the Council defines the job by occupation, which can be very misleading. For example, a steel worker, whose occupational category is production worker or operator (at a good $18 per hour), has an upgraded occupational category when fired and then hired at a McDonald's hamburger stand as a director or assistant manager (paid only $9 an hour) (91).

This situation in the U.S. labor market questions the position that "insiders," those who have work (and their representatives, the unions), are actually responsible for the situation of "outsiders," those who do not have jobs. The assumption made by neoliberal and conservative authors is that unions' defense of good, high-paying jobs with good social protection makes it difficult for employers to hire new workers. Thus, highly protected workers are insensitive to the plight of those who cannot get jobs because workers are too strongly defended by the unions. This argument, however, assumes a clear-cut separation between insiders and outsiders, with the former responsible for the plight of the latter. But as the U.S. experience shows, insiders and outsiders are not independent of each other. The fate of the insider is closely linked to the situation of the outsider. Experience in the United States shows that the weakening of insiders does not automatically benefit the outsiders; the growth of instability among those who have work does not improve conditions for the majority of the labor force, both insiders and outsiders. To the contrary, instability may just become more widespread.

Another lesson that can be learned from the U.S. experience is that the proposal in some E.U. circles to diminish wages and social protection for entry-level positions so as to facilitate the integration of youths into the labor force may condemn these new entrants to unattractive jobs, either permanently or for very long periods, rather than providing them with stepping stones to better jobs. These low-level jobs become the only ones available to these workers, keeping them stuck in such occupations for the rest of their working lives. The great mobility of the U.S. labor market, so often extolled, is not upward but downward or sideways. Actually, the percentage of young workers with low-wage jobs (65 percent of the median worker's wage) that move to better jobs is smaller in countries with deregulated labor markets than in those with highly regulated labor markets (31, p. 31). Thus there is no evidence that the lowering of wages and social protection facilitates the entrance and integration of young workers into the labor market. In the United States, temporary, low-paying jobs easily become the only type of jobs these workers will ever have. This experience has forced the latest OECD report on employment to recognize that "the reduction of wages and social protection cannot be considered an effective measure to facilitate the integration and mobility of the young into the labor market" (31, p. 45).

All this evidence demonstrates the highly questionable nature of the recommendation that the best way of creating jobs is to deregulate labor markets. Deregulation, labor mobility, and labor flexibility are terms and concepts that are constantly treated as interchangeable, but they are not. Countries with more regulated labor markets than the United States have greater labor flexibility and geographical mobility (Sweden, Japan, and Norway), occupational mobility (Belgium and Great Britain), and sectional mobility (Denmark) than the United States (31, p. 49). Countries having the greatest labor flexibility have been those, such as Sweden, with highly regulated labor markets.

REFERENCES

1. Declaration of Congressman Gingrich. *New York Times*, October 13, 1995, p. A1.
2. Armstrong, P., Glyn, A., and Harrison, J. *Capitalism Since 1945*. Blackwell, Oxford, 1991.
3. Godley, W. America's unaccountable admiration for Mrs. Thatcher's economics. In *Global Unemployment: Loss of Jobs in the 90's*, edited by J. Eatwell, p. 21. Sharpe, Armonk, N.Y., 1996.
4. Glyn, A. Stability, inegalitarianism, and stagnation: An overview of the advanced capitalist countries. In *Macro-economic Policy after the Conservative Era*, edited by G. D. Epstein and H. M. Gintis. Cambridge University Press, Cambridge, England, 1995.
5. Mishel, L. Behind the numbers. Capital gains. *The American Prospect*, July-August 1997, pp. 71–73.
6. Gordon, D. Putting the horse (back) before the cart: Disentangling the macro-relationship between investment and saving. In *Macro-economic Policy after the Conservative Era*, edited by G. D. Epstein and H. M. Gintis, p. 57. Cambridge University Press, Cambridge, England, 1995.
7. Botwinick, H. *Persistent Inequalities, Wage Disparities under Capitalist Competition*. Princeton University Press, Princeton, N.J., 1993.

8. Blanchflower, D. G., and Oswald, A. J. *The Wage Curve*. MIT Press, Cambridge, Mass., 1994.
9. Marimon, R. *La Economía Española*, p. 296. 1995.
10. Navarro, V. La economía y el estado de bienestar. *El Socialismo de Futuro*, No. 9, 1994.
11. McFate, K., Lawson, R., and Wilson, W. N. (eds.). *Poverty, Inequality, and the Future of Social Policy: Western States and the New World Order*. Russell Sage Foundation, New York, 1995.
12. Marglin, S., and Schor, J. (eds.). *The Golden Age of Capitalism*. Oxford University Press, Oxford, 1990.
13. Audretsch, D. B. *Industrial Policy and Competitive Advantage*, Vol. III. Edward Elgar, 1998.
14. Hooks, G. The rise of the Pentagon and U.S. state building: The defense program as industrial policy. In *Industrial Policy and Competitive Advantage*, edited by D. B. Audretsch, Vol. III, pp. 358–404. Edward Elgar, 1998.
15. Eatwell, J. (ed.). *Global Unemployment: Loss of Jobs in the 90's*. Sharpe, Armonk, N.Y., 1996.
16. Eatwell, J. Unemployment on a world scale. In *Global Unemployment: Loss of Jobs in the 90's*, edited by J. Eatwell. Sharpe, Armonk, N.Y., 1996.
17. Gordon, D. Growth, distribution, and the rules of the game: Social structuralist macro-foundations for a democratic economic policy. In *Macro-economic Policy after the Conservative Era*, edited by G. D. Epstein and H. M. Gintis, p. 335. Cambridge University Press, Cambridge, England, 1995.
18. Rifkin, J. *The End of Work: The Decline of the Global Labor Force and the Dawn of the Post-Market Era*. Putnam's Sons, New York, 1995.
19. International Labor Organization. *World Employment, 1996–1997: National Policies in a Global Context*. Geneva, 1996.
20. Wood, A. *North-South Trade, Employment and Inequality: Changing Fortunes in a Skill-Driven World*. Clarendon Paperbacks, Oxford, 1994.
21. Dicken, P. *Global Shift*. Guilford Press, New York, 1992.
22. Gordon, D. Underpaid workers, bloated corporations. *Dissent*, Spring 1996, p. 33.
23. Cline, W. R. *Trade and Income Distribution*. Institute for International Economics, 1997.
24. Bowles, S., and Boyer, R. Wages, aggregate demand and employment in an open economy: An empirical investigation. In *Macro-economic Policy after the Conservative Era*, edited by G. D. Epstein and H. M. Gintis, p. 143. Cambridge University Press, Cambridge, England, 1995.
25. Skott, P. Financial innovation, deregulation and Minsky cycles. In *Macro-economic Policy after the Conservative Era*, edited by G. D. Epstein and H. M. Gintis, p. 255. Cambridge University Press, Cambridge, England, 1995.
26. Thurow, L. The crusade that's killing prosperity. *The American Prospect*, March-April 1996, p. 54.
27. Organization for Economic Cooperation and Development. *Income Distribution in OECD Countries*. Paris, 1995.
28. Learning to cope. *The Economist*, April 6, 1996, p. 13.
29. Organization for Economic Cooperation and Development. *Jobs Study: Facts, Analysis, Strategies*. Paris, 1994.

30. Nickell, S. Unemployment and labor market rigidities: Europe versus North America. *J. Econ. Perspect.* 3(Summer): 55–74, 1997.
31. Organization for Economic Cooperation and Development. *Employment Outlook 1997*. Paris, 1997.
32. Organization for Economic Cooperation and Development. *Implementing the OECD Job Strategy: Member Countries' Experiences, 1997*. Paris, 1997.
33. Organization for Economic Cooperation and Development. *Labor Statistics, 1974–1995*. Paris, 1996.
34. Mitchell, S. *The Collapse in Demand for Unskilled Labour: What Can Be Done*. Institute of Economics and Statistics, University of Oxford, Oxford, England, 1995.
35. Organization for Economic Cooperation and Development. *Employment Trends, 1996*. Paris, 1996.
36. Nickell, S., and Bell, B. The collapse in demand for the unskilled and unemployment across the OECD. *Oxford Rev. Econ. Policy* 11: 40–62, 1995.
37. Buchele, R., and Christiansen, J. Do employment and income security cause unemployment? A comparative case study of the U.S. and the E-4. *Cambridge J. Econ.* 22(1): 117–136, 1998.
38. Esping-Andersen, G. *Unemployment and Employment Refutations: A Review of the Evidence from Comparative Research.* University of Trento, Italy, 1997.
39. Atkinson, A., and Micklewright, Unemployment compensation and the labor market transitions. *J. Econ. Lit.* 29: 1679, 1991.
40. Organization for Economic Cooperation and Development. *Making Work Pay*. Paris.
41. Schmitt, J. *Job Market Flexibility and Job Creation in the U.S.* Economic Policy Institute, Washington, D.C., 1997.
42. Organization for Economic Cooperation and Development. *Employment Outlook*, July 1997. Paris, 1997.
43. Rasell, E., Bluestone, B., and Mishel, L. (eds.). *The Prosperity Gap. A Chart Book of American Living Standards*. 1997.
44. Atkinson, A. B., Rainwater, L., and Smeeding, T. M. *Income Distribution in the OECD Countries*. OECD, Paris, 1995.
45. Maher, V. A., Jesuit, D. K., and Roscoe, D. D. *Exploring the Impact of Trade and Investment on Income Inequality: A Cross-National Sectoral Analysis of the Developed Market Economy Countries*. Working Paper No. 159. Luxembourg Income Study, 1997.
46. Gottschalk, P., and Joyce, M. *Cross-National Differences in the Rise of Earning Inequality. Market and Institutional Factors*. Working Paper No. 160. Luxembourg Income Study, 1997.
47. Gottschalk, P., Gustafsson, B., and Palmer, E. *Changing Patterns in the Distribution of Economic Welfare*. Cambridge University Press, Cambridge, England, 1997.
48. Smeeding, T. M. *Financial Poverty in Developed Countries: The Evidence from L.I.S.* Working Paper No. 155. Luxembourg Income Study, 1997.
49. *World Development Report 1997*. Oxford University Press, Oxford, 1997.
50. Mishel, L., Bernstein, M., and Schmitt, J. *The State of Working America, 1996–1997*. Economic Policy Institute, Washington, D.C., 1997.
51. Korpi, W. *Democratic Class Strategies*. Sharpe, Armonk, N.Y., 1988.

52. Hanke, B. *Labor Unions, Business Coordination and Economic Adjustment in Western Europe, 1980–90.* Research Unit, Economic Change and Employment, W.Z.B.F.S. 196-309, August 1996.
53. Mishel, L., and Schmitt, J. (eds.). *Beware of the U.S. Model: Jobs and Wages in a Deregulated Economy.* Economic Policy Institute, Washington, D.C., 1996.
54. William, W., and Colamosa, A. *The Judas Economy: The Triumph of Capital and the Betrayal of Work.* Addison, Reading, Mass., 1997.
55. Navarro, V. Production and the welfare state: The political context of reforms. *Int. J. Health Serv.* 21(4): 585–614, 1991.
56. Organization for Economic Cooperation and Development. *Globalization of Industry.* Paris, 1996.
57. European Commission. *Growth, Competitiveness and Employment.* December, 1993.
58. Schwab, K. *Redefining the Basic Assumption of Mankind.* United Nations, New York, 1996.
59. Schmitt, J. *Inequality and Globalization.* Economic Policy Institute, Washington, D.C., 1996.
60. Organization for Economic Cooperation and Development. *Globalization of Industry.* Paris, 1997.
61. Wade, R. Globalization and its limits. In *National Diversity and Global Capitalism,* edited by S. Berger and R. Dore. Cornell University Press, Ithaca, N.Y., 1996.
62. Greider, W. *One World, Ready or Not: The Manic Logic of Capitalism.* Simon and Schuster, New York, 1997.
63. Lipsey, R. E., Blomsten, M., and Ramstetten, F. *Internationalized Production in World Output.* National Bureau of Economic Research, 1997.
64. Lee, E. Globalization and employment: Is anxiety justified? *I.L.O. Rev.* 5: 488.
65. Gordon, D. *Fat and Mean.* Free Press, New York, 1996.
66. Glyn, A. Egalitarianism in a global economy. *Boston Rev.* 22(6), 1997–1998.
67. Hirst, P., and Thomson, G. *Globalization in Question.* Polity Press, Cambridge, England, 1996.
68. Tyson, L. They are not US: Why American ownership still matters. *The American Prospect,* Winter 1991, pp. 37–49.
69. Tyson, L. *Capital Flows in the 1980s: A Survey of Major Trends.* B.I.S. Economic Papers. Bank for International Settlements, April 1991.
70. Hagland, J. Surrender to the money men. *Washington Post,* December 10, 1995.
71. Faux, T. *The Party Is Not Over: A New Vision for the Democrats.* Basic Books, New York, 1997.
72. Aschauer, D. A. *Public Investment and Private Sector Growth.* Economic Policy Institute, Washington, D.C., 1991.
73. Eisner, R. The misunderstood economy. In *What Counts and How to Count It.* Howard University Press, Washington, D.C., 1994.
74. Fazzari, S. *Investments and U.S. Fiscal Policy in the 1990s.* Economic Policy Institute, Washington, D.C., 1993.
75. Blecker, R. *Are Americans on a Consumption Binge?* Economic Policy Institute, Washington, D.C., 1990.
76. International Labor Organization. *Can Expansionary Policies Raise Growth?* I.L.O. Report, Geneva, 1996.

77. Roosevelt, F. D. Inaugural Address, The White House, Washington, D.C., 1937.
78. Helliner, E. Post-globalization: Is the financial liberalization trend likely to be reversed? In *States Against Markets*, edited by R. Boyer and D. Drache. Routledge, New York, 1996.
79. Glyn, A. Capital flight and exchange controls. *New Left Rev.* 155: 37–49, 1986.
80. Tobin, J. A proposal for international monetary reform. *Eastern Econ. J.* 4: 153–159, 1978.
81. Center for Economic Research. *Unemployment Choices for Europe*. 1995.
82. Boeri, T. *On the Job Search and Unemployment Duration.* Working Papers in Economics, No. 95/38. European University Institute, 1995.
83. Health Services Research Agency. *Facts and Figures of the U.S. Medical Care Sector.* U.S. Government Printing Office, Washington, D.C., 1997.
84. Organization for Economic Cooperation and Development. *Investment, Productivity and Employment.* OECD Job Study. Paris, 1995.
85. Princeton Survey Research Associates. *Survey of Labor Force in the U.S.* Princeton, N.J., August 1997.
86. Bernstein, J., and Schmitt, J. The sky hasn't fallen: An evaluation of the minimum wage increase. *Working U.S.A.*, September-October 1997, p. 88.
87. Brand, H. Global capitalism and the decay of employment policy. *Dissent*, Autumn 1997.
88. Schmitt, S., and Sworny, S. V. Recent trends in job security and stability. *J. Labor Res.*, 1998, in press.
89. Council of Economic Advisors. *Job Creation and Employment Opportunities: The United States Labor Market, 1993–1996.* U.S. Government Printing Office, Washington, D.C., 1996.
90. Bernstein, J. Anxiety over wages is justified. *Challenge*, July-August 1996.
91. Faux, L. The American model exposed. *The Nation*, October 1997, p. 18.

CHAPTER 3

HEALTH AND EQUITY IN THE WORLD IN THE ERA OF "GLOBALIZATION"

Vicente Navarro

Since the late 1970s and early 1980s, a new position has become dominant in the world's major economic and political circles that assumes we are witnessing a new and unprecedented situation, referred to as the "globalization" of the economy. According to this position, the globalization of commerce, investments, and finance has become a major force behind the setting of public policies, including health policies. The power of governments to shape national policy is being considerably limited and diminished by an increasingly competitive international economy. The only choice of governments is to join in and facilitate the process, to open up their countries to globalization, since any resistance to doing so will be penalized. According to a 1998 World Health Organization (WHO) document, countries that resist globalization "will find themselves marginalized in the world community and in the world economy" (1). Indeed, we have seen how much pressure the U.S. government and the International Monetary Fund (IMF) have been putting on Russia and the Southeast Asian and Latin American countries to open up their economies, to help them integrate into the global economy and thus solve their economic and financial crises.

To that effect, in order for their countries to participate in the welfare and well-being assumed to result from integration into the global economy, governments must create conditions favorable to the mobility of commerce, investments, and financial transactions. They should achieve this through policies that include, among other things, lowering taxes on capital investments and transactions; reducing public deficits through a decrease in public and social (including health care) expenditures; deregulating financial and labor markets; privatizing public enterprises and programs (as in the proposals put forward by the World Bank and IMF to privatize social security systems); and developing fiscal policies that favor high-income sectors of the population, which are assumed to be those most able to save and therefore to invest (with the supposition that the riches at the top will "trickle down" to the rest of the population). Such public policies have been the most strongly supported by prominent international financial agencies such as the IMF and the World Bank and by governments of major countries, including the United States.

CONSEQUENCES OF PUBLIC POLICIES THAT BENEFIT GLOBALIZATION

One consequence of public policies that benefit globalization has been an unheard of growth of inequalities in today's world, with the net worth of the 358 richest people equaling the combined income of the poorest 45 percent of the world's population—2.3 billion people (2). These inequalities are growing at an unprecedented rate, not only among countries but also within most of the developed and developing countries. This situation is the primary reason for the slowing down of the health improvements that occurred worldwide in previous decades, causing stagnation and even declines in the levels of health and well-being in many regions of the world (3). This growth in inequalities has resulted from (*a*) the unprecedented growth in wealth and income derived from capital versus that derived from labor, (*b*) the growing polarization of wages with a consequent increase in wage dispersion, and (*c*) the diminishing impact of the redistributive effect of the welfare state and the fast deterioration of the public infrastructure, particularly notable in the less developed countries (4–6) (see Chapters 2 and 4).

REVOLTS AGAINST "GLOBALIZATION"

Not surprisingly, we are seeing large mobilizations by those who are being harmed by the globalization process. In the late 1990s there have been labor strikes, with fears of popular uprisings, in many of the Southeast Asian countries once seen as success stories, examples of globalization (but where average wages have declined spectacularly). Such mobilizations have been particularly strong in South Korea, Malaysia, and Indonesia. There have also been mobilizations of the unemployed, with substantial popular support, in France and in Germany (where unemployment has reached unheard of levels), and mobilization of Indians in Chiapas and worker unrest elsewhere in Mexico (where average wages have declined since 1994). In the United States (where median hourly wages have declined in the 1980s and 1990s), popular rejection forced the withdrawal of President Clinton's proposal to expand the terms of free trade to many Latin American countries.

All these mobilizations have one thing in common: they are popular protests against globalization. To dismiss these protests as "isolationism," "protectionism," "xenophobia," "nationalism," or whatever—as the above mentioned WHO document (1) implies—is to ignore this fact: while, for some, the globalization they extol has meant an enormous growth in wealth and income, for others the process has meant an enormous deterioration in their standard of living, health, and well-being. Not only in developing but also in developed capitalist countries we have seen an increasing aggression against the welfare state, justified by the argument that globalization and competitiveness require such structural adjustments in both developed and developing countries. Here, I would like to reply to those who assert that the popularity of the welfare state in developed capitalist countries is such that no government—not even the Reagan and Thatcher governments—would dare touch it. Those supporting this argument point out that countries governed by quite different political parties, such as Sweden, Germany, Great Britain, and the United States, have all maintained their levels of social transfers (measured by social expenditures as percentage of GNP) (7). But it is misleading to present this as an indication of the resilience of the welfare state. Social transfers are more difficult to cut back than social services because the impact of their reduction is more immediate (pensioners very soon notice any reduction in their Social Security checks) than is the reduction of social services (it takes longer for users of these services to notice any declines in funding). This is why cutbacks in expenditures on services are more doable politically than cutbacks in social transfers. And this is what has been happening. The rate of growth in spending on services per user and in public employment per user has been declining in developed capitalist countries in the 1980s and 1990s, even though the need for such services has been increasing due to the growth of unemployment, demographic changes (with growth of the elderly population), growing inequalities, and increasing poverty (8).

Another factor ignored by those certain of the resilience of the welfare state is that the rate of growth of social transfers and social expenditures has been declining during the 1980s and 1990s—even as human needs (for the reasons noted above) have been increasing substantially. The decline in the rate of growth of public employment has been particularly accentuated in countries within the liberal tradition such as the United States, Great Britain, and Canada, with declines also occurring in continental countries in Europe such as France, Germany, Italy, Belgium, and the Netherlands. Countries with social democratic traditions and strong labor movements such as Sweden, Norway, Denmark, Finland, and Austria have been better able to resist the declines, although some reductions have occurred (see Chapter 4).

A similar situation is evident in public consumption, which includes the costs of goods and services provided by the public sector, of which the welfare state makes up the majority. We can see a very accentuated decline of public consumption over the 1980s, although here again, social democratic countries have had higher rates of growth in public consumption than the continental European and liberal countries. Other changes have also occurred in the welfare states of developed capitalist countries as a result of the liberal avalanche, such as (*a*) the transformation of some universal benefits into means-tested benefits, (*b*) the greater role of the private sector in the funding and provision of services, and (*c*) lessening of the intensity of care through the reduction of employment and/or expenditures per user or beneficiary, a general phenomenon that has occurred everywhere—although its implementation has varied with the political context, again being more accentuated in liberal and continental European countries than in social democratic countries (see Chapter 4).

A far more dramatic situation has arisen in the developing countries. Today, every two seconds a child dies of hunger. A total of 14 million children die of hunger every year, a number of children's deaths equivalent to 60 Hiroshima bombs—bombs that explode every year without producing a sound. These deaths are not even "news" in our press. They are part of the normal international order. And the situation for many parts of the world is getting worse. The percentage of the population in developing countries with access to drinking water, for example, has been declining since the mid-1970s, and the standards of what the United Nations defines as decent housing have also worsened. Income and wealth inequalities in these countries have reached unprecedented levels, with Latin America breaking all records in the inequalities league.

RESPONSES TO THE GLOBALIZATION PHENOMENON BY THE HEALTH POLICY COMMUNITY

Much has been written in policy circles about globalization, and much scholarly work has been done and continues to be done on its health consequences. With very few exceptions (such as WHO EURO), WHO (Geneva) has been a latecomer in adding its interest in studying this phenomenon. Actually, one important response to globalization by major sectors of the international health establishment has been that this process is a necessary part of progress: part of the internationalization of commerce, finance, culture, and ideas that is making all of us part of the global village. The WHO document (1) reproduces this message. Examples also appear in the Milton Roemer editorial introducing the WHO document in the *American Journal of Public Health* (9). In this theoretical scenario, the role of progressive forces is to minimize the costs—including the social and human costs—of globalization while optimizing the benefits: reduction of prices, internationalization of the division of labor, international cooperation and scientific development, and other benefits. Any reading of WHO or U.S. Agency for International Development (AID) (or even World Bank and IMF) documents reveals a list of good and bad things about globalization, usually with the conclusion that the process has more positive than negative consequences. I am aware, of course, of the meaningful differences among the various agencies, as well as among the major western academic centers, regarding globalization. I am aware, for example, that the IMF's position that the current financial and economic crisis in the less developed countries requires further opening up of their economies (until recently, a position shared by the World Bank; we now see some distancing from that position) differs from WHO's more balanced position in its recent documents, in which the costs of such liberalization are questioned, when not denounced. An interesting report along these lines is the recent 1998 report of the United Nations Development Program (UNDP) (10), which thoroughly documents the nature of the growing inequalities. It shows how unequal are the patterns of consumption in today's world: 20 percent of people in the high-income countries account for 86 percent of private consumption, while the poorest 28 percent of the world's people consume only 1.3 percent of the global pie. The report lists, commodity by commodity (beef, rice, oil, etc.), how much more the rich consume than the poor. It indicates, for example, the amounts consumed by Americans in cosmetics ($8 billion) and by Europeans in ice cream ($11 billion), amounts equivalent to what it would cost to provide basic education ($6 billion) or water and sanitation ($9 billion) to the more than 2 billion of the world's people who go without schools and toilets. And yet the reports making these denouncements, however shocking, are spectacularly insufficient, when not plain wrong. They never touch on the real causes of these inequalities. Why?

Here we have to realize that however meaningful and important the differences among the various international agencies may be, there are important similarities. Among these similarities, three are of critical importance. One is the confusion in identifying the concept and reality of globalization with the concept and reality of internationalization. This explains why the 1998 WHO report (1) dismisses those who oppose globalization as "isolationist," "protectionist," "xenophobic," "nationalist," or whatever. These agencies present themselves as the true internationalists: the international agencies as components of the international government that guarantees the international order.

The second characteristic shared by these agencies (very clear not only in the IMF and World Bank but also in WHO, UNICEF, and UNDP) is the complete absence in their analysis of globalization of the role of power and politics. This observation does not imply that these agencies are apolitical—far from it. It means simply that they never appear to be political. In their analysis and their recommendations, power is not mentioned. Their discourse and their recommendations appear to be "value free," guided primarily by scientific and technical considerations, with conclusions and recommendations that tend to coincide with the conventional wisdom of the dominant establishment centers of power in today's world. This discourse and practice (which I will provisionally define as technocratic) quickly becomes the accepted discourse in academia and the guiding force for all the systems of rewards that exist for intellectuals in our societies. One part of their strategy of reproduction, incidentally, is that all critical views are excluded, usually by being ignored. Any reader of most WHO publications, for example, knows how rare it is to find in these forums any voices that are truly critical of that conventional wisdom. And multiple examples exist of professionals being vetoed by and excluded from such forums. Hopefully, we will see changes under the new leadership of WHO. But there are too many examples of critical views being excluded, which should be cause for alarm in the health policy community. The conservatism that one detects, for example, in western economic and academic circles—broken by a few, very isolated voices—is constantly reproduced not only in the World Bank and the IMF, but also in many U.N. agencies.

A third characteristic, which appears primarily in the humanitarian agencies such as UNDP, is the way in which these inequalities are presented, suggesting that the primary conflict in the world today is between the North (the ice cream eaters) and the South (those who do not even have safe drinking water). The message is one of inducing guilt in those who eat ice cream in the North: if they would just stop eating ice cream, it seems, those in the South would have safe drinking water. This approach, incidentally, is also appearing as a new fad in U.S. academia: the establishment of human rights courses, all of which are characterized by a profound humanism and a profound apoliticism.

ALTERNATIVE VIEWS

It needs to be stressed that the discussion of globalization is not neutral and that the views of globalization theorists are not value-free. There is nothing intrinsically good or bad in the flow of capital, labor, and knowledge around the world; its goodness or badness depends on who governs the flow, which determines who benefits from it. *Globalization is a specific form of internationalization that responds to specific financial and economic interests that are articulated in the class relations of each society.* There are other forces and expressions of internationalization that do not respond to and are not a part of globalization. The issue, therefore, is not "internationalization or not," but rather, "what type of internationalization are we talking about?" The WHO document celebrates the process of globalization by celebrating the liberalization of health services under the provision of the General Agreement on Trade in Services, because it will "blur the boundaries between the national and 'globalized' health sectors . . . generating 'powerful transitional dynamics' . . . [with] national health systems . . . becoming transnationalized" (1). This liberalization, however, is facilitating the penetration of commercial health insurance into health care all over Latin America (and in many other parts of the world as well), weakening or dismantling long-established government national health services, replacing them with a dynamic in which profit maximization is the major guide to health policies—as has already occurred in the United States. And the World Bank, Pan-American Health Organization, and U.S. AID are actively promoting managed care and managed competition in Latin America today.

The majority of people in the United States have already experienced such a health care model, and they do not like it. According to a report on a nationwide poll by the American Hospital Association (11):

> the majority of the people in the U.S. see [in the health services they receive] neither a planned system nor a consumer-oriented organization except

> one devoted to maximizing profit by blocking access, reducing quality, and limiting spending. . . . They blame most of it on the pursuit of profits by health insurance companies. . . . Americans believe that their health insurance companies have too much influence and exert too much control over their care.

The deregulation, liberalization, and transnationalization of health services is hurting the families of the United States, as well as those of countries where for-profit, insurance-driven medical care is now being imposed, with the assistance of the IMF, World Bank, and WHO. So, when WHO supports the recommendations of the Institute of Medicine's influential report *America's Vital Interests in Global Health* (12), which calls for rich countries such as the United States to help in globalizing health policies, the question that must be raised is: *whose health policies?* Those of the commercial health insurance companies, or those of average families in the United States and other countries? They are not one and the same. They are in conflict. Too frequently, the interests of the health insurance companies prevail—in which case, opposition is necessary and justified, and it is wrong to define such opposition as isolationism.

In the fall of 1998, polls showed that the majority of the U.S. population followed the lead of the labor and ecological movements in opposing the free trade, fast-track proposal put forward by President Clinton and the Republican-controlled Congress. They were against the proposal unless the tariffs were conditional on an increase in the minimum wage and an increase in occupational and environmental regulations in the Latin American countries with which the United States would sign the agreement. It has not escaped people's notice that the increase in wages and improvements in working and environmental conditions promised by the U.S. government on signing the North American Free Trade Agreement have not materialized on either side of the Rio Grande.

It is also wrong to see this as a conflict between North and South. This dichotomy, put forward by the governing elites in the South, ignores the fact that each country is divided into classes (of which those elites are a part) and that class interests are more powerful than national interests. The United States' so-called medical care model is not benefiting the majority of the working class and lower middle class (60 percent of the U.S. population): it benefits only the top 20 percent as well as the large employers and financial interests that control the system. Similarly, export of the U.S. medical care model will benefit 20 percent of the Latin American population but hurt the majority. It is the alliance of the top elites on the two continents that is responsible for that predicament. (This, incidentally, is one reason why the change in composition of leadership of the international agencies to include individuals from developing countries has not had any effect on their policies.) A similar situation is appearing with the privatization of social security. This reality, based on class power, is completely ignored in the globalization discourse.

DEMYSTIFYING GLOBALIZATION

We need to demystify globalization and what it stands for. And we need to realize that it is not as new or as "unprecedented" or even as irreversible as some would claim. Many thorough and rigorous scholarly studies now show that the processes of internationalization of commerce and production has not been so intensive as has been claimed. It would be wrong to suggest that there has been no change in the development and reproduction of capitalism, of course. But the evidence that has accumulated questions the extent and novelty of the process (see 4 for a review of this literature). The only exception is the internationalization of finance, with a daily transaction of $1.7 trillion, mostly of a speculative character—as the Southeast Asian crisis testifies. Governments are cutting public health expenditures in response to pressures from financial markets whose objective is to facilitate the penetration of financial interests into those countries.

What now passes as globalization is a specific type of internationalization of capital, labor, and knowledge, characterized by an unrestrained and unregulated search for profits and greatly enhanced by the public policies initiated by the governments of President Reagan and Prime Minister Thatcher and continued by their successors. Actually, many of the pro-globalization arguments were made years ago by President Hoover, whose policies led to the Great Depression. As President Franklin Roosevelt (who reversed those policies) indicated, "We have always known that heedless self-interest was bad morals; we know now that it is also bad economics" (13). We should add, "and poor public health."

Why has that process been heightened today? To explain this we need to understand the nature of class relations in each country. As I mentioned before, we cannot explain this reality by focusing on the conflict between North and South. We must look at the conflict between capital and labor, with financial capital being the major force of that mobilization. Let's not forget that within each country, the growth in inequalities means that the owners of capital (and high skills) are doing much better, and all others are doing much worse. We can therefore see that class relations, and the expression of these relations through the political, economic, and cultural institutions, are at the root of our understanding of current realities.

The discourse of globalization and its economic determinist message is being reproduced because it serves a class purpose. But it is important to realize that politics and the state continue to play a critical role. Politics and class politics are key elements in understanding what happens in our health policy.

We have seen that, contrary to globalization theory, some of the most globalized countries are those with the most extensive welfare states. In developed capitalist countries, those in which labor is stronger have been more equitable (with larger welfare states) and more efficient (with lower unemployment and more economic growth) than those where capital is stronger. And even under attack by neoliberalism, the former countries have been able to respond much better than the latter. In Chapter 4 I document how the countries with strong labor and social democratic movements—such as Northern European countries—and with a strong commitment to equity have also been those with, during the 1960–1995 period, the most efficient economies: greater economic growth, higher rates of job production, higher occupational rates, lower unemployment, lower inequalities, and better health indicators. To the contrary, countries in which capital has been stronger, and which have followed neoliberal policies, have had lower economic growth, higher unemployment, and worse health indicators.

Which leads me to another observation: the enormous importance of including political categories of power in our analysis so as to understand the impact of inequalities on health. The failure to do so is precisely the main weakness of most studies on the impact of income distribution on the health of populations. They deal with the symptoms rather than the causes. Looking at how health and income are generated leads to an understanding of exploitation and domination, the roots of the unjust international order in which we live, and also to an understanding of the effects of change.

OBSERVATIONS ON THE SCHOLARSHIP ON INEQUALITIES AND HEALTH

Given what I have indicated so far, I should conclude with some observations about the current studies on inequalities and health. Indeed, the fantastic growth of scholarship in this area has been a most welcome development. Most of these studies—although not all—have taken income inequalities as the point of departure for understanding the health of our populations. Among these researchers, Richard Wilkinson has been the most influential on this topic. He takes income inequality as an indicator of social cohesion (a somewhat vague concept that means participation, togetherness, support, and community), which is the actual determinant of the level of population health (3). In Wilkinson's position, the theoretical frame linking income inequality, social cohesion, and health is based primarily on the understanding of income as a consumption category, enabling individuals to articulate themselves with their society mainly through the world of consumption. It is important, however, to emphasize that in these studies, income inequality is used as an indicator of the degree of cohesion. Wilkinson therefore conceptualizes income as an intermediary variable for measuring cohesion, with social cohesion as the critical factor in understanding the level of health and well-being.

As Muntaner and Lynch (14) have indicated, though, the concept of social cohesion has serious problems, both conceptually and empirically. For example, Nazi Germany was a very cohesive society with high levels of participation, sense of togetherness (denying the existence of class divisions, with employers and workers militating in the same trade organizations), and community. Thus, social cohesion per se cannot be chosen as a healthy objective. Similarly, the enormous decline in health indicators in the former Soviet Union cannot be explained by a collapse of its social cohesion. It is certainly more than that. (See Chapters 14–16 for more on the Wilkinson–Muntaner and Lynch debate.)

Furthermore, societies and communities can be highly cohesive while reproducing exploitative relations. Actually, the emphasis on cohesion may be presented as an alternative to policies aimed at reducing income inequalities. The Reagan administration put great emphasis on community and participation while carrying out clearly regressive incomes policies. And today, both the Clinton and Blair administrations emphasize social cohesion and community, divorced from any redistributive concerns.

The limitation of this approach is that the linkage between income, cohesion, and health is not based on how income results from particular power relations in the worlds of production and distribution of resources. It is this absence of concern about how power relations (including class, gender, and race relations) exist and are reproduced that leaves these researchers unable to explain the roots of the problem: how and why income inequalities are produced and reproduced. Different positions in power relations generate various sources and types of economic, political, social, and cultural power, including income. Moreover, these relations are based on relations of exploitation and domination that play a key role in explaining the level of health of our populations. And by power relations, I mean the overall distribution of power in society based on how people own and produce the means of generating that power (from physical to non-material, such as knowledge) (15).

In that respect, income distribution, social cohesion, and other such concepts are symptoms rather than causes. Looking at relations of exploitation and domination, and understanding how exploitation and domination occur and are reproduced, is of paramount importance to understanding the growth of inequalities and the deterioration of health. This means that our research agenda should include the analysis of class, gender, and race power and how it is manifested in political, economic, social, and scientific terms. We can see that neoliberalism and globalization, for example, are the political and ideological instruments of class domination. Demystifying them, and introducing an analysis of the power relations in our society, is of the utmost urgency. It is not just insufficient but wrong to analyze the determinants of our populations' health without analyzing the reproduction of power relations (exploitation and domination), of which class, gender, and race relations are of overwhelming importance (e.g., 16; see 17 for a critique).

I invite you to study, for example, how different power relations configure societies and the level of well-being of their populations, and how labor movements and other allied forces in both developed and developing countries are the most important forces in improving the health and well-being of much of the human race. (See Chapter 4 for empirical studies along these lines (see also reference 18).) I am aware that neither the international agencies nor the research-funding agencies will be willing to fund this type of research, and it is quite likely that those daring to engage in such research will be ignored or silenced. But you should remember that Galileo, a great son of your country, Italy, was also once silenced. Science and the scientific project require integrity and courage, and we owe it to the millions of people who do not have health and remain voiceless to proceed with both.

Note — This chapter is based on a paper presented at the International Symposium on Health and Illness, Perugia, Italy, October 24–27, 1998.

REFERENCES

1. Yach, D., and Bettcher, D. The globalization of public health: Threats and opportunities. A World Health Organization report. *Am. J. Public Health* 88(5), May 1998.
2. United Nations Development Program. *Human Development Report 1996,* p. 13. New York, 1996.
3. Wilkinson, R. G. *Unhealthy Societies: The Afflictions of Inequality.* Routledge, London, 1996.
4. Navarro, V. Neoliberalism, "globalization," unemployment, inequalities, and the welfare state. *Int. J. Health Serv.* 28(4): 607–682, 1998.
5. Navarro, V. The political economy of the welfare state in developed capitalist countries. *Int. J. Health Serv.* 29(1): 1–50, 1999.
6. Navarro, V. *Neoliberalismo y Estado del Bienestar.* Ariel, Barcelona, 1998.
7. Pearson, P. *Dismantling the Welfare State?* Cambridge University Press, Cambridge, England, 1994.
8. Clayton, R., and Pontusson, J. *The New Politics of the Welfare State Revisited.* Cornell University Press, Ithaca, N.Y., 1998.
9. Roemer, M. Editorial. *Am. J. Public Health* 88(5), May 1998.
10. United Nations Development Program. *Human Development Report 1998.* New York, 1998.
11. American Hospital Association. *The State of American Opinion on the Medical Care of the U.S.* July, 1997.
12. Institute of Medicine. *America's Vital Interests in Global Health. 1997.*
13. Roosevelt, F. D. Inaugural Presidential Address. Washington, D.C., January 1937.
14. Muntaner, C., and Lynch, J. Income inequality, social cohesion, and class relations: A critique of Wilkinson's neo-Durkheimian research program. *Int. J. Health Serv.* 29(1): 59–81, 1999.
15. Navarro, V. The labor process and health: A historical materialist interpretation. *Int. J. Health Serv.* 12(1), 1982.
16. Evans, R., et al. *Why Are Some People Healthy and Others Not? The Determinants of Health of Populations.* Aldine de Gruyter, New York, 1998.
17. Poland, B., et al. Wealth, equity and health care: A critique of population health perspective on the determinants of health. *Soc. Sci. Med.* 46(7), 1998.
18. Navarro, V. Has socialism failed? An analysis of health indicators under socialism. *Int. J. Health Serv.* 22(4): 583–601, 1992.

CHAPTER 4

THE POLITICAL ECONOMY OF THE WELFARE STATE IN DEVELOPED CAPITALIST COUNTRIES

Vicente Navarro

I. INTRODUCTION: UNDERSTANDING THE WELFARE STATE—THE NEED TO BREAK WITH ECONOMIC DETERMINISM

One of the most constantly repeated messages in major political and economic circles of the developed capitalist countries is the need to reform their welfare states. In the United States, for example, both the Republican Party and the Democratic Party have made specific proposals for reforming some of the key components of the welfare state such as Medicare and Social Security. The Clinton administration, on the other hand, has claimed that its main social policy proposals (to reform Social Security and the welfare services) represent a "Third Way" between the market-oriented reforms put forward by the right and the public sector reforms advocated by the left.

In western Europe, the call for reforms—many of them triggered by the impending European monetary union—has not been limited to particular political parties or countries. Indeed, there is a continent-wide call for welfare reforms, although the meaning of these reforms varies considerably with the political party calling for them and the country in which the welfare state is to be reformed. A new position has also developed in the European Union, represented by the Blair government in the United Kingdom—and also referred to as the "Third Way"—whose aim is to depart from both the left's and the right's solutions to social problems. This position presents itself as the "radical center," as realized primarily in its approach to the welfare state. It would seem, then, that the issue under contention is not so much whether the welfare state needs to be reformed, but rather what type of reform is needed.

But before addressing this question, let's focus on what social, economic, political, and cultural changes are occurring in the developed capitalist countries and how they are affecting the welfare state. These changes can be grouped into five categories: changes in the family, changes in people's life cycles, changes in the economic and social structures of the developed capitalist countries, changes in their labor markets, and, most importantly, changes in their political contexts. As I will show in this chapter, each of these changes is having a most dramatic impact on the welfare states of the developed capitalist countries. But how these changes take place and how various countries respond to them depend primarily on the correlation of forces (of which class forces continue to have great importance) and their expression in the political space. I will show how countries respond to these changes differently, depending on who is in government. In that respect, I will question those theories and positions—such as the globalization theories—that assume an economic determinism which eliminates or substantially reduces the importance of politics in explaining current changes in the welfare state.

An aim of this chapter is to recover the importance of politics, to put politics at the center of the explanation of what is now happening in the welfare states of the developed capitalist countries. The position presented here is therefore anti-determinist, in both the economic and technological sense. It questions the dominant theoretical frame (reproduced by many international institutions and national governments) that assumes all governments, regardless of who governs, are forced to follow the same policies because of the need to be competitive in the globalized economy, where international markets (whether financial or commercial markets) determine what governments can and must do. But let's not move ahead too fast. We should first focus on the changes that are affecting the welfare states of the developed capitalist countries.

II. CHANGES IN THE FAMILY

Families in the developed capitalist countries are changing markedly. These changes result from many different factors, one of the most important being the increasing involvement of women in the labor force. In all OECD countries, we have seen an increase in the percentage of women participating in the labor market: Table 1 shows the evolution of women's labor force participation from 1979 to 1996. As is evident from the table, while the percentage of men who are working has been declining in most OECD countries, the percentage of women working has been increasing, except in Sweden (where the percentage of women working is the second largest, 54.2 percent, after the United States, 56 percent). It is also important to note that in some countries, such as the United States, the increase in the percentage of women in the labor market has been much more accentuated and has occurred much faster than the decline in the percentage of men in the labor market. Consequently, the percentage of people in the labor force has actually increased rather than decreased in those countries. This means, among other things, that more, rather than fewer, people are paying payroll taxes now than 20 or 30 years ago. But, before elaborating on the meaning of this

Table 1

Total employment as percentage of working-age population[a]

	Employment, %		
	1979	1989	1996
Men			
Japan	78.2	75.1	74.9
United States	73.8	72.5	70.9
Australia	75.3	71.9	67.9
Netherlands	74.3	65.0	66.9
Great Britain	74.5	70.4	65.7
Canada	73.4	71.4	65.2
Sweden	73.7	70.9	61.8
Spain[b]	75.1	66.2	60.7
Germany	69.8	65.9	60.1
France	69.6	61.2	57.6
Italy	66.3	59.9	56.6
Women			
United States	47.5	54.3	56.0
Sweden	57.2	61.7	54.2
Canada	45.3	53.7	52.1
Australia	40.7	48.6	50.4
Great Britain	45.3	49.1	50.1
Japan	45.7	47.4	47.7
Netherlands	29.2	37.4	44.9
Germany	38.4	39.7	41.2
France	40.5	41.2	40.3
Spain[b]	28.6	32.5	38.4
Italy	27.3	28.6	28.4

[a]Source: reference 1, Table 8.17, p. 381.
[b]Information for Spain is from the EPA, Series homogéneas, in reference 2, p. 12.

important point for the funding of the welfare state, let's consider the reasons for the growth of women's participation in the labor force.

There are several such reasons. Among the most important are (*a*) the growing consciousness among women, inspired by the women's liberation movement, of their need and desire for autonomy and self-realization through integration in the labor market; (*b*) the decline of wages among men (either an absolute decline, as in the United States, or a relative decline, as in the majority of E.U. countries), forcing wives or partners into the labor market to maintain the family's standard of living; and (*c*) the growth in the services sector of the economy, which offers the supply of jobs needed for women's integration into the labor force (a point I will expand on later).

The primary cause, the liberation of women, is a positive and irreversible change—part of human progress toward full liberation and full realization of potential. It is therefore predictable that women's labor force participation is much higher in countries where consciousness of women's need for autonomy is more highly developed, for example northern European countries such as Denmark, Sweden, Norway, and Finland (of social democratic tradition) and Anglo-Saxon countries such as the United States, Canada, and the United Kingdom (of liberal tradition), than in central and southern Europe where the Catholic tradition is stronger and the women's liberation movement is weaker (as well as in Japan). For example, the percentage of women in the labor force in 1996 was 56 percent in the United States and 54.2 percent in Sweden, but only 38.4 percent in Spain and 28.4 percent in Italy (Table 1) (1, 2).

The second reason for the growing participation of women, the decline of men's wages, is particularly accentuated in the United States, where men's hourly wages were lower in 1996 than in 1972, forcing more women to enter the labor force. This explains why income levels for U.S. families could be maintained until the end of the 1980s; since then, however, the continuing growth in women's labor force participation has not been able to prevent the decline in family income for the lower 60 percent of U.S. families. In the European Union, men's wages have not undergone an absolute decline, but their rate of growth has decreased significantly; this has led to (besides a growth in men's unemployment) a growing need for women to participate in the labor force (1; see also 3).

The integration of women into the labor force has many implications for family structure and functions. We are witnessing, for example, a growth in the number of families with more than one breadwinner, as well as single-parent families and families headed by a single, female breadwinner. The traditional type of family, with the male head of household as the only breadwinner and the wife working at home, and taking care of grandparents and children, is quickly becoming a minority in the developed capitalist countries (with the exception of southern European countries). The family is thus constantly being redefined. It is wrong to assume, however, as do conservatives, that the decline of the *traditional* family means the decline of the family. All empirical evidence shows the family to be one of the most important points of reference for the citizenry. According to the most recent E.U. polls on people's attitudes toward the family, 78 percent of adults indicated that the family is the most important point of reference, the same percentage as in 1977; and in U.S. polls the percentage is even larger at 82 percent (4). And, although families in the United States are less stable than those in the European Union, 82 percent of divorced people in the United States remarry, creating new families—thus demonstrating the importance of family on both continents (5, 6).

It is also wrong to assume, as do many conservatives and Christian democrats, that the integration of women into the labor force weakens the family; in fact, the evidence shows that such integration may strengthen the family. For example, the fertility rate in the northern European countries is almost double that in the southern European countries, where we find (in Spain and Italy) the lowest fertility rates in the world today (7). Why? The answer demonstrates the importance of understanding the relationship between women, the labor market, and the welfare state. Table 2 shows the relationship between women's participation in the labor force, unemployment among adult and young women, and the fertility rate. As shown in the second column, there was a spectacular decline in the Italian and Spanish fertility rates (from 2.21 in 1975 to 1.25 in 1992 in Italy, and from 2.79 to 1.23 during the same period in Spain). This decline has been attributed to the increased participation of women in the labor force (women working and women looking for jobs) in these two countries during the years 1975–1992, from 37 to 46 percent in Italy, and from 32 to 42 percent in Spain (8). This explanation, however, is unconvincing. The majority of OECD countries have larger female

Table 2

Statistical synopsis of women's labor force participation, fertility, and unemployment[a]

	Female participation rate (ages 15–64), %		Fertility rate, no. of children per woman		Female unemployment rate, %	Female unemployment rate (ages 15–24), %
	1975	1992	1975	1992	1980–92	1980–92
United States	53	68	1.77	2.07	7	12.7
Japan	51	62	1.91	1.53	2.4	4.3
Austria	49	62	2.22	1.91	8	13.8
Belgium	42	54	1.74	1.57	15	22.5
Denmark	63	79	1.92	1.76	9	15.3
France	51	58	1.93	1.73	11.7	26.0
Germany	50	58	1.45	1.40	7.8	8.6
Ireland	34	39	3.40	2.02	12.2	18.9
Italy	37	46	2.21	1.25	16.6	37.6
Netherlands	31	55	1.66	1.59	10.7	15.9
Norway	53	70	1.98	1.88	3.5	8.6
Spain	32	42	2.79	1.23	22.7	42.7
Sweden	67	79	1.78	2.09	2.6	5.8
Great Britain	55	64	1.81	1.79	6.8	13.6

[a]Source: adapted from reference 7, p. 139.

participation in the labor market yet higher fertility rates. Actually, the northern European countries—Norway, Sweden, and Denmark, for example—have among the largest female participation rates and the highest fertility rates (Table 2). It is therefore not the participation of women in the labor market per se that creates lower fertility, but rather the way in which that participation takes place—that is, the security, stability, and support experienced by women when they enter paid work. A major source of insecurity and instability is unemployment, one of the main reasons for women's concerns and anxieties and resistance to having children. In this regard, Table 2 shows the high unemployment among women in general and young women in particular in Italy and in Spain: 37.68 percent among young women (16.60 percent among adult women) in Italy and 42.71 percent among young women (22.70 percent among adult women) in Spain. These numbers compare with only 5.81, 8.64, and 15.33 percent among young women (2.6, 3.5, and 9 percent among adult women) in Sweden, Norway, and Denmark, respectively.

Another source of instability and uncertainty among women interested in working is the number of jobs available to them. For the most part, the job supply for women is very much related to the extent of services employment since most women work in this sector. Indeed, Table 3 shows a clear relationship between the extent of the services sector (as percentage of the total working population) and the percentage of women working.

The low participation of Spanish and Italian women in the labor force is due in large part to the limited development of the services sector in these countries, which explains the scarce supply of jobs for women. Why are these services undeveloped in the southern European countries? The answer to this question is rooted in the role of the family, which in these countries is responsible for services provided, in other countries, by either the private sector or the welfare state. Major family responsibilities lead to a minor services sector, as Table 3 shows.

This assignment of responsibility for services to families, in particular to women, charging them with the provision of personal services (such as laundry, house cleaning, nutrition) and social services (such as care of children, elders, and the disabled), reduces the demand for personal and social services and at the same time overburdens women. The overburdened southern European woman, wanting to enter the labor market, postpones marriage and childbearing because of the lack of supportive services; she is also fearful and anxious about the paucity of jobs available to her, and aware of the high unemployment among women. This is why, in order to increase fertility, these countries need to develop a social services structure that enables women to combine work and family, and to increase the overall number of services jobs for which women may apply and find stable employment.

We are now in a better position to understand why the countries of northern Europe have higher fertility than those of southern Europe. A major reason is the

Table 3

Extent of the services sector and women's participation in the labor force[a]

	Employment in the services sector, as % of total working population (1992)	Women's participation in the labor force, % (1992)
Sweden	38	79
Denmark	37	76
Norway	36	72
United States	36	72
Canada	34	68
Great Britain	32	66
France	28	58
Germany	29	58
Austria	28	57
Netherlands	32	58
Belgium	25	54
Italy	22	48
Spain	18	42
Greece	16	41
Ireland	17	39
Correlation coefficient = 0.89		

[a]Source: OECD, 1992.

wide availability in the northern European countries of services, such as child care and domiciliary care for the elderly and the handicapped, that assist families (and women) in taking care of the young and the old. The availability of such services facilitates the entry of women into paid jobs. In the central and southern European countries, however, the scarcity of these services means that families, and very much in particular women, are overburdened with responsibility for the care of family members—children, adolescents, adults, and the elderly—besides (for the 36 to 38 percent of women in the labor force) their own paid work. This large dependency of the entire family on women (most frequently on the woman of the family) is certainly not good for women or for other family members. The data in Table 4 indicate the overburdening of women in families in various countries of the OECD. We can see how women in Italy and Spain perform more housework than do their counterparts in northern European and other countries. Also evident in Table 4 is the percentage of young people living with their parents: as high as 63 percent in Spain and 81 percent in Italy, compared with

Table 4

The overburdening of families (especially of women)[a]

	Percent of elders living with children	Percent of adolescents living with parents	Weekly hrs of household work (by women)
Northern European countries			
Denmark	4	8	24.6
Norway	11	–	31.6
Sweden	5	–	34.2
Southern European countries			
Italy	39	81	45.4
Spain	37	63	45.8
Other countries			
United States	15	28	31.9
Great Britain	16	35	30
Japan	65	–	33

[a]Source: adapted from reference 19.

28 percent in the United States and only 8 percent in Denmark. This "retention" of the young in southern European families also explains the considerable delay in the process of family formation and the consequent lower fertility. Parents in southern European countries are older at the birth of their first child, and have fewer children, than those in northern European countries.

To the degree that women everywhere are becoming integrated into the labor market, the need for family-support services is increasing. Consequently, such services are the fastest growing sector of the labor force, except in southern European countries. In these countries, conservative and Christian democratic forces call for civil society rather than the welfare state to take care of and assist families. In this political discourse, the welfare state is replaced by the welfare society, a division and substitution of responsibilities that further weakens rather than strengthens families: voluntary associations and other forms of organizations in civil society should complement rather than replace the services of the welfare state. And the experience of the southern European countries shows that in reality, the lack of family-supportive services means an overburdened family (see section V for an expansion of this point).

In summary, then, changes in the family are greatly affecting the welfare state, creating a need for an expansion of its services.

III. CHANGES IN THE LIFE CYCLE

The preceding discussion of changes in the family and their impact on the welfare state can also help us to understand the evolution of people's life cycles in the developed capitalist countries. During the "golden age of capitalism," the period from World War II to the late 1960s, the traditional family was the dominant type of family in the western world: the husband as the breadwinner and the wife working primarily in the home, taking care of the family. Within this social model, the life cycle was predictable. The citizen would attend school until approximately 16 years of age. A young man would then start work in the labor force, where he would remain, usually in the same or similar type of work, for 45 to 50 years of working life. He would then retire around his 65th birthday, and enjoy his retirement for approximately seven years until his death at about 72 years of age. In this way, the typical worker contributed to the Social Security fund for 45 to 50 years, paying for his own seven years of pension and for his wife's four or five years of widow's pension, since she would likely survive him for several years (life expectancy—the number of years a person expects to live—being four or five years longer for women than for men). The entire edifice of the Social Security system rested on the contributions of working men. Employers' contributions were basically deducted from wage earners' pay, as several historical studies have concluded (see 9 for a review of the literature; see also 10). Workers' wages, incidentally, were determined primarily by wages in the manufacturing sector (where most salaried workers were employed), whose high productivity allowed for high wages guaranteed by strong unions.

The changes in the family described earlier, along with other social changes, have substantially modified this life cycle. At the first stage, adolescence and youth, the young in most OECD countries now attend school until at least 18 years of age, rather than 16. Thus a delay in the young person's entry into the labor force results from an expansion of the period of education. This explains why young persons' participation in the labor force, in most OECD countries, is lower than in earlier cohorts. In Spain, for example, labor force participation for young men under 20 years of age was 61 percent in 1977 but only 25 percent in 1997. Participation also declined for young women of the same age group, from 55 percent to 20 percent during the same period (2, p. 46).

A consequence of this delay in the entry of the young into the labor force is a shortening of the total working life of the average worker. And this shortening has been further accentuated, at the other end of the life cycle, by early retirement. The early retirement of older workers has been stimulated by public policies aimed at creating new jobs for the young and increasing overall productivity (under the erroneous assumption that the young are more productive than the old). In Spain, again, the labor force participation rate among men in the age group 55–59 fell from 85 percent in 1977 to 75 percent in 1997, while for men in the age group 60–64 it fell from 40 to 20 percent during the same period. A somewhat similar situation has occurred among working women, although that change has been less dramatic because women's rate of participation, for both age groups, was already rather low in 1977—25 percent for ages 55–59 and 20 percent for ages 60–64. In 1997, the rate for the first group remained practically the same, while declining to 15 percent for the second group (2, p. 46). Most OECD countries have witnessed similar changes.

As a consequence of these changes in the life cycle—the expansion of education for the young and early retirement for the old—the total working time per person has decreased. This situation has been interpreted as a negative development for maintenance of the welfare state, and very much in particular for the Social Security system, which is supported by contributions from working persons. Indeed, contributing time (the period in people's life when they work) has decreased while consuming time (the period when people consume public resources, such as education for the young and pensions for the old) has increased. Those who are inclined to see continuous crisis in the welfare state view this development as the cause of yet another crisis. These alarmist voices, however, have confused the variable "working time in the life cycle" with the variable "overall income generated by that working time." In reality, the contribution to the welfare state depends more on the overall level of income generated from labor than on the number of workers or overall time of work per person or by all workers. And the overall amount of income generated by work has been rising in the majority of OECD countries due to the large increases in productivity (which have permitted increases in wages) and in many countries due to the increased number of workers (due primarily to the growing entry of women into the labor force). Moreover, the growing autonomy of women and their demands for wage equity have led to a rise in women's wages, so as to reduce and eliminate the historically inherited wage differences between women and men. This wage growth due to the reduction of gender inequalities has also increased the contributions to the welfare state. In the United States, for example, it has been calculated that if women were to earn the same wages as men, the resulting overall increase in state revenues would be sufficient to eradicate the deficit predicted for Social Security by 2030, delaying that deficit for another 20 years.

These facts question the claim that the welfare state is in crisis owing to the demographic and social changes occurring in our societies. To the contrary, these changes require and favor an expansion of the welfare state. The demographic transition is not a cause for alarm; there is no scarcity of young and adult persons in today's world. It is not the number of the young and adult that determines the level of state revenues, but rather the number of workers, their productivity, and the level of wages—these determine the contributions to the Social Security system. Moreover, there is nothing sacred about funding Social Security with payroll taxes (based on labor); it can be funded by general revenues as well. And it is difficult to argue—as do liberals—that our societies have reached a level of tax exhaustion. The overall level of taxation has been declining rather than increasing in most OECD countries in the last 20 years (11).

The evolution of the life cycle has had enormous consequences for the welfare state, requiring an expansion of educational services on the one hand and an increase in social transfers and services for the elderly on the other. Whether or not those needs are met depends, as I will show later, on the political conditions in each country.

IV. CHANGES IN ECONOMIC STRUCTURE AND IN EMPLOYMENT

Another type of change occurring in the second half of the 20th century that has affected the welfare states of the developed capitalist countries is the transformation of industrial societies (with the largest percentage of employment in industry) into service societies (with the largest percentage of employment in services). These changes, occurring in different time periods in different countries, have frequently been compared with the transformation in the 19th and early 20th century from agricultural societies (with the largest percentage of employment in agriculture) to industrial societies. Even though these transitions have many elements in common, the differences are greater than the similarities. One difference, for example, is that while the flow of agricultural workers to the industrial sectors meant an increase in wages and/or income, the movement from industrial to service work has usually meant a *decline* in wages and/or income and in workers' standard of living. Wages in the services sectors are lower than those in the industrial sectors, in part because productivity is, on average, greater in industry.

Another difference between the transition from agricultural to industrial societies and from industrial to service societies is that, while it was relatively easy for peasants and agricultural workers to become industrial workers, it is not so easy for industrial workers to become services workers such as programmers or home caregivers. There are more differences between industrial and services jobs than between industrial and agricultural jobs. This explains why it is difficult for industrial workers to find jobs in the services sectors, particularly jobs that pay as well as their previous jobs in industry. Complicating matters for these ex-industrial workers is that, in looking for services jobs, they are competing with a growing number of women who also want to participate in the labor market and for whom services jobs are the most—and sometimes the only ones—available. Thus we see a growing demand for services jobs that requires a growing supply of such jobs in order to avoid unemployment. Actually, the ability of an economy to produce services jobs is a primary determinant of the level of unemployment in a country.

The other determinant of unemployment rate, besides the supply of jobs, is the *demand* for jobs. This simple fact is constantly overlooked: the rate of unemployment is frequently taken as an indicator of a country's economic efficiency, but it is not. Actually, two countries can be equally efficient in producing jobs (have the same rate of job production) and yet have very different unemployment rates if they have different rates of demand for jobs. This is precisely the reason for the difference in unemployment rates in the European Union and the United States. As I have shown elsewhere, both the U.S. and the E.U. economies have, on the whole, very similar rates of job production (12). The European Union, however, has a much larger demand for jobs than does the United States due to (*a*) a larger growth in the number of women who want to work and (*b*) a greater destruction of jobs in agriculture and in industry (primarily because of a larger growth of productivity) in the European Union than in the United States.

The large increases in agricultural productivity, with massive destruction of jobs in that sector, occurred much earlier in the United States than in the European Union, and thus the decline in agricultural employment took place much earlier in the United States. Employment in agriculture declined from 25 percent of the U.S. labor force in 1935 to 8 percent in 1960. In Europe that transformation took place later and has been slower. In France, for example, agricultural employment declined from 38 percent of the labor force in 1962 to 9 percent in 1982; in Italy, from 32 percent in 1952 to 7 percent in 1993; and in Spain, from 25 percent in 1970 to 9.8 percent in 1996 (13). This process of job destruction in agriculture has also been responsible in western Europe for the huge demand from job seekers, much higher than in the United States, since the pool of jobs to be destroyed and the growth of productivity have been much larger in Europe than in the United States (14, 15).

A similar situation has occurred in the industrial sectors, although the percentage of the labor force working in industry has always been somewhat smaller in the United States than in the major economies of Europe (Germany, France, Great Britain, and the Scandinavian countries). The growth in productivity, however, has been more pronounced in western Europe than in the United States, which explains the greater destruction of jobs in the western European industrial sectors than in U.S. industry.

This greater destruction of jobs in the European Union does not, therefore, result—as many liberal authors claim—from "eurosclerosis": inefficient E.U. economies, stuck with excessive social protection and rigid labor markets. To the contrary, these changes are the result of very efficient economies whose productivity has been growing faster than that of the U.S. economy for a long time, such that today, France and Germany have an overall level of productivity exceeding that of the United States (1).

In both the United States and western Europe the growth of the services sector has been absorbing workers whose jobs in agriculture and industry have been destroyed. The rate of job production in services, as indicated earlier, has been very similar on both continents. In the European Union, however, the growth in the services sectors has not been sufficiently fast or large to absorb both workers expelled from agriculture and industry as well as new entrants into the labor market. This is the reason for the large unemployment in the European Union. It is important to repeat, however, that the rate of job production (most net production of new jobs on both continents is in services) is very similar on both sides of the North Atlantic, although the growth varies within the broad category of services, as I will describe in the next section. But first, we need to understand why the services sectors are growing so rapidly and so considerably. To answer this key question, we must disaggregate the highly cumbersome, complex, and sometimes baroque structure of the services sectors.

The Services Sectors

The category "services" covers many different types of activities; they include:

1. *Business services*. These include primarily services provided to the business community, such as marketing, accounting, engineering, design, and other services that used to be conducted by the firm itself on its own premises but are increasingly provided on a contractual basis by outside enterprises—part of the process of "outsourcing." Such business services, when provided on its own premises by the business itself, were counted as part of industrial employment; now, when provided by entities other than the contracting firm, they are counted as services. This explains the large growth in business services, which have doubled in the OECD in just 30 years. Part of this "growth" is therefore the result of new ways of counting rather than a real growth in these activities. They are just counted differently.

Besides the services provided primarily to the business sector, there are other services in this category that serve the population at large; I am referring to financial services such as insurance and banking, real estate, and others.

2. *Distribution services*. These services help to distribute what is produced in society, whether material or nonmaterial, such as information or knowledge. They include commerce and communications (whose workforce is predominantly female) and transport (whose workforce is predominantly male). Distribution services represent approximately 20 percent of all employment in the OECD, although the percentage is much larger in the United States (32 percent) where consumerism is more highly developed than in other OECD countries. This services sector is particularly small in southern European countries, where the infrastructure of commercial services is still underdeveloped.

3. *Personal services*. These services include work in restaurants, cleaners, barbershops, domestic services, and others. For the most part they do not require a high skill level and, until recently, many of these services were primarily provided in the household by housewives. The incorporation of women into the labor force has escalated the demand for and growth of these types of services. Actually it has been estimated that the integration of one woman into the labor market creates a demand for services equivalent to one new job (cited in 16).

This has been one reason for stimulating women's entry into the labor market: it creates a new demand for services, which creates new jobs. In short, working women create jobs. The personal services have been growing in all OECD countries, and are most highly developed in the United States, which has one of the highest rates of women's labor force participation in the OECD (Table 1).

The United States is also the country using the greatest degree of technology in these services. If we compare, for example, an average southern European kitchen with an average U.S. kitchen, we can see that the latter is more mechanized and technologically advanced. However, the higher mechanization of these services in the United States does not mean fewer people working in them—to the contrary. Increased mechanization of the kitchen, for example, facilitates women's integration into the labor force and, as a result, stimulates the creation of jobs to provide the services she is no longer providing for the family. It is therefore erroneous to assume that technology destroys jobs. The United States has the most technologically advanced personal services and has the largest employment in personal services of all OECD countries. This reality contradicts the frivolous claims of Rifkin and many other futurologists who assert that workers will be replaced by machines, creating a jobless future (17). Such an assumption not only ignores the reality around us but also supposes that human needs are limited. The destruction and creation of jobs and the ongoing redefinition of human needs are a constant in the human project.

4. *Social services*. These services are provided collectively and can be funded and/or delivered by the public or the private sectors. They include health and medical care, education, and services to vulnerable populations (such as children, the elderly, and the disabled), among others. They are the services of the welfare state, and the services that have grown most rapidly in the OECD since World War II. This growth has resulted from social changes in the developed capitalist countries (such as the changes in the family analyzed earlier), demographic changes (such as the growth of the elderly population), and, very much in particular, political changes. The political changes include a development of democratic institutions that has permitted the expansion of human needs by the popular classes, especially the working and middle classes, calling for an expansion of social and political rights as part of the full realization of their citizenship. It is not a mere coincidence that the E.U. countries with the least developed welfare states—Spain, Greece, and Portugal—are also those that endured class dictatorships which repressed the expression of popular demands.

Within social services, two types require separate consideration. One type includes those services, such as health and medical care and education, that serve the whole (or most) of the population. We may call them *universal services*. The other type includes those that serve only vulnerable populations (such as children, the elderly, and the disabled) and are of particular assistance to families, and primarily to women. The great variability among the developed capitalist countries in the percentage of the working population occupied in social services is due to differences in the number of people working in these *family-oriented social services*. For the most part, the developed capitalist countries do not differ greatly in the percentages of people working in medical care and in education; the percentage does vary from country to country, but not dramatically or substantially. Where the difference is much larger is in family-oriented social services: the percentage of services workers employed in these services ranges from 30 percent in the Scandinavian countries and 28 percent in France and Belgium to 8 percent in Italy and Spain. The average for the OECD is 15 to 20 percent (14). Actually, the primary reason for the very high percentage of women working in the Scandinavian countries (Table 1) is the advanced development of family-oriented services: this helps women move into the labor market and stimulates the demand for services (thus creating jobs) in response to the new human needs created in the household as women enter paid work. For the same reason, the very low percentage of women working in southern European countries results from the underdevelopment of family-oriented social services.

Another element of the social services that varies markedly among the OECD countries is the type of funding: public in most E.U. countries and private in the United States (except for primary and secondary education, which are mainly public in the United States). The main, but not exclusive, reason for this funding difference is the relative strength of the social democratic movement, much weaker in the United States than in the European Union.

It is also important to note that, in general, the social services that are privately funded are systematically less efficiently run than those that are publicly funded, even though units within the system may operate more efficiently in the private than in the public realm. One example, among many others, is health and medical care services, which are funded publicly in the E.U. countries and privately in the United States. The latter country spends 14 percent of its GNP (the largest in the OECD) on health and medical care, while covering only 82 percent of its population. This means 18 percent of the U.S. population is not covered by any type of health services, a situation that is responsible for 100,000 deaths a year, three times the number of deaths caused by AIDS.[1] And this occurs even though specific components of the health services, such as hospitals, may be very efficient—demonstrating that a system can be very inefficient even though some of its parts are very efficient: the whole is more than the sum of its parts.

Actually, in analyzing the efficiency of the welfare state, it is important to look at what people contribute to the financing of services versus what they receive in return. Comparing the United States with Sweden, for example, we see that the amount paid for health and medical care, education, pensions, and child care by the average U.S. family, directly (in direct, out-of-pocket expenses) and indirectly (through taxes and insurance premiums), is very similar to the amount paid by the

[1] All these data are analyzed and discussed in reference 18.

average Swedish family for the same services: 39.6 percent of its income for the U.S. family and 41.2 percent for the Swedish family (19). Despite the similar level of payment, however, the U.S. family receives much less coverage by these services and benefits than does the average Swedish family. The difference between the families is not so much in what they pay but rather in what they receive. The Swedish welfare state (public) is far more complete and comprehensive than the U.S. welfare state (private), even though the costs for both families are practically the same. The reason for the difference in coverage resides in the institutions that channel the funds. In Sweden, payments are made to the state, which manages the funds and provides the services and transfers. In the United States, however, payments are made to private institutions (with the exception of schools), which manage the funds and provide the services, with much larger administrative and overhead costs, among other types of inefficiencies. For example, 25 percent of expenditures on health and medical care in the United States goes into administration, compared with only 6 percent in the Swedish National Health Service.

Regardless of their mode of financing, the social services are growing rapidly in response to the social, demographic, and political forces detailed in this section, and are the fastest growing employment sectors in the OECD.

V. POLITICAL CHANGES

The most important causes of the evolution of the funding and organization of the welfare state are political. Although the basis for establishing the welfare state preceded World War II, its full development took place after the war, in the golden age of capitalism. This development varied with the political tradition that became dominant in each country. Of these political traditions, four were particularly important: the social democratic, the Christian democratic, the fascist, and the liberal. Each of these is discussed in the following sections.

PUBLIC POLICIES IN THE SOCIAL DEMOCRATIC COUNTRIES

Social democratic public policies were for the most part developed in the northern European countries (Sweden, Norway, Denmark, and Finland) and in Austria. In these countries the labor movement had two instruments to defend its interests: the unions and the social democratic parties. The very strong and powerful trade union movements enrolled, on average, 75 percent of the labor force, both blue-collar and white-collar workers. The unions were mainly centralized and established the framework for collective bargaining agreements, which were later developed further at the branch and lower levels. The degree of enrollment was very high, ranging in the 1980s from 59 percent of the labor force in Norway to 82 percent in Sweden.

The other instrument of the labor movement, the social democratic parties, had a privileged relationship with the unions. These parties saw themselves primarily as the parties of the working class. They governed during most of the years from 1945 to 1980, alone or in coalition with other parties. The average duration of social democratic governments in that period was 23 years, ranging from 14 years in Finland to 30 years in Sweden. In all these countries (except Sweden), the employers' associations were relatively weak and the conservative and liberal parties were small and divided. Only the rural parties (representing the interests of farmers) had some political strength, although never comparable to that of the social democratic parties. On several occasions the rural parties shared government with the social democrats (20).

The objective of the social democratic policies was to expand political and social rights to the entire population as a way of protecting citizens throughout their life cycle. Consequently, one aim of these policies was to achieve material security of the population through solidarity, universalizing such rights. It was for this reason that the social democratic parties identified workers' interests with citizens' interests, demanding the universalization of social and political benefits. Moreover, the alliance of the labor movements with other sectors and classes (especially the middle class, whose expectations exceeded those of the working class) facilitated the establishment of high-quality universal systems. In this way most of the programs instituted by social democratic governments were based on proof of citizenship (universal programs) rather than on means (means-tested programs). As a way of achieving such universality, the objectives of the social democratic movement's economic and social policies were to achieve full employment and to establish a welfare state that protected citizens throughout the entire life cycle and (through redistributive policies) reduced the social inequalities created by the market. Achievement of these objectives required a high employment rate in the population, based on the active participation of both men and women in the labor force. To that effect, the state had to provide a series of services to families (and particularly to women) to enable women to enter paid employment. Women's participation took place primarily through the services of the welfare state.

These policies required a social pact among the trade union movement, the employers' associations, and the government, with a commitment to full-employment and incomes policies. In this social pact, the trade unions accepted the rights to property (with some reservations in the case of Norway, Finland, and Austria), while employers accepted the criteria for developing incomes and the full-employment policies, guaranteed by social democratic parties that had accepted capitalism and thus the need to support the process of capital accumulation and production. These governments saw their function as defending the interests of citizens, in particular their major social base, the working class (21).

Table 5, from the Comparative Social Policy Project directed by Huber and Stephens, summarizes the economic and social indicators outlined above. We can

Table 5

Political characteristics, policy outcomes, and the welfare state (circa 1980s)[a]

	Yrs of social democratic government, 1946–80[b]	Yrs of Christian democratic government, 1946–80[b]	Union density[c]	Social pact[d]	Social Security expenditures[e]	Total taxes[f]	Public employment in health, education, and welfare[g]	Redistributive effect of the state[h]	Women's participation[i]
Social democratic political economies									
Sweden	30	0	82	4	31	56	20	53	74
Norway	28	1	59	4	20	53	15	40	62
Denmark	25	0	70	3	26	52	18	39	71
Finland	14	0	73	3	17	36	9	35	70
Austria	20	15	66	4	21	46	4	–	49
Mean	23.5	3.2	70	3.6	23.2	48.8	13.2	41.8	65.2
Christian democratic political economies									
Belgium	14	19	72	3	21	43	7	47	47
Netherlands	8	22	38	4	27	53	4	41	35
Germany	11	16	40	3	23	45	5	38	51
France	3	4	28	1	25	45	9	35	54
Italy	3	30	51	2	20	33	5	29	39
Switzerland	9	10	35	3	13	33	7	19	54
Mean	7.8	16.7	43.9	3.0	21.6	41.8	6.2	34.8	46

Liberal Anglo-Saxon political economies									
Canada	0	0	31	1	13	36	4	25	57
Ireland	3	0	68	3	19	39	–	34	36
Great Britain	16	0	48	2	17	40	8	36	58
United States	0	0	25	1	12	31	5	26	60
Mean	4.7	0.0	43.0	1.8	15.2	36.5	5.7	30.3	52.8
Conservative-fascist dictatorships									
Spain	0	3	0	0	9	18	3	15	28
Greece	0	2	0	0	6	16	2	18	24
Portugal	2	3	0	0	8	15	3	16	26
Mean	0.7	2.6	0	0	7.7	16.3	2.6	16.3	26

[a]Source: reference 20; for conservative dictatorship countries, my own elaboration.
[b]Years in Cabinet, scored 1 per year, less for coalition (reference 20).
[c]Union density as percentage of the labor force.
[d]Scale of 1 to 4 used to measure social pact (reference 20).
[e]Social security as percentage of GDP.
[f]Total taxes as percentage of GDP.
[g]Public employment in health, education, and welfare as percentage of working-age population.
[h]Percentage reduction of income inequality effected by direct taxes and transfer payments.
[i]Percentage of working-age women in the labor force.

see that the social democratic countries had a high commitment to social pacts, with an average score of 3.6, on a scale of 0 to 4—the highest among developed capitalist countries. Among the countries in which Christian democrats had been dominant during that period, only The Netherlands reached a level of commitment to social pacts similar to that of the social democratic countries. Table 5 also shows the expansion of social transfers of the welfare state (primarily Social Security funds), representing on average 23.2 percent of the GDP. These large social transfers existed alongside extensive welfare state services such as health care, education, and social services to vulnerable populations (children, the elderly, and the disabled), which primarily assisted families. As a consequence of the highly developed welfare state services, a large percentage of the working-age population (13.2 percent) worked in the services sector of the welfare state. The exception here was Austria. The involvement of the working-age population in welfare state services was 20 percent in Sweden, 15 percent in Norway, 18 percent in Denmark, and 9 percent in Finland, but only 4 percent in Austria. This low percentage in Austria was similar to that in countries governed by Christian democratic parties, all of which had very low percentages due to their emphasis on the family as the unit responsible for providing family-oriented services—a result of the Catholic influence. In social democratic countries, family-oriented social services facilitated the entry of women into the labor force, with rates of participation reaching 65.2 percent on average (and 74 percent in Sweden). Here, again, Austria was the exception, with a rate of women's participation (49 percent) comparable to that of the Christian democratic countries.

The extensive development of the welfare state in the social democratic countries required large taxes (Table 5). On average, taxes represented 48.8 percent of GDP (ranging from 36 percent in Finland to 56 percent in Sweden). Most of these taxes were progressive, hence the large redistributive effect of the state in these countries (Table 5).

In social democratic countries the state has played a key role in reaching full employment (a situation that has changed somewhat in the 1990s, as I will discuss later) through its economic and social policies. Pension funds, for example, were used to provide credit to employers who made the commitment to create jobs. Also, the state favored an enlargement of the services sector of the welfare state to employ large percentages of the labor force. But before analyzing and detailing the state interventions to guarantee full employment, several questions need to be addressed.

Are Social Democratic Policies Still Possible?

The Errors of the Globalization Thesis. One thesis that has reached the level of dogma in most economic and social policy circles is that the process of economic globalization has dramatically weakened states, making it impossible for them to follow redistributive and full-employment policies. As confirmation of this thesis, its proponents have used the current high unemployment rates in the social democratic countries as proof of the "failure" of the social democratic model, with a new globalized economic context in which international market forces and the need for increasing competitiveness have forced these countries to abandon their full-employment policies.

I will show later that the high unemployment in the social democratic countries responds more to changes occurring within those countries (of which political changes have been the most important) than to their integration into the "global economy." Actually, all the social democratic countries have been highly integrated in the international economy for many decades now. All have had export-oriented economies, a result in part of their small size. Table 6 shows that as early as the 1960s, exports represented 40 percent of GNP in Norway, 30 percent in Denmark, 27 percent in Austria, and 22 percent in Sweden and Finland. Indeed, these percentages were the highest among the developed capitalist countries, contrasting with only 5 percent in the United States, 11 percent in Japan, 13 percent in France, and 15 percent in Italy. Clearly, the social democratic countries were already, in the 1960s, the most "globalized" economies—the most integrated into international markets. Moreover, the period of maximum expansion of the welfare states in the social democratic countries (1970–1990) coincided with the expansion of their exports and commerce. The importance of exports in their economies increased, on average, from 28.2 percent of GNP in the period 1960–1973 to 35.8 percent in the period 1980–1989—again, some of the highest percentages (representing a high dependency on international markets) among the developed capitalist countries. This high percentage, incidentally, has varied very little during the 1990s, when, for the first time, these countries have experienced unemployment as a mass phenomenon. Thus we cannot consider the unemployment in these countries to result from an increased economic integration during the 1990s: there has been no such increase in economic integration into the global economy in this decade. The argument that these countries should dismantle or reduce their welfare states and their commitment to full employment because of the need to become more competitive in the globalized economy is not sustainable. As shown in Table 6, the social democratic countries were competing very successfully indeed (as shown by their exports and trade balances) during the golden age of capitalism, when they were already highly integrated into world markets. High unemployment rates in the 1990s did not coincide with a change in integration into world markets, as globalization theory maintains.

In summary, reality is exactly opposite to the assumptions of globalization theorists. *The social democratic countries were able to compete successfully in international markets precisely because of their social pacts, which required a strong state, actively intervening in the areas of production and distribution.* The experience in these countries shows that, contrary to the proposition that

Table 6

Globalization, export dependency, budget deficits, economic growth, and unemployment[a]

	Exports, % of GNP			Budget surpluses, % of GNP			Economic growth, %				Unemployment, %					
	1960–73	1974–79	1980–89	1960–73	1974–79	1980–89	1960–73	1974–79	1979–89	1989–95	1960–73	1974–79	1980–88	1990	1993	1995
Social democratic political economies																
Sweden	22	29	33	2.8	–0.4	–3.1	3.4	1.5	1.8	–0.1	1.9	1.9	2.5	1.6	8.2	7.7
Norway	40	43	43	3.3	1.4	4.9	3.5	4.3	2.3	2.9	1.0	1.8	2.5	5.2	6.0	4.9
Denmark	30	29	35	1.4	0.6	–3.4	3.6	1.6	1.8	1.6	1.4	6.0	8.1	8.3	10.7	7.0
Finland	22	27	30	2.0	1.1	–1.0	4.5	1.8	3.2	–1.1	2.0	4.6	5.3	3.6	17.9	17.1
Austria	27	33	38	–0.1	–2.3	–3.7	4.3	3.0	2.0	1.3	1.7	1.6	3.3	3.2	4.2	3.8
Mean	28.2	32.2	35.8	1.9	0.1	–1.3	3.9	2.4	2.2	0.9	1.6	3.2	4.3	4.4	9.4	8.1
Christian democratic political economies																
Belgium	38	50	67	–1.8	–4.2	–8.8	4.4	2.1	1.8	1.3	2.2	5.7	11.5	8.8	12.0	12.9
Netherlands	46	49	57	–0.3	–5.7	–6.9	3.6	1.9	1.1	1.8	1.3	5.0	10.0	7.5	6.7	7.1
Germany	21	27	32	0.3	–1.6	–2.6	3.7	2.5	1.7	1.3	0.8	3.4	6.7	6.2	7.9	8.1
France	13	20	22	–0.3	–2.5	–3.8	4.3	2.3	1.6	0.8	2.0	4.6	9.0	9.1	11.7	11.5
Italy	15	20	20	–3.2	–9.2	–11.6	4.6	3.2	2.4	1.1	5.3	6.3	9.1	10.5	10.6	12.0
Switzerland	30	34	36	4.6	3.7	3.7	3.0	–0.1	1.7	–0.5	0.0	0.4	0.6	0.5	3.8	3.3
Mean	27.2	33.3	39	–0.1	–3.2	–5.0	3.9	2.0	1.7	1.0	1.9	4.2	7.8	7.1	8.7	9.2

Liberal Anglo-Saxon political economies																
Canada	20	24	27	−1.6	−3.3	−6.2	3.6	2.9	1.8	−1.0	5.0	7.2	9.5	8.1	11.2	9.5
Ireland	35	45	54	−3.8	−9.2	−11.7	3.7	3.3	2.7	5.8	5.2	7.6	14.2	13.7	15.6	12.1
Great Britain	20	27	27	1.8	−5.8	−3.7	2.6	1.5	2.2	0.7	1.9	4.2	9.9	5.4	10.2	8.6
United States	5	8	8	1.7	−3.6	−4.3	2.6	1.4	1.5	0.9	5.0	7.0	7.8	5.6	6.8	5.5
Mean	20	26	29	2.2	−5.5	−6.5	3.1	2.3	2.1	1.6	4.3	6.5	10.3	8.2	11.0	8.9

[a]Source: reference 20, Tables 2 and 3.

globalization is weakening states and diluting their importance, integration into international markets *increases* the importance of the state, requiring an active state intervention in production and distribution.[2]

The Error of Identifying Keynesianism with Social Democracy. A characteristic of the economic policies of the social democratic countries is that they have not relied on public deficits to stimulate demand. Actually, their policies are not, for the most part, demand oriented. In contrast to most countries with Christian democratic and liberal governments, they did not run large public deficits during most years of the period 1960–1989 (Table 6); in fact they ran surpluses in most of these years. Thus they did not manipulate the level of demand by running large deficits. They achieved full employment through state interventions primarily on the supply side, facilitating and stimulating the production process and capital accumulation. This was achieved through public policies that included *credit policies* providing low-interest credit to enterprises committed to creating employment and *fiscal policies* that prioritized investment over consumption—policies that supported the process of capital accumulation without prioritizing the interests of the capitalist class. In that respect, the social democrats' position on capital differed from the Christian democratic and liberal positions, which saw the interests of the capitalist class as identical to those of the economic system. Such an understanding led Christian democrats and liberals to favor the growth of profits as a condition for investment and for the growth of capitalist production. The social democrats, however, made a distinction between profits and investments. Indeed, as Table 7 shows, the income delivered from capital (corporate profits, plus profits of unincorporated business, including the earnings of self-employed persons) as percentage of national income in the social democratic countries was the lowest in the OECD during the period 1960–1989, while the rate of investments was among the highest. During the years 1960–1973, 1974–1979, and 1980–1989, total profits as percentage of national income in the social democratic countries (averaging 28.1, 21.4, and 22.8 percent in the three periods) was, in general, lower than in Christian democratic and liberal countries during the same periods (33.3, 23.5, and 25 percent in the Christian democratic and 25.7, 23.5, and 25 percent in the liberal countries). The only exception occurred in 1960–1973 when the total profits as percentage of national income were lower in the liberal than in the social democratic countries. Nevertheless, the investment rate was higher in the social democratic countries than in the Christian democratic and liberal countries. Gross fixed capital formation as percentage of GDP was 25.6, 25.9, and 21.8 percent for the periods 1960–1973, 1974–1979, and 1980–1989, respectively, in the social democratic countries, higher than in

[2] The reader is referred to the excellent work by Huber and Stephens for an expansion of this point (20, 22). See 23 for a discussion of the relationship between states and international markets.

Table 7

Total profits and gross fixed capital formation, 1960–1989[a]

	Operative surplus (corporate profits, including state enterprises) and profits from unincorporated business (including earnings of self-employed persons), % of national income			Gross fixed capital formation, % of GDP		
	1960–73	1974–79	1980–89	1960–73	1974–79	1980–89
Social democratic political economies						
Sweden	21	15	17	23	21	19
Norway	27	20	27	28	33	25
Denmark	30	24	24	24	22	17
Finland	32	24	22	25	27	24
Austria	30	23	24	27	26	24
Mean	28.1	21.4	22.8	25.6	25.9	21.8
Christian democratic political economies						
Belgium	34	25	29	22	22	18
Netherlands	32	25	29	24	21	20
Germany	30	23	23	25	21	21
France	32	25	24	24	24	20
Italy	41	28	40	25	24	21
Switzerland	31	38	23	28	23	25
Mean	33.3	23.5	25	24.4	22.4	20.8
Liberal Anglo-Saxon political economies						
Canada	26	25	26	22	24	21
Ireland	31	29	33	20	26	20
Great Britain	21	18	20	18	19	17
United States	25	22	21	18	19	17
Mean	25.7	23.5	25	19.4	21.9	18.8

[a]Source: reference 20, Table 4.

countries with Christian democratic (24.4, 22.4, and 20.8 percent) and liberal (19.4, 21.9, and 18.8 percent) governments.

It is therefore important to differentiate the interests of the production process and of the process of capital accumulation from the interests of the capitalist class (whether in production or finance): they do not necessarily coincide. As the chief economist of *Business Week* recently indicated, the U.S. capitalist class is too powerful for the good of the reproduction of the U.S. capitalist system (24). The Christian democratic and liberal parties assumed that both interests are the same. The social democratic parties did not necessarily assume so. This is why the social democratic governments did not see a conflict between redistributive public policies and public policies that supported the production process (via credit and fiscal policies), the growth of competitiveness, and the growth of the economy. As Table 6 shows, during the period 1960–1989 the rate of economic growth in these countries was larger than that of the Christian democratic and liberal countries.

Besides the policies outlined above, social democratic policies included other state interventions in the labor market aimed at achieving full employment, which successfully integrated women into the labor market through (*a*) active labor policies, including occupational training, (*b*) labor flexibility and other labor mobility measures, and (*c*) public employment.

The first type of intervention is revealed by the high expenditures on labor training (up to 3 and 4 percent of GNP). The second type has successfully achieved greater geographical, occupational, and sectoral labor mobility, among the largest in the OECD. Denmark, for example, has a higher rate of occupational mobility than the United States, the country constantly said to have the most flexible labor force (14). These two types of policies were complemented by measures aimed at creating public employment either continuously and structurally (by expansion of the services sectors of the welfare state) or conjuncturally (by allowing public investments at the local and regional levels in times of recession).

This spectrum of state interventions supported the process of production and capital accumulation, helping employers maintain their competitiveness while protecting the rights of workers and preventing unemployment through full-employment and redistributive policies.

An indispensable condition for the implementation of these policies was the social pacts, in which labor agreed to moderate its salary demands and facilitate labor flexibility, employers agreed to invest and to provide employment, and government agreed to assist the process of production and to create employment. These policies were most highly developed in Sweden, in large part because it had the smallest public sector of the northern European countries. Indeed, because of the strength of employers (stronger than in the other countries), public enterprises played a smaller role in Sweden. In Norway (and in Austria, another country having a long experience with social democratic governments) the public sector was more developed than in Sweden, enabling these governments to rely more extensively on public investments and employment in public enterprises to cope with the unemployment crisis of the 1990s. This explains why Norway and Austria had the lowest unemployment rates of all developed capitalist countries (4.9 and 3.8 percent, respectively)—*proving that a large public sector may be more of a help than, as neoliberals suggest, a handicap in responding to external shocks*. Sweden, with a smaller public sector, had to rely more actively on cooperation with the private sector, achieved through social pact arrangements.

As indicated earlier, a condition for the development of social democratic public policies was the existence of strong representative institutions that enabled the various social agents (in particular unions and employers) to negotiate and defend their interests at the national level. This required (*a*) unions to be representative of the majority of the labor force, and their leadership to have wide support among the different sectors and locals of the labor movement; (*b*) employers' associations to be authentically representative of large and small employers; and (*c*) governments to have strong popular support and the collaboration of both unions and employers. These three conditions fostered the establishment of tripartite arrangements—among government, unions, and employers—coordinated centrally by the leadership of these institutions. Central coordination did not necessarily preempt the possibility of establishing local and regional collective bargaining agreements (as occurred in Norway), but such agreements had to follow the framework and objectives set up at the national level. The national negotiations intrinsic to social pacts required strong representative institutions, which is why social democratic governments encouraged the strengthening of these institutions, actively favoring, for example, workers' syndicalization. It is the social pacts, based on these centralized negotiations and agreements, that underlay the success of full-employment and incomes policies.

Have Social Democratic Policies Failed?

There has been an obvious and deliberate effort to discredit social democratic public policies that are based on an expansion of the welfare state. According to this scenario, the high unemployment in the social democratic countries proves the failure and irrelevance of such policies. Before I address this argument, I would like to emphasize that Norway and Austria, two countries within the social democratic tradition, have had some of the lowest unemployment rates in the OECD while following social democratic public policies. The success of the Norwegian experience has been credited mainly to its oil revenues, minimizing the importance of its social democratic policies. However, this argument ignores the fact that Great Britain, which has followed neoliberal policies, also has large oil revenues but has worse economic and social indicators than Norway.

The growth of unemployment in the social democratic countries is not due to a growing globalization but rather to political developments within these countries that are changing and weakening the social pacts that have governed their economies. In Sweden, for example, the labor movements have been weakened over the last 15 years, with internal division in the trade union movement, strengthening of employers, and growing collaboration between employers' associations and the conservative and liberal parties. The weakening of the labor movement is partly due to changes in the processes of production and consumption. Among the changes in production is the disaggregation of the production process, dividing and atomizing the labor force, and a growing hierarchical specialization that establishes wider demarcations between blue-collar and white-collar workers. This explains why Sweden's metal workers, clearly supported by their employers, broke the social pact, which they saw as constraining their demands, and called instead for more decentralized and autonomous negotiations. Increases in white-collar employment and in particular in the professional and technical strata, whose growth has depended in part on the expansion of the welfare state and whose interests frequently conflict with those of blue-collar workers, have also contributed to the challenge to the social pact. All these factors explain why the employers' association (S.A.F.) abandoned the social pact, with the support and encouragement of the conservative and liberal parties. This breakdown was the main reason for the growth of unemployment, by undermining the coordinated public policies of the preceding period.[3]

Contributing to the end of the social pact was deregulation of the financial markets, breaking with a major element of social democratic policies: government control of credits, interest rates, and the price of currencies. Indeed, one condition for the success of the opening up of economies to the international markets was the regulation and control of financial markets, which enabled them to follow the credit and fiscal policies indicated above. Deregulation of the financial markets disrupted these policies, allowing each employer to be completely autonomous in its access to credit—a policy favored by large employers but having an enormously negative effect on small employers. The breakdown of the social pact clearly benefited financial interests (interest rates doubled during the 1980s), large employers, and skilled workers, who could negotiate better terms outside the social pact. Those most hurt by the breakdown were unskilled workers, small employers, and, of course, the unemployed.

In summary, the growth of unemployment was a result of political rather than economic factors. Deregulation of the financial markets, for example, was carried out by the Swedish Finance Minister K. O. Feldt, who was convinced of the superiority of financial markets in determining the country's credit needs.

Korpi (26) has detailed how this deregulation of the financial markets came about, showing the ideological rather than scientific bases on which the policies were established. These neoliberal policies were carried out despite the fact that the assumptions that guided them were empirically incorrect and proven false even at the time they were chosen. Korpi also convincingly shows how the data presented by the influential Lindbeck report (27)—which justified the deregulation of the financial sector—were erroneous and simply manipulated. Korpi's detailed critical analysis of what became the conventional wisdom has, for the most part, been ignored due to the powerful image of "Swedish sclerosis"

[3] See 25 for different interpretations of the growth of unemployment in Sweden.

put forward by the economic forces that promote the liberal discourse. These forces include the Nobel Prize Committee on Economics, many of whose members were also members of the Lindbeck Commission, including Lindbeck himself. It speaks of the highly ideological nature of this debate that in spite of Korpi's very complete and rigorous analysis of the "social democratic failure" thesis proposed by Lindbeck and others, his critique has basically been ignored. For example, in a recent analysis of the Swedish experience Weiss (25) uncritically repeats the Lindbeck Commission findings, without once mentioning Korpi's article.

It is important to emphasize that deregulation of the financial markets, while carried out by the Swedish Finance Minister K. O. Feldt, was opposed by most members of the social democratic party and by the trade unions, who thought that such deregulation would lead to a large speculative boom, hurting the country's productive capacity and economic growth. The realization of these predictions led to the electoral losses of the Social Democratic Party. Mr. Feldt abandoned that party and his policies are those advocated by the Liberal Party. Also, Lindbeck and Ståhl—the main liberal voices of the Nobel Prize Committee on Economics—were forced to resign from that committee, which explains why Amartya Sen received the 1998 Nobel Prize in economics.

PUBLIC POLICIES IN THE CHRISTIAN DEMOCRATIC COUNTRIES

Having analyzed the social democratic public policies on the welfare state, we are in a better position to understand Christian democratic public policies, the policies of the conservative parties based in the Christian tradition. It is important to clarify that included under the rubric "Christian democratic" are other parties that do not carry this name. I will focus on the countries where such parties have governed for long periods of time during the years 1960–1980. Needless to say, these parties on occasion have had to govern in coalition with other parties, including social democratic parties (as in Belgium, Germany, and The Netherlands), which left their mark on the public policies. But, even if these alliances did occur, conservative parties of Christian tradition and/or influence governed for longer periods of time, which explains their common characteristics. *One such characteristic is assigning to the family the tasks carried out by the state in the social democratic countries.* In the Christian democratic countries, the family and the life cycle have defined the welfare state. The male was the head of the family, the breadwinner responsible for the family's economic stability, which depended on his wages and his pension. The housewife took care of elders and children, all of whom lived at home. Within this scenario, the key economic element for the family was the salary and the pension of the family member working in the labor force: the male breadwinner. He was the guarantor of the family's welfare.

The male worker followed the traditional life cycle as outlined in section III, working 40 to 50 years, contributing to the Social Security that later funded his seven years of pension plus four to five years of his widow's pension. Pensions (retirement and widow's pensions) and wages were the key determinants of the social welfare of the family and of the population. It is therefore understandable that the major social debates in these societies focused on the level of wages and pensions.

On the other hand, women in the Christian democratic countries continued to work at home: in the 1980s only 46 percent of women worked in the labor market (compared with 65 percent in the social democratic countries) (Table 5). The housewife took care of children and elders living at home. Child care services or domiciliary home care services for the elderly (or disabled) were practically unknown or were poorly developed, which explains why employment in welfare state services remained very low (Table 5). Only 6.2 percent of the working-age population was occupied in the services sector of the welfare state, working primarily in health care (mainly in hospitals) and education, in contrast to 13.2 percent in the social democratic countries.

These two circumstances—the heavy reliance on families for the care of family members and the importance of wages and pensions for the welfare of the family and the population—explain why the welfare states of Christian democratic countries have underdeveloped family-supportive social services but large social transfers (mainly in pensions). Their average social transfers expenditure is 21.6 percent of GDP, only slightly lower than in social democratic countries (23.2 percent), but much higher than in countries governed by liberal parties (15.2 percent). This large expenditure in social transfers is based on large fiscal revenues, which in Christian democratic countries in the 1980s represented 41.8 percent of GDP, lower than in social democratic countries (48.8 percent) but much higher than in liberal countries (36.5 percent).

The underdevelopment of social services for families (such as child care services and domiciliary services for the elderly and disabled) created a burden for families (especially women). In the 1980s women in the age group 30–55 had the largest number of stress-related conditions. A woman's welfare was related to her husband's income, such that divorce or separation could result in sudden poverty. In the 1980s poverty among single, divorced, or separated women was five times higher in Christian democratic countries (28 percent in Germany, 23 percent in Italy) than in social democratic countries (6 percent in Denmark, 5 percent in Sweden) (19).

Dependency on the family means dependency on women. It is not surprising, therefore, that the changes in the family and the life cycle described earlier are having an enormous impact on the welfare states of the Christian democratic countries. *These welfare states are precisely the ones facing the greatest changes and convulsions*. Women are rebelling and do not want to have the same family responsibilities their mothers had for decades and women have had for centuries.

They want to become active members of the labor force, with the same rights as men. This positive and irreversible change, one of the most important revolutions in the 20th century, is also occurring in the Christian democratic countries, challenging the power relations within traditional families and societies. It is important to stress again that this redefinition of family responsibilities does not mean the end of the family as a key unit of our society (as conservatives fear), but rather a redefinition of the family! Women in social democratic countries are integrated into the labor force in much higher percentages (74 percent in Sweden) than in Christian democratic countries (39 percent in Italy). And yet, fertility rates (the number of children per woman) in Sweden are double those in Italy, which (with Spain) has the lowest fertility rate in the world today. As noted in an earlier section, integration of women into the labor force does not have to weaken the family if it is accompanied (as in northern social democratic countries) by the wide availability of family-oriented services. Opposition (or resistance) to the development of such services, characteristic of Christian democratic social policies, is anti-family: such policies make it difficult for families to survive and grow and for new families to be established.

Welfare State versus Welfare Societies?

A characteristic of Christian democratic public policies has been to counterpoise the concepts of the welfare society and the welfare state; in this position, responsibilities for care are assigned to different agents of civil society, with dependence on societal mobilization to provide care services. *Voluntarism* is the key ingredient in this mobilization, calling on people's altruism and/or compassion, as well as their sense of family duty and responsibility, on which the Christian democratic discourse relies. It is important to clarify that much can be done by mobilizing civil society to help those in need. But it is profoundly wrong to try to replace the welfare state by voluntarism and calls for family responsibility. The welfare state and the welfare society should be complementary rather than mutually exclusive. The relationship between the state and civil society is not a zero sum relationship: expansion of one does not necessarily mean shrinkage of the other—quite the contrary. Goran Therborn (28), in his detailed study of European societies, has shown that societies with more developed welfare states (with more extensive development of civil, political, and social rights) also have richer civil societies (measured by the number of associations, networks, and forms of voluntary organizations). As I will show later in analyzing southern European societies (all of which endured long periods of dictatorship), undeveloped welfare states existed side by side with great poverty in the associative life. In these societies, women carried most of the care responsibilities within the family, with very little assistance from either the state or civil society.

Thus we cannot find any evidence to support the Christian democratic dictum that there are no major differences between women's burdens in Christian democratic and social democratic countries, with civil society helping women in the former and the state helping them in the latter. The data presented in this article challenge this interpretation of who carries family responsibilities in both types of societies. Indeed, in the absence of family services, women—as wives, mothers, and daughters—do the entire job. This is an enormous burden, and underlies the low fertility and delay in family formation in the Christian democratic countries.

There is, paradoxically, an element of the Christian democratic call for the mobilization of civil society that could be of great assistance to families and women. I am referring to the civil mobilization that is required to change cultural norms and social values, transforming, reducing, and finally eliminating the sexism that is so dominant in Christian democratic societies (in particular in Catholic countries). The values and roles within families and within societies need to change, stimulating men to share in what has been called "women's work." But it is in the Christian democratic countries that these conservative, sexist values have changed the least; the average man spends only three hours per week in domestic work in Italy and Spain, and five hours in France, compared with 20 hours in Sweden (19, p. 28). Unfortunately, the Christian democratic and conservative parties and institutions have not provided much leadership in this cultural and social mobilization that is so much needed to help women and families. *In the absence of this and other types of mobilizations to help families, the Christian democratic calls for civil mobilization seem to be more a justification for cutting the welfare state than a serious attempt to help families.*

The Political Economy of Christian Democratic Public Policies

The Christian democratic parties were heavily influenced by the Catholic Church and its economic and social policies. Their primary objective was to achieve social stability within the existing social order (threatened by the labor movement and its social agitation in the 19th and early 20th century). To reach these objectives, the parties focused on the family unit as the guarantor of the social order and carrier of social responsibilities. The male wage earner was head of that unit, and the standard of living and the welfare of the family were based on his wages and on the pensions that he and his wife received after his retirement. According to the defense of the social order that such public policies aimed to maintain, the pensions and other benefits that workers received depended on their status within the hierarchy in the production process and in society. This status also determined the level of contributions made by employers and employees to the different Social Security funds (with each hierarchical level having different funds). It is this intent to divide the working class that underlies one characteristic of Social Security in these Christian democratic countries: its stratification, with benefits dependent on the type of work and a worker's position in the social order.

It was Bismarck (the founder of German Social Security) who explicitly referred to the need to divide benefits in order to disarticulate the working class. He wrote in a letter to Herman Vagener that (quoted in 29):

> the containment of the Social Democratic Party can not be realized simply by the repression of Social Democratic excesses, but that this must be accompanied by the positive enhancement of workers. . . . the development of the Bill on workers' insurance introduced by the Federal Government . . . will establish separate corporate associations under the State protection that will satisfy the different needs of the different sectors of the working population. This arrangement will render possible a solution to the tasks which the State alone would be unable to handle to the same degree.

The enormous fear generated in the German establishment by the Paris Commune had motivated this proposal for a highly stratified Social Security system. Later, to the degree that the power and influence of the German labor movement increased, those benefits tended to become less unequal, although the perceptive observer can see even in the current German system the historical roots of the Social Security stratification.

In the Christian democratic countries the power and organization of the labor movements varied with the degree of unionization, which ranged from 72 percent in Belgium to 28 percent in France (Table 5). Belgium, Germany, and The Netherlands were the Christian democratic countries with the greatest social democratic influence, with Christian democrats forced to include the social democratic parties in the government. These Christian democratic countries therefore had public policies with more redistributive effects, as shown in Table 5. In general, though, Christian democratic countries had less redistributive public policies than social democratic countries. The rate of state redistribution in the former countries was 34.8 percent and in the latter was 41.8 percent; the degree of redistribution was related to the strength of the labor movement and the social democratic parties.

Christian democratic parties clearly favored the interests of the capitalist class (Table 7). The total profits were larger than in social democratic and liberal countries, although higher profits did not mean higher investments, higher economic growth, or lower unemployment than in social democratic countries. To the contrary, as shown in Tables 6 and 7, in the years 1960–1989 the average investment rate was lower in the Christian democratic countries (24.4 percent of GDP in 1960–1973, 22.4 percent in 1974–1979, and 20.8 percent in 1980–1989) than in the social democratic countries (25.6, 25.9, and 21.8 percent in the same three periods). For the 1960–1989 period, economic growth was practically identical (3.9 percent) in 1960–1973 for Christian democratic and social democratic parties, but in 1974–1979 and 1979–1989 was lower for the Christian democratic countries. For the period 1989–1995, economic growth in the Christian democratic countries (1 percent) was slightly above that in the social democratic countries (0.9 percent).

A similar situation is evident when we analyze unemployment (Table 6). It was higher in the Christian democratic countries in 1960–1973 (1.9 percent), 1974–1979 (4.2 percent), 1980–1988 (7.8 percent), 1990 (7.1 percent), and 1995 (9.2 percent) than in the social democratic countries for the same periods or years (1.6, 3.2, 4.3, 4.4, and 8.1 percent, respectively). In 1993 unemployment was lower in the Christian democratic countries (8.7 percent) than in the social democratic countries (9.4 percent). This was primarily due to the very high unemployment in Finland resulting from the collapse of Finland's main trading partner, the Soviet Union. But with this exception, we see better economic efficiency indicators and greater state redistributive effects in the social democratic than in the Christian democratic countries.

The larger unemployment in the Christian democratic countries in those years was due to several factors. One of them was the lack of full-employment policies, which are not a trademark of the Christian democrats and have not received high priority in these countries. Nor have Christian democratic parties prioritized expansion of the labor force; these countries had percentages of the adult population working that were among the lowest in the OECD countries (after Spain, Greece, and Portugal) in the period 1945–1980, a result of women's very low participation rate in the labor market. The absence of full-employment policies and the poor development of the social services sectors are responsible for the scant supply of employment, clearly insufficient to respond to the increased demand resulting from women's growing desire to enter the labor market.

The current unemployment problem in the Christian democratic countries is not due to a supposed "eurosclerosis" or economic inefficiency, but rather to an inadequate response to a new and massive phenomenon—entry of women into the labor force—for which these countries are not prepared. *This is why women's unemployment (especially among unqualified female workers) is much higher than in the social democratic countries.* Particularly worrisome is unemployment among the young (both women and men), who seem to be unemployed for long periods of time in these countries. Only 30 percent of unemployed youth in Germany and France moved out of unemployment at the end of 1989–1990, compared with 65 percent in Denmark (15). *The Christian democratic countries are clearly ill-equipped to respond to one of their greatest challenges: the liberation of women and their integration into the labor market. Their welfare states have been dramatically affected by the social and family changes discussed here.*

PUBLIC POLICIES IN THE FORMER FASCIST DICTATORSHIPS OF SOUTHERN EUROPE, 1945–1975/1980

The welfare states in the southern European countries—Spain, Greece, and Portugal—have been heavily influenced by long periods of dictatorship. Because they share several characteristics with the Christian democratic countries, as I will show, some authors have erroneously grouped them with those countries. Both types of countries have welfare states that focus primarily on social transfers, with poorly developed social services. But the 40 years or so of dictatorship puts the three southern European countries in a separate group, since they have very low social transfers as well: although most welfare state expenditures do focus on social transfers, the transfers and expenditures are at a very low level. In 1980 (three years after the end of the dictatorship in Spain), for example, Social Security expenditures represented 9 percent of GDP, much less than the average for the Christian democratic countries (21.6 percent) (Table 5). Thus these countries not only had poorly developed services sectors in the welfare state (with only 2.6 percent of the working-age population employed in health services, education, and social services, compared with 6.2 percent in the Christian democratic and 13.2 percent in the social democratic countries), but also had poorly developed social transfers such as pensions. Needless to say, in the new democracies populations could express their wishes and demands (long prohibited and repressed under the dictatorships) and press for a major expansion of the welfare state. But even now, after a considerable welfare state expansion, these countries have the least developed welfare states in the developed capitalist countries.

The dictatorships were highly repressive class dictatorships with low social conscience and low social expenditures. In Spain in 1960, for example, the spending on health care and education by the central government amounted to 60 percent of the spending on the armed and police forces. It is important to stress this reality since Spain underwent the transition from dictatorship to democracy without a rupture with the previous regime (as occurred in Germany and Italy after the defeat of Nazism and fascism). The transition in Spain left many elements of the previous regime untouched, allowing the economic and social agencies that had dominated in the dictatorship to continue and indeed to flourish in the new democratic institutions. The state—including the universities—was not purged of personnel who had supported the previous regime and remained dominant in the state institutions. This explains the relatively successful project to present the Spanish dictatorship as a mildly conservative, authoritarian regime, not very repressive and certainly not fascist.[4] This definition has been reinforced by those who see that regime as a personal dictatorship centered on the figure of Franco, referred to as *regime Franquista*. The Barcelona paper *La Vanguardia*, owned and controlled by the Godo family (major supporters of the Franco regime), has been the main proponent of such a reading of the Spanish dictatorship. It has published many articles by the Italian journalist Montanelli, who has even claimed that Franco saved Spain from a worse fate: becoming a Stalinist dictatorship. The reality, however, shows the erroneousness of this interpretation.

[4] A prominent spokesman for this position is J. Lintz; see 30 for a critique of Lintz's position.

The regime was not a dictatorship around a *caudillo*; it was far worse than that. It was dictatorship by a class that reproduced itself through enormously repressive interventions, becoming one of the most repressive regimes in Europe. Its extensive support for financial and industrial interests with the most regressive fiscal policies in Europe reveals the class character of that dictatorship. This class character is also evident in the prohibition of trade unions or any other organization that defended workers' interests, and in the highly selective repression against the working class.

As indicated earlier, with the transition to democracy (including Spain's) many of the dictatorships' class-oriented policies were changed, with considerable expansion of the welfare state and the introduction, for the first time in Spain, of income taxation. Yet despite these expansions, the social expenditures and taxation levels remain among the lowest in the developed capitalist countries (Table 5).

Another characteristic of the dictatorship in Spain was the great scarcity of public resources, except in the apparatuses of repression. (Even today, Spain has more police per 1,000 inhabitants and fewer social community workers per 1,000 elders than most other European countries.) The scarcity of resources is responsible for the enormously rigid state apparatus and the poorly developed sensibility toward users of the welfare state. This characteristic has persisted into the democratic period because of the lack of any profound reforms in public administration. Such rigidity appears in both health care and education, in which the majority of personnel are functionaries, working for the public administration for fewer hours than their counterparts in the Christian democratic and social democratic countries. This is the reason for the low productivity of the public sector and the consequent growth of the private sectors of the welfare state. In the three former dictatorships, the private sector in both health care and education is among the largest in the developed capitalist countries.

A characteristic that these countries share with the Christian democratic countries is their emphasis on the family (and on women) as responsible for the care of children and the elderly, at a considerable cost to women. This family focus is even more accentuated than in the Christian democratic countries due to the strong influence of the Catholic Church during the dictatorships, an influence that is still considerable today. In these countries, the liberation of women, although still a slow process, has had a marked impact on the welfare state, on women, and on the labor market. As we saw in the Christian democratic countries, increasing numbers of women (and young of both sexes) are looking for jobs, which is one of the primary causes of the high unemployment in Spain: the economic machinery cannot produce enough jobs to absorb this increased demand.

Another similarity with Christian democratic countries is the massive destruction of jobs in the agricultural sector (still a very large percentage of the labor force.) This destruction of jobs and agricultural workers' need for other types of work adds to the demand for new jobs, further increasing the rate of unemployment.

PUBLIC POLICIES IN THE LIBERAL COUNTRIES

This is a varied group of countries, including those that have never been governed by social democratic parties (such as Canada and the United States) and those governed by such parties for as long as 14 years during the period 1960–1980 (such as Great Britain). Some authors, for this reason, group Great Britain with the social democratic countries. Despite these differences, however, all the countries in this group share some common features of their public policies that distinguish them from the social democratic and Christian democratic countries. Their social policies, for example, are residual and assistential; that is, their welfare states provide benefits and services based on proven financial need (means-tested programs) rather than as a matter of citizens' or workers' rights. There are, of course, exceptions such as the universal health services in Canada and Great Britain. But the exceptions only confirm the rule. The majority of these Anglo-Saxon countries follow the liberal model, in which the social transfers of the welfare state are supplemented by benefits acquired through the labor market by collective bargaining. Public expenditures tend to be concentrated on the needy, with need defined according to political-administrative criteria.

Some readers will probably be surprised to see the British welfare state defined as an assistential—rather than universal—welfare state. The comparative political literature commonly refers to the Beveridge model (named for the intellectual architect of the British welfare state) as a universal model (distributing benefits to all citizens and residents as a matter of rights), contrasting it to the Bismarck model (named for the intellectual architect of the German welfare state) referred to as a contributive or Social Security model, in which benefits depend on the contributions of workers (and their employers) to the welfare state.[5] Actually, neither the Bismarck nor Beveridge models are universal, as is rightly pointed out by some British observers who have taken the trouble to read the Beveridge plan in its entirety. The Beveridge plan was a liberal response to the authentically universalistic proposal put forward by the left of the Labour Party. The latter was a truly universalistic proposal guaranteeing social rights to the entire population, as is characteristic of the social democratic model. However, Beveridge (a profoundly conservative employer, anti-trade-unionist, and writer for the *Morning Post*, whose proprietor was the pro-fascist coal-mine-owning Duke of Northumberland) called for the welfare state to provide a minimum set of benefits to be supplemented by benefits acquired through collective bargaining agreements and administered by the private sector.[6] This description characterizes most social transfers and some services of the welfare state in Great Britain and other Anglo-Saxon countries. Prime Ministers Margaret Thatcher and John Major

[5] See 31 for an example of this error.

[6] See 32 and 33 for critiques of the Beveridge report.

claimed that their liberal proposals did not represent a break with the Beveridge philosophy. They were right.

As a consequence of this lack of universalization of welfare state benefits (except the minimum set of benefits), we see in these Anglo-Saxon liberal countries a marked commodification of benefits with very extensive private expenditures. The percentage of GDP spent on Social Security is relatively low, the lowest of the developed capitalist countries (15.2 percent of GDP) except for the southern European countries that suffered long periods of dictatorship. The percentage of public spending on Social Security (the largest component of social transfers) in liberal countries is much lower than in Christian democratic countries (21.6 percent of GDP) and social democratic countries (23.2 percent).

A similar situation occurs in the services sector of the welfare state. Public social services occupy only 5.7 percent of the labor force in the liberal countries, compared with 13.2 percent in social democratic and 6.2 percent in Christian democratic countries. Consequently, their taxes are much lower, representing only 36.5 percent of GDP, compared with 41.8 percent in Christian democratic and 48.8 percent in social democratic countries.

It is important to stress that the liberal model, unlike the Christian democratic model (which assigns welfare state responsibilities to the family) and the social democratic model (which assigns these responsibilities to the state), assigns welfare state responsibilities to the private sector (and very much in particular to a highly decentralized collective bargaining process), once the minimums are guaranteed by the state. For this reason, the liberal model does not burden the family and women. Consequently the percentage of women integrated into the labor force in these countries is, on average, very high at 52.8 percent (but only 36 percent in Ireland). Women and families are assisted by family-oriented services provided by the private sector and purchased at market prices. Because of this market provision, availability depends on price and on the salary and wage levels prevalent in the private services sector. In none of these liberal countries do these services have high costs because they are provided by cheap, unskilled labor. The McDonald's restaurants in the United States typify this sort of service. The cheapness of labor in these services is a primary reason for the higher wage polarization in these countries, condemning large sectors of the labor force (in particular the young) to very low wage jobs in the family-oriented services (34).

The Political Economy of the Liberal Model

This liberal model translates into a situation in which capital is strong and labor is weak, compared with Christian democratic and social democratic countries. The level of unionization in the liberal countries (except Ireland) tends to be very low (Table 5). This class relation of forces explains the limited redistributive effect of the state (Table 5) and the large total profits (Table 7), much larger than in social democratic countries though somewhat smaller than in Christian democratic countries. It is important to stress that despite the sizable mass of profits (as percentage of national income), the investment rate during the period 1960–1989 was lower in these liberal countries than in the social democratic and Christian democratic countries (Table 7). The liberal countries also had lower economic growth during the years 1960–1995 (with the exception of 1989–1995, when their economic growth was the highest).

The liberal countries are also characterized by a limited state intervention in the labor market (they have the most unregulated labor markets) and in economic development, and at the same time are the countries with the highest unemployment (Table 6). This situation proves the erroneousness of the liberal position that stresses the need to deregulate labor markets as a way of reducing unemployment. Actually, the countries with less regulated labor markets had higher rates of unemployment during the period 1960–1995.

The countries with liberal governments have also had larger public deficits (Table 6)—proving that in the absence of state interventions on the supply side (as in social democratic countries), there is a need for intervention on the demand side. This is achieved by manipulating the public deficit as a way of either stimulating (or slowing down) internal demand and the economic growth that such demand stimulates. Thus Keynesianism is an economic policy primarily of the neoliberal countries with weak states. In the absence of strong states and social pacts, large public deficits have been the most effective interventions to stimulate demand and economic growth. Keynesianism, therefore, is not a component or characteristic of a strong state but rather an indicator of state weakness. This reality is what makes the European process of monetary union, with its austere criteria for reducing and even eliminating public deficits, a particular economic obstacle for the liberal E.U. countries (and to a lesser degree for the Christian democratic countries). The social democratic countries have the most effective public instruments and mechanisms for coping with the enormous task of eliminating their public deficits. The social pact enables them to establish incomes policies that can better respond to the austerity measures imposed by the process of monetary union. It is precisely because of this that the process requires strong states rather than the weak states advocated by neoliberals.

VI. POLITICAL RESPONSES TO THE GROWTH OF INEQUALITIES

The most important determinants of social inequalities are (*a*) the distribution of wealth and income derived from property or capital versus that derived from labor; (*b*) the internal distribution of wages—that is, wage dispersion; and (*c*) the redistributive effect of the welfare state.

Each of these variables depends primarily on the political context of a country: the strength of the different political and social instruments of the various agents and classes. Table 8 shows, for example, how wage growth during 1979–1996

Table 8

Characteristics of the labor market: Wages, family income, hours of work, and poverty[a]

	Wage growth[b]		Relative hourly compensation of manufacturing production workers, 1979–96, U.S. = 100[c]			Earnings inequality growth, 1979–97[d]		Household income inequality relative to national median incomes, ratio 90th to 10th percentile[e]	Annual hrs of work per worker[f]		Poverty[g]		
	1979–89	1989–96	1979	1989	1996	1980	1990	1990–91	1979	1995	Total	Elderly	Children
Social democratic political economies													
Sweden	1.3	0.8	125	123	139	2.04	2.21	2.78	1,451	1,544	6.7	6.4	3
Denmark	0.3	1.6	116	102	137	2.14	2.18	2.86	–	–	7.5	11.3	5.1
Norway	0.4	1.4	114	128	142	2.06	–	2.80	1,516	1,424	6.6	13.5	4.9
Finland	3.0	2.3	77	118	133	2.46	2.34	2.75	1,868	1,775	6.2	14.4	2.7
Mean	1.25	1.5	108	117	137	2.17	2.24	2.79	1,611	1,581	6.75	11.4	3.92
Christian democratic political economies													
France	1.1	1.1	85	90	120	3.24	3.06	3.48	1,813	1,631	7.5	4.8	7.4
Germany	1.2	–0.1	125	124	180	2.69	2.32	3.21	1,764	1,559	7.6	7.5	8.6
Belgium	0.9	1.7	131	108	146	–	2.07	2.79	–	–	5.5	11.9	4.4
Netherlands	0.0	0.4	126	105	131	–	2.59	3.05	–	–	6.7	4.1	8.3
Italy	1.4	0.7	78	101	99	2.94	2.80	3.14	1,788	–	6.5	4.4	10.5
Mean	0.9	0.7	109	105	135	2.95	2.56	3.14	1,788	1,595	6.7	6.54	7.84

Liberal Anglo-Saxon political economies														
United States	–0.3	0.1	100	100	100	3.65	4.43	5.78	1,905	1,952	19.1	19.6	24.9
Canada	–0.5	0.5	87	103	94	4.01	4.20	3.90	1,802	1,737	11.7	5.7	15.3
Great Britain	2.1	0.5	63	74	80	2.79	3.37	4.67	1,821	1,735	14.6	23.9	18.5
Ireland	1.6	1.4	54	67	78	–	–	4.18	–	–	11.1	7.6	13.8
Mean	0.9	0.6	76	86	88	3.48	5.47	4.63	1,842	1,808	14.25	14.2	18.1

[a]Source: reference 1.
[b]OECD Statistical Series, analyzed by the Economic Policy Institute, from reference 1, Table 8.5.
[c]U.S. Bureau of Labor Statistics and OECD Statistical Series, from reference 1, Table 8.6.
[d]Measured as the ratio of the earnings of the 90th percentile of workers to those of the 10th percentile of workers; adapted from reference 1, Table 8.9.
[e]Adapted from reference 1, Table 8.11.
[f]OECD, 1996; adapted from reference 1, Table 8.18.
[g]Smeeding, T. M. *Financial Poverty in Developed Countries: The Evidence from L.I.S.* Working Paper No. 155. Luxembourg Income Study, 1997; adapted from reference 1, Table 8.14.

was, on average, higher in social democratic than in Christian democratic countries (except during the years 1989–1996) and much higher than in the liberal countries. Taking the level of wages in the United States as 100, the average wage level in the social democratic countries was 108 in 1979, 117 in 1989, and 137 in 1996. Wage levels have been higher in social democratic than in Christian democratic countries, and much higher than in liberal countries. Another indicator of labor weakness in liberal countries is longer working hours (Table 8): 1,842 hours a year in 1979 and 1,808 hours in 1995, compared with 1,788 hours and 1,595 hours, respectively, in Christian democratic countries, and 1,611 hours and 1,581 hours in social democratic countries.

These and other data in Table 8 also show that labor strength translates into less wage dispersion, less income inequality, and less poverty (except for the elderly). The table shows that in the liberal countries in 1980, the average wage of the upper decile was 3.48 times that of the lower decile, increasing to 5.47 times larger in 1998. In 1986 these were almost double, and in 1990 more than double, the wage differentials in the social democratic and Christian democratic countries.

A similar situation appears in the analysis of family income differentials. As Table 8 also shows, in 1990–1991 the average income of the richest families was 4.63 times that of the poorest families in liberal countries, almost double the difference in social democratic countries (2.79 times). It is important to emphasize that while the wage differentials were somewhat larger in Christian democratic than in social democratic countries, family income differentials were far larger in the Christian democratic countries, reaching levels similar to those in liberal countries. This is the result of much more family income coming from capital in the Christian democratic and liberal countries than in the social democratic countries (Table 8). The family income differentials between Christian democratic and social democratic countries are explained by income from capital and the way in which that income is treated by the state. And these two factors, together with wage differentials, explain the family income differentials between the liberal and the social democratic countries.

These differences in income and wage inequalities are largely responsible for the variability in poverty levels among the developed capitalist countries. The other reason for the variability is differences in the redistributive impact of the welfare state, in particular in social transfers and in taxes and state fees. Table 9 shows how the poverty reduction effect of the welfare state is much greater in social democratic than in Christian democratic and liberal countries. The only exception is reduction of poverty among the elderly, which is greater in the Christian democratic than in the social democratic countries; thus poverty among the elderly is somewhat lower in Christian democratic than in social democratic countries, but is much higher in liberal countries. Almost one of every four elders in Great Britain and one of every five in the United States live in poverty. Liberalism is not kind to elders. The lower poverty among elders in Christian democratic countries is partly due to the role played by the family, which also explains the low poverty rate among elders in Ireland, a country that in all other aspects is representative of liberal countries.

We should note that the low poverty among the elderly in the Christian democratic countries contrasts with the high poverty among children. Italy and Spain, two of the most Catholic countries, have higher percentages of children living in poverty than any other Christian democratic countries. But it is in the liberal countries that poverty among children is most accentuated: 24 percent of children in the United States and 18.5 percent in Great Britain live in poverty. As shown by these figures, and others presented in this chapter, liberalism is not kind to workers, elders, and children.

The Liberal Attack on the Welfare State

The political triumph of neoliberalism, under President Reagan in the United States and Prime Minister Thatcher in the United Kingdom, as well as the collapse of the Soviet Union, led to the expansion and international dominance of the liberal model, behind which lie the class interests described in this chapter. Liberal countries are those in which the capitalist class is very powerful and the working class is less so: the opposite pole from social democratic countries in which labor is strong and capital less so. I have shown in this chapter that, for the most part, social democracy has been more equitable and efficient than liberalism. Despite this reality, the liberal model has become the most dominant in the world today. This model and the forces behind it are also responsible for the deregulation of markets, including financial markets, that has led to the process referred to as globalization. This process and the promotion of the liberal model have been assisted by the U.S. government and by international agencies such as the International Monetary Fund and the World Bank, which are heavily influenced by the U.S. government. In this liberal discourse and practice, the interests of the dominant classes are presented as universal interests. The expansion of the liberal model has had a most negative impact on the welfare state of the developed capitalist countries. The weakening of the labor movement and the strengthening of the business community (and very much in particular, the financial community) have undermined the welfare state in these countries.

I am aware of the argument, widely presented by social policy analysts, that the popularity of the welfare state is such that no government—not even the Reagan and Thatcher governments—would dare to touch it. In support of this thesis, Pearson and others have shown that countries governed by quite different political parties, such as Sweden, Germany, Great Britain, and the United States, have all maintained their level of social transfers (measured by social expenditures as percentage of GNP) (35).

It is misleading, however, to present these indicators as proof of the resilience of the welfare state. Social transfers, for example, are more difficult to cut back than social services, because the impact of their reduction is more immediate

Table 9

The impact of the welfare state (taxes, fees, and social transfers) in reducing poverty, 1990–1991, percent[a]

	All people			Elderly			Children		
	Pre	Post	Change, %	Pre	Post	Change, %	Pre	Post	Change, %
Social democratic political economies									
Sweden	34	6.7	−80.4	68.2	11.4	−83.3	18.4	3.0	−83.7
Norway	21.8	6.6	−69.7	68.0	13.5	−80.1	12.7	4.9	−61.4
Denmark	26.9	7.5	−72.1	69.9	11.3	−83.8	17.1	5.1	−70.2
Finland	15.6	6.2	−60.3	43.8	14.4	−67.1	11.6	2.7	−76.7
Mean	–	–	−70.6	–	–	−78.5	–	–	−73
Christian democratic political economies									
Belgium	28.4	5.5	−80.6	88.9	11.9	−86.6	17.2	4.4	−74.4
Germany	22	7.6	−65.5	65.8	7.5	−88.6	11.7	8.6	−26.5
Netherlands	22.8	6.7	−70.6	65.5	4.1	−93.7	15.2	8.3	−45.4
France	21.6	7.5	−65.3	79.9	4.8	−94.0	27.4	7.4	−73.0
Italy	18.4	6.5	−64.7	55.7	4.4	−92.1	11	10.5	−4.5
Mean	–	–	−69.3	–	–	−91	–	–	−44

Former dictatorship countries									
Spain	28.2	10.4	–63.1	68.2	11.4	–83.3	20.7	12.8	–38.2
Portugal	–	–	–	–	–	–	–	–	–
Greece	–	–	–	–	–	–	–	–	–
Liberal countries									
Great Britain	29.2	14.6	–50	68.5	23.9	–65.1	28.7	18.5	–35.5
Ireland	30.3	11.1	–63.4	54.9	7.6	–82.2	30.3	13.8	–54.5
United States	26.7	19.1	–28.5	58.7	19.6	–66.6	28.7	24.9	–13.2
Canada	23.4	11.7	–50	58.2	5.7	–90.2	22.7	15.3	–32.6
Mean	–	–	–43	–	–	–76	–	–	–33.9

[a]Source: Smeeding, T. M. *Financial Poverty in Developed Countries: The Evidence from L.I.S.* Working Paper No. 155. Luxembourg Income Study, 1997.

(pensioners notice immediately any reduction in their Social Security checks) than is the reduction of social services (it takes longer for the users of these services to notice any reductions in the funding of services). This is why the cutback in expenditures on services is more doable politically than cutbacks in social transfers. And this is what has been happening. The rate of growth in spending on services per user and in public employment per user has been declining in developed capitalist countries in the 1980s and 1990s, even though the need for such services has been increasing due to the growth of unemployment, demographic changes (with growth of the elderly population), growing inequalities, and increasing poverty (36).

Another factor ignored by those certain of the resilience of the welfare state is that the rate of growth of social transfers and social expenditures has been declining during the 1980s and 1990s, a decline that has occurred even as human needs (for the reasons noted above) have been increasing substantially. Regarding public employment, Table 10 shows the decline in the rate of growth of public employment from the 1980s on, although the growth continues to be higher in social democratic than in Christian democratic countries and much higher than in liberal countries (except in 1989–1994, when the growth was higher in the Christian democratic than in the social democratic or liberal countries).

A similar situation is evident regarding public consumption (Table 10), which includes the costs of goods and services provided by the public sector, of which the welfare state makes up the majority. We can see a very accentuated decline of public consumption over the 1980s, although here again, social democratic countries had higher rates of growth in public consumption than Christian democratic (except for 1989–1994) and liberal countries.

Other changes have also occurred in the welfare states as a result of the liberal avalanche, such as (*a*) the transformation of some universal benefits into means-tested benefits, (*b*) the greater role of the private sector in the funding and provision of services, and (*c*) lessening of the intensity of care through reduction of employment and/or expenditures per user or beneficiary, a general phenomenon that has occurred everywhere—although its implementation has varied with the political context, being more accentuated in liberal and less accentuated in social democratic countries.

The changes in the welfare state respond primarily to political rather than economic forces, as has been shown in this chapter. The current emphasis on globalization as the cause of these changes has an apologetic function, defending the inevitability of such changes. Yet globalization is not a cause but a symptom of the state of class relations in the developed capitalist countries. As I have shown, the social democratic countries have actually been among the most integrated internationally, without "globalization" being a handicap for the extensive development of their welfare states. Actually, the extensive welfare state development was a *condition* for their competitiveness and integration into world markets. This chapter has demonstrated this, as well as providing empirical

Table 10

Growth in public employment and public consumption, 1960–1994[a]

	Annual changes in public employment, %				Growth of public consumption, %			
	1960–73	1973–79	1979–89	1989–94	1960–73	1973–79	1979–89	1989–94
Social democratic countries								
Sweden	5.6	4.9	1.3	–2.1	4.9	3.7	1.6	0.9
Denmark	–	4.8	1.7	–0.4	5.8	4.1	1.5	0.8
Norway	–	5.4	2.5	2.6	5.9	5.3	3.5	3.1
Finland	4.6	4.8	2.7	–1.2	5.4	4.8	3.5	–0.1
Mean	5.1	4.9	2.05	–0.2	5.5	4.4	2.5	1.1
Christian democratic countries								
Belgium	2.1	3.3	0.7	–0.5	5.5	3.7	0.5	0.9
Germany	3.7	2.3	1.0	0.2	4.5	3.0	1.3	1.7
Netherlands	1.7	2.3	0.5	–0.8	2.8	3.5	2.0	1.2
France	–	2.8	1.7	1.4	4.0	3.4	2.3	2.6
Italy	–	2.7	1.4	0.0	4.0	2.7	2.6	0.9
Mean	2.5	2.68	1.06	0.06	4.1	3.2	1.7	1.4
Liberal countries								
Great Britain	1.7	1.5	–0.2	–6.1	2.7	1.8	1.0	1.5
Ireland	–	–	–	–	–	–	–	–
United States	2.7	1.5	1.2	1.2	2.5	1.7	2.7	0.1
Canada	–	2.0	2.3	1.8	6.1	3.5	2.5	1.1
Mean	2.2	1.6	1.1	–1.03	3.7	2.3	2.0	0.9

[a]Source: OECD, *Historical Series,* 1960–1994.

evidence that the state should take a leading role in developing economic and social policies that better respond to the growing internationalization of the economy. And it is for these reasons that we need to recover the important elements of the social democratic model, clearly under attack these days. The countries where such models have been most closely followed have been better able to resist the liberal avalanche and its economic and social consequences, such as lower economic growth and higher unemployment. The social democratic model, with active state intervention in economic and fiscal policies, and with active full-employment and redistributive policies, continues to be of great relevance in the developed capitalist countries today.

REFERENCES

1. Mishel, L., Bernstein, J., and Schmitt, J. International comparisons. In *State of Working America 1998–99*, Chapt. 8. Economic Policy Institute, Washington, D.C., 1998.
2. Toharia, L., et al. *El mercado de trabajo en España*. McGraw Hill, New York, 1988.
3. Mishel, L., and Bernstein, J. *The State of Working America, 1994–1995*. Economic Policy Institute, Washington, D.C., 1995.
4. Eurostat. 1997.
5. Kiernam, K., and Mueller, G. *The Divorced and Who Divorces?* ERSC Research Center, May 1998.
6. White, L. K. Determinants of divorce: A review of research in the eighties. *J. Marriage Fam.* 52(4): 904, 1990.
7. Bettio, F., and Villa, P. A. Mediterranean perspective on the breakdown of the relationship between participation and fertility. *Cambridge J. Econ.* 22: 137–171, 1998.
8. Delgado, M., and Bacci, L. Fertility in Spain and in Italy: The lowest in the world. *Fam. Plann. Perspect.* 24(4): 167–171, July-August 1992.
9. Moody, K. *Workers in a Lean World.* Verso, London, 1997.
10. Galbraith, J. K. *Created Unequal.* Free Press, New York, 1998.
11. Organization for Economic Cooperation and Development. *Historical Series*. Paris, 1960–1992.
12. Navarro, V. Eurosclerosis versus U.S. dynamism. *Challenge*, July 1998, p. 52.
13. Organization for Economic Cooperation and Development. *Historical Series*. Paris, 1960–1990.
14. Organization for Economic Cooperation and Development. *Employment Outlook, 1997*. Paris, 1997.
15. Organization for Economic Cooperation and Development. *Employment Outlook, 1998*. Paris, 1998.
16. Economic Policy Institute. *State of Working America, 1995*. Washington, D.C., 1995.
17. Rifkin, J. *The End of Work*. Putnam's Sons, New York, 1995.
18. Navarro, V. *The Politics of Health Policy*. Blackwell, Cambridge, Mass., 1994.
19. Esping-Andersen, G. *The Social Foundations of Post-Industrial Economies*. Oxford University Press, Oxford, England, 1999.

20. Huber, E., and Stephens, J. D. Internationalization and the social democratic model: Crisis and future prospects. *Comp. Polit. Stud.* 13(3): 353–397, 1998.
21. Korpi, W. *The Democratic Class Struggle*. Routledge and Kegan Paul, London, 1983.
22. Huber, E., and Stephens, J. D. Politics of the welfare state after the Golden Age. In *Social Democratic Welfare State: Origins, Achievements, Crisis and Future*. 1998, in press.
23. Collins, S. M. *Exports-Imports*. Brookings Institution, Washington, D.C., 1998.
24. Wolman, W., and Colamosa, A. *The Judas Economy: The Triumph of Capital and the Betrayal of Work*. Addison, New York, 1997.
25. Weiss, L. Limits of the distributive state: Swedish model on global economy. In *The Myth of Powerless State*, Chapt. 4. Polity Press, Cambridge, Mass., 1998.
26. Korpi, W. Eurosclerosis and the sclerosis of objectivity: On the role of values among economic experts. *Econ. J.* 106: 1727, November 1996.
27. Lindbeck, A., et al. *New Conditions for Economic Policy*. 1993.
28. Therborn, G. *European Modernity and Beyond: The Trajectory of European Societies, 1945–2000*. Sage, London, 1995.
29. Therborn, G. When, How, and Why Does a State Become a Welfare State? Paper presented at the ECPR Workshop on Comparative Study of Distribution and Social Policy in Advanced Industrialized Nations, Freiburg, March 20–25, 1983.
30. Preston, P. *Franco*. Gujalbo, 1993.
31. Rieger, E., and Leibfried, S. Welfare state limits to globalization. *Polit. Sociol.* 26(3): 363, September 1998.
32. Miliband, R. *Parliamentarian Socialism*. Merlin Press, 1973.
33. Navarro, V. *Class Struggle, the State and Medicine*. Martin Robertson, 1978.
34. Palley, T. I. *Plenty of Nothing*. Princeton University Press, Princeton, N.J., 1998.
35. Pearson, P. *Dismantling the Welfare State?* Cambridge University Press, Cambridge, England, 1994.
36. Clayton, R., and Pontusson, J. *The New Politics of the Welfare State Revisited*. Cornell University Press, Ithaca, N.Y., 1998.

PART III
Critique of International Agencies: WHO, PAHO, World Bank, IMF, UNICEF, and UNDP

CHAPTER 5

RAVAGING THE POOR: THE INTERNATIONAL MONETARY FUND INDICTED BY ITS OWN DATA

Gabriel Kolko

For the first time since its creation a half-century ago, the International Monetary Fund (IMF) is being subjected to severe criticisms from establishment sources that may profoundly alter its future role in guiding the world economy.

The IMF's failure to reverse the economic crisis in Thailand, Indonesia, and South Korea, which is now spreading throughout Asia, is producing unprecedented condemnations from powerful voices within business and policy circles who believe that the Fund's conservative strategy, with its insistence on slashing government spending to balance budgets, is endangering the stability of the entire world economy. Since the beginning of the year (1998), Harvard Professor Martin Feldstein, former chair of Reagan's Council of Economic Advisers and arguably the single most influential U.S. economist, the prestigious *Financial Times*, billionaire speculator George Soros, and many others have raised fundamental questions about the IMF's direction of the world economy. In March, the World Bank formally withdrew from joint sponsorship of the quarterly *Finance & Development,* which for 34 years had reflected the profound consensus between the two institutions, and Bank officials have publicly attacked the IMF's core policies in Asia.

Far less powerful critics have long condemned the IMF on a different score. They have contended that IMF "structural adjustment" programs, imposed on dozens of poor Third World nations, perpetuate and even intensify poverty. The IMF always admitted that adjustment may involve short-term social costs for vulnerable groups, but asserted that this short-term pain would ultimately benefit the poor themselves, since Fund-spurred economic growth would solve the basic problem of underdevelopment. Well before the economic storm in East Asia began to rage, the IMF was under mounting attack.

THE IMF IMPOSES RULES

In December 1987, the IMF expanded its existing structural adjustment program to create an "Enhanced Structural Adjustment Facility" (ESAF). It invited "low-income developing nations" to borrow from it. By August 1997, 79 countries were eligible to join ESAF but only 36, with a combined population of around 670 million, had done so. In order to receive ESAF loans, countries must agree to the IMF's "conditionality" and make "general commitments to cooperate with the IMF in setting policies to the formulation of specific, quantifiable plans for financial policies."

These conditions include fundamental domestic and external policies that, depending on the IMF's intentions, can effectively control a state's crucial social and economic priorities. Among the standard IMF prescriptions for developing countries: reducing government spending and involvement in the economy; promoting exports and removing trade restrictions; deregulating the economy; privatizing government-run enterprises; eliminating price subsidies, including on essentials like food and housing; and imposing consumption taxes. The IMF reviews country compliance with "performance criteria" designed to measure adoption of these policies on a semi-annual or even monthly basis. Countries that fail to pass the test are denied additional drawings on previously agreed-to loans.

Most World Bank aid, and much of the development aid that nations give, is dependent on a country satisfying IMF criteria. The Fund therefore serves as a gatekeeper to official loans and aid, and has far more power than the funds it provides directly would suggest.

The IMF has always defended its draconian demands as the essential preconditions to economic growth, without which poverty and stagnation will continue. But growth in the developing nations under IMF tutelage has either not occurred or occurred only very unevenly. Indeed, a number of national economies following IMF prescriptions have even shrunk. In the face of mounting criticism of its performance, in 1996 the IMF initiated a review of its impact "in strengthening economic performance in ESAF countries." On July 28, 1997, the IMF issued a laudatory summary, but postponed releasing a carefully edited complete text until late February.

The policy implications of this review are very profound; the IMF cannot allow the data it gathers to be used to prove that a major aspect of its work is useless, much less harmful, to the nations accepting its guidance. Not surprisingly, the IMF interpreted the data it released as vindication of its success. But no amount of statistical manipulation can reverse the fact that the majority of those nations that have followed the IMF's advice have experienced profound economic crises: low or even declining growth, much larger foreign debts, and the stagnation that perpetuates systemic poverty. Carefully analyzed, the IMF's own studies provide a devastating assessment of the social and economic consequences of its guidance of dozens of poor nations.

ASSESSING POOR NATIONS

The July 28, 1997, IMF release of the preliminary results of its internal review of all 79 low-income developing nations gave the best possible interpretation of the ESAF nations' performance, but it was unconvincing. Even on the basis of the data as the IMF presented them, countries that stayed out of ESAF began and remained better off by not accepting its advice. The value of all such comparisons is limited by the fact that most of the poor countries not participating in ESAF chose nonetheless to adopt IMF-preferred policies, though often not as fully as the Fund would like.

The IMF claimed per capita annual gross domestic product (GDP) growth for ESAF countries declined 1.1 percent in 1981–1985, before the ESAF program began, and rose to zero growth during 1990–1995. Non-ESAF developing nations rose from 0.3 percent in 1981–1985 to 1.0 percent in 1991–1995.

ESAF failed at one of its key, ostensible purposes: reducing poor countries' foreign debt. External debt as a percentage of gross national product (GNP) for the ESAF nations grew from 82 percent in 1980–1985 to 154 percent in 1991–1995. Non-ESAF nations were far less encumbered: their external debt grew from 56 to 76 percent of their GNP.

The biggest difference between ESAF and non-ESAF country performance was in exports, not surprising since maximizing exports and integrating developing countries into the world economy is the ultimate objective of all IMF programs. The annual export growth of the ESAF nations increased more than four times, according to the August 5, 1997, *IMF Survey* (the IMF's biweekly publication reporting on Fund activities, policies and research), from 1.7 percent in 1981–1985 to 7.9 percent in 1991–1994, while the non-ESAF nations' exports grew modestly, from 4.4 percent to 5.7 percent.

To assess the impact of the IMF's structural adjustment programs accurately, however, a different methodology than the IMF's should be used: only nations that are economically similar should be compared. Some of the non-ESAF nations had 1995 per capita incomes of $3,000 or more, and should not be compared to countries with per capita incomes roughly a tenth as large. There are 23 nations under ESAF for which data exist (with approximately 436 million population) with a per capita income below $400, and 13 non-ESAF nations (with 1.2 billion population) with similarly low incomes. These are the countries that should be studied to evaluate the IMF's ESAF program.

There are also limits in comparing the two groups of states under $400 annual per capita income, however. Significantly, averaging the 22 poorest ESAF nations for which there are sufficient data against the 13 that were independent fails to weight them by population size, which varies enormously; but to weight them introduces other distortions. The vast bulk of the non-ESAF population lived in India, while Pakistan and Bangladesh accounted for about half those under the ESAF.

Ignoring population, during 1985–1995 the poorest ESAF nations had a negative growth of 0.1 percent annually, while the 11 poorest non-ESAF nations declined 0.4 percent annually. The external debt of ESAF countries as a percent of the GNP grew from 52 percent in 1980 (in the 16 countries for which there are data) to 154 percent in 1995 (23 nations). For 11 non-ESAF nations it increased three times, to 117 percent—about the same for both groups. Debt service (interest payments on foreign debt) as a percentage of exports of goods and services over the same time grew from 16 percent to 21 percent for ESAF countries, 11 to 23 percent for the others.

On the basis of these data, there was no great difference between these two groups—all were in severe economic difficulty. But if India is assigned its importance by population, the non-ESAF poor nations as an aggregate performed far better. India had an annual growth rate from 1985 through 1995 of 3.2 percent, nearly three times that of Pakistan and one-half more than Bangladesh. Although it has begun to move to implement IMF-style liberalization in the 1990s, India remains far less dependent on exports than other low-income nations, and this has insulated it from external pressures and made stable, steady growth possible. More important, unlike its two large neighbors, its terms-of-trade (the relative value of the goods and services a nation imports compared to its exports) since 1985 have not varied greatly, further protecting it from the fluctuations of the world economy. Given the experience of these three nations only, there is a powerful argument against integrating a nation into the world economy and linking its development more than is absolutely essential into an inherently unstable export system.

Increasing exports is an absolute condition for IMF loans and ESAF nations embarked on an export-led development strategy. This decision was a recipe for stagnation and explains one crucial reason for the decline in growth for most of those who pursued it. Between 1985 and 1995 the terms-of-trade for the 18 very poor ESAF nations for which data exist fell 27 percent, according to the World Bank's *World Development Report 1997*, the basic source for the IMF's reviews and this article. This emphasis on exports in the face of declining prices was a disastrous strategic choice for development, because it is highly unlikely for a nation to export its way out of poverty in the face of falling prices for its goods. The result was that the states that the IMF directed, containing 670 million people, continue on a cycle that produces growing debts and sustains human deprivation. India chose another course, and notwithstanding its other difficulties, it averted many of the grave problems existing elsewhere.

Despite some modest differences, all very poor nations have fared badly, and debts have aggravated rather than cured their basic problems. Indeed, it is the very fact they become indebted that compels many of them to submit to the IMF's control, creating a vicious cycle of yet greater obligations—and poverty.

SEVERELY INDEBTED

Nothing proves the danger of excessive reliance on exports more than the World Bank's list, published in the *World Development Report 1996*, of 25 countries that are "severely indebted exporters of nonfuel primary products." These are among the world's poorest nations, and 16 of them (with a 1995 population of 217 million) were under the IMF's ESAF guidance; nine (with 143 million persons) were not. Of the 23 nations under IMF control with per capita income below $400, 13 were in the especially troubled economy category.

The 10 highly indebted ESAF nations under $400 per capita for which data exist during 1985–1995 had an average per capita GNP decline of 0.6 percent (compared to 0.2 percent for all ESAF nations together). For the seven non-ESAF states for which there are data, the average annual decline was 1.4 percent. What united all of these nations was that their external debt as a percentage of the GNP increased about three times between 1980 and 1995, their debt service consumed about a quarter of their exports of goods and services, and they became more deeply mired in debt. The terms-of-trade for their exports fell 23 percent between 1985 and 1995. Although nine were not under direct IMF supervision, they all nonetheless pursued its program for export-oriented development and staked their economic future on exports. The gamble failed: they stagnated and became poorer.

THE IMF'S SOCIAL COSTS

It is, above all else, the human and social consequences of the IMF's structural reform programs that has evoked the most condemnation, compelling the IMF to embark on an aggressive defense of its crucial role in the Third World. But the emerging IMF data only confirm that IMF policies have eroded existing social services and aggravated the poverty and suffering of hundreds of millions of people.

One IMF structural reform program demand that directly affects the poor is the forced reduction of government deficits. This comprises everything from slashing price subsidies for rice and fuel—which, as in Indonesia last May, often produces social disorder where implemented—to health clinics and public works. "Due regard needs to be paid to the cost-effectiveness and financial viability of these safety nets," stated the Fund in the December 15, 1997, *IMF Survey*—which means reducing them for the sake of a prosperous future which, so far, has never arrived.

As a companion to its defense of the ESAF, the IMF's Fiscal Affairs Department in November 1997 produced a study, "The IMF and the Poor," which reported health and education spending in 23 ESAF-supported nations for which it had data, comparing the three years before each nation accepted the ESAF to 1994 or 1995. On balance, the IMF concluded, ESAF countries increased health and education spending after adopting structural adjustment programs.

However, six of the 23 countries examined, containing 122 million people—one-fifth of the ESAF nations' population—reduced the proportion of their GDP allocated to health and education. And the report does not include the 13 countries under ESAF for which it did not have data. Those excluded have a combined population of one-third of the 620 million persons in the ESAF countries in 1994. The report's optimistic conclusions therefore applied, at most, to slightly under half of the people under ESAF programs—but even here the IMF distorted the data.

The IMF report averaged real per capita spending for health and education in its 23 nations. But averages are wholly misleading; the real issue is which class within each nation's population gains most from socially sponsored health and education programs—that is, whether the benefits are spread evenly. In a sample of eight ESAF nations, the IMF study found that the wealthiest fifth of the population received 32 percent of the education benefits, and the poorest 13 percent. For five nations where health data existed, the wealthiest quintile received 30 percent of the allocations, the poorest 12 percent. In Vietnam, an ESAF nation whose relative spending on health and education has dropped, the wealthiest fifth receives 45 percent of the public subsidies for health and education, according to the World Bank's January 1995 "Viet Nam: Poverty Assessment and Strategy."

The IMF's own evidence shows that the poorest three-fifths of these nations are being largely excluded from whatever social "safety net" exists for education, health, housing, and social security and welfare; their position has either not changed or, for many, become worse.

In some ways, focusing on health and education spending is misleading. IMF conditionalities affect the population's economic security considerably more than does spending on health and education. ESAF programs routinely cut government wages and salaries and facilitate private sector wage cuts and layoffs, so that each nation becomes "cost-effective" in the world export market. Price subsidies on basic commodities like bread and cooking oil—most critical for the poor—are cut. The higher value-added taxes it advocates are regressive on income distribution.

Ignoring the fact that it did not benefit the poorest, the nominal increase for health and education as a percentage of GDP in its 23 nations was only one-seventh of the reduction in wages, salaries, subsidies, and transfers that the ESAF program imposed on the total population, with the worst impact felt by the poorest. (The net decline for these functions combined was 1.8 percent of GDP.) The IMF's own data confirm that structural adjustment programs made the poor even poorer.

Unfortunately for the IMF, just as it was preparing its rebuttals of the widespread belief that its strategy hurts the poor, the World Bank, its sister institution, published a comprehensive analysis of poverty in the developing nations since 1980 which provides further evidence on how the IMF's programs have helped to sustain and create it. The Bank's study, published in the May 1997 *World Bank Economic Review*, traces poverty rates in 42 nations, divided by regions. It found that trends in living standards and absolute poverty are linked, above all else, to economic growth. No region displayed a consistent pattern, but Eastern and Central Europe, Latin America and Sub-Saharan Africa—regions where the IMF was most active—generally had a higher incidence of poverty since 1980, while poverty declined in East and South Asia, the Middle East, and North Africa.

THE IMF BURDEN

Most of the nations whose economic destinies the IMF has guided have not grown; they have either stagnated or declined economically, and the poor have suffered both in the short and long run in the name of the Fund's socially dangerous ideological mystifications. Save for India, which alone confirms the value of independent strategies, most of the poor nations which remained outside the ESAF program did not do much better, but they certainly did not do worse than the IMF-led countries.

The causes of the sustained crisis of development in the Third World are extremely complex, but it is certain that excessive reliance on export-led growth in an unstable world economy creates major structural problems that all growth strategies must avoid. But exports are at the core of the IMF philosophy, and its guidance has gravely hindered the struggle of innumerable poor nations to escape their suffering.

Note — This chapter is adapted from a report published in *Multinational Monitor*, June 1998, pp. 20–23.

CHAPTER 6

WORLD BANK EDUCATION POLICY: MARKET LIBERALISM MEETS IDEOLOGICAL CONSERVATISM

Adriana Puiggrós

The theme of the Fifth Ibero-American Summit, held in the Argentine resort of Bariloche in October 1995, was "Education and Development." The 22 heads of state who were present at the gathering painted an imaginary portrait of progress and good pedagogical intentions toward the region's excluded majorities. They reflected on the need to improve the quality and effectiveness of education, and to make primary schooling universally available. The whole event had a strangely surreal air. At the same time that the presidents were extolling the importance of education, most of their administrations were chopping away at their public education systems.

The region's governments are taking their cue from the World Bank, which has been in the vanguard in defining social policy in the neoliberal era. The Bank recommends drastically reducing public investment in education through privatizing and breaking up school systems, and nullifying teachers' contracts. Such a restructuring of the education system is part of a larger effort to wipe out the remnants of the region's so-called "paternalistic" states.

The Bank's education policy has an exclusively economic logic. It is based on a short-term cost-benefit analysis. As a researcher from the Fundación Mediterránea, a think tank affiliated with Argentina's Minister of Economics Domingo Cavallo, put it, "What we try to measure is how well the training provided by each school fits the needs of production and the labor market" (1). The World Bank advocates reducing all investment in education that does not generate direct income or cannot be recouped right away. Only educational spending that is immediately profitable is considered justifiable. Disciplines like anthropology and cultural studies, for example, are considered irrelevant.

This concept of "profitability" needs to be scrutinized. In the 1960s and 1970s, economists tried hard to come up with a formula for measuring the value which education contributes to labor, and education's role in the rate of return on investment. They never found a mathematical formula that worked, much less anything capable of becoming the basis for a universally applicable model. The reason for that failure is rooted in the fact that the logic of economic discourse is different from the logic of pedagogic discourse. To educate, you have to be looking toward the future and believe in a better world. Better worlds, however, aren't necessarily profitable in the short term.

The World Bank's current education policy is the reverse of the traditional liberal thinking that characterized U.S. education policy with respect to Latin America since the end of the Second World War. Liberalism and "development theory" encouraged investment in public education so that Latin America's citizens would become productive participants in the institutions of capitalism. U.S. policy makers viewed public education in Latin America as a key component of the social peace which was needed to guarantee the security of U.S. investments in the region.

Today, the bottom line is most important. The Bank's education policy is part and parcel of a larger neoliberal economic program whose overarching goal is to reduce state spending so that governments are able to continue making payments on their foreign debt.

Latin America's public school systems have developed quite unevenly over the past century. The quality and availability of public education varies considerably between different regions and countries, and also within each country. Because of the concentration of poverty in the countryside and the concentration of economic and political power in the urban centers, public school systems have traditionally been highly centralized with a top-down pyramidal structure. School curricula generated by central-government offices have rarely reflected the diversity and vitality of popular cultures.[1]

The World Bank has taken up these real concerns, criticizing the traditional education systems' bureaucracy, excessive centralization, poor quality, and uneven development. In terms of solutions, the Bank rightly recognizes that "it's impossible to come up with universal formulas, since the steps to be taken must be adapted to the situation of each country." No single model of a school system can be universally applicable in a region as socially and culturally diverse as Latin America. Yet the Bank adds that there is "a group of general policies that could be useful basic guides for all countries" (2, p. 19). In the end, the World Bank has a single prescription for all countries.

One of the principal recommendations of the World Bank's education policy is that governments focus on improving primary education. To achieve this goal, the Bank does not recommend increasing public spending on education; rather, it

[1] Education, however, was not entirely homogeneous as programs were reinterpreted by teachers in each locality and region. During the military dictatorships in Argentina and Uruguay in the 1970s, for example, many teachers taught a very different curriculum than that imposed by the governments. Some paid with their lives for this act of liberty.

proposes diverting money that used to go toward financing high schools and universities in order to expand access to primary schooling. The Bank recognizes that its plan will meet with fierce opposition from the many people who will be hurt by this redistribution of scarce funds. So for marketing purposes, the Bank makes highly dubious use of terms like "equity."

Its arguments are simple and direct. "Although public spending on primary education generally benefits the poor," one Bank report claims, "total public spending on education in low- and middle-income countries often favors the affluent" (3, p. 62). The same argument in favor of a focus on primary schooling is also made on the grounds of economic efficiency. "The high rates of return estimated for basic education in most developing countries," says the same report, "strongly suggest that investments to improve enrollments and retention in basic education should generally have the highest priority" (3, p. 9). There is no question that some groups are more in need of state-sponsored education than others, and compensatory programs must exist. But the word "equity" has been manipulated to cover up the attempt to eliminate free public schooling beyond the primary level. The Bank's rhetoric about the need to distribute free services more "equitably" deflates when we take into account that these services are administered at the whim of corrupt functionaries as part of broader structural adjustment programs that impoverish the population as a whole.

Members of the Menem administration parroted the World Bank's claims during Argentina's National Constituent Assembly in 1994, when they defended the neoliberal reform of the constitutional provisions for education on the grounds that the government wanted to distribute free educational services more equitably. In practice, the reform restricted guaranteed access to free education to the primary level. The student movement is currently fighting the government's attempt to impose university tuition fees in the wake of the reform. Where these fees have been imposed, large sectors of Argentina's impoverished middle class have been pushed out of the post-secondary education system.

It is open to question whether primary education really is a priority of the World Bank. Shifting funds from one level to another won't do the job. You can't broaden access to primary education unless you have enough teachers trained to teach primary school. You can't train these teachers in isolation, without raising the educational and professional levels of the entire society. Far from acknowledging the need for more teachers, the Bank recommends cutting back the number of primary school teachers as well as government-funded teacher-training and education programs.

Universal access to primary education will only be achieved if more money is invested in educating rural, indigenous, and poor urban children, as well as adults who never attended school. Such programs, however, would raise the average cost per student, which is contradictory to the goals of structural adjustment (4). Since neoliberal governments are loath to spend a penny more on education, educational services for the poor get reduced to a few small-scale efforts such as the educational components in Argentina's Social Plan and Mexico's Solidarity Program. Both of these social investment funds were designed in concert with structural adjustment programs.

Aside from redistributing educational funds, the World Bank also calls for the privatization of the school system under the guise of decentralization and modernization. In Peru, the national government is handing elementary schools over to local jurisdictions as part of its larger efforts to shrink the purview of the state. Following the World Bank's advice, President Alberto Fujimori passed a series of new laws which regulate the transfer of control of schools from the national government to Community Boards of Education that have been set up in each municipality. These boards have legal standing as private entities. Only some of them receive state financing to cover part or all of their monthly expenses. The new laws also allow the state to transfer school facilities to teachers, parents, and religious institutions, among others (5).

Decentralization of primary school systems without accompanying state financial support is producing greater inequality in educational services. While a handful of provinces and municipalities may be able to assume this new economic burden, other localities simply will not be able to sustain an elementary-school system on their own. The Bank recommends eliminating poorly functioning schools altogether, which will make the system even more elitist. As schools are passed from hand to hand, the transfer process results in further closings and the deterioration of school infrastructure.

Making matters worse, neoliberal governments have started handing schools over to local governments and private interests at a time of economic catastrophe. The World Bank agreed to provide loans to several countries to cover the administrative expenses of the transfer itself. But loans—which are always limited and temporary—will not make up the shortfall in educational spending that already exists and has simply been passed from the national government to local municipalities.

The Bank favors running education on the model of the free market under the premise that competition will stimulate better quality schooling. According to neoliberal pedagogical theory, parents and students can "freely" choose among the different options offered in the educational marketplace: they can foot their children's tuition fees if they have the money, they can go into debt, or they can give up altogether on educating their children.

Nicaragua offers a preview of what this new educational marketplace will look like. In a letter dated October 8, 1992, the Nicaraguan finance minister promised the president of the World Bank "to continue promoting the private provision of educational services at the primary and secondary levels" and "to remove restrictions on licenses and tuition charges" (quoted in 6). Nicaragua's public high schools now have obligatory tuition payments, and the elementary schools have "voluntary" ones. Schools charge rent on required textbooks. They have to raise funds to pay for their own water, electricity, and telephone. Subsidies for hot

EDUCATION REFORMS ADVOCATED BY TEACHERS

Educators International and the Confederation of American Educators—the two organizations to which the majority of teachers in the Western world belong—met on October 14–16, 1995 in Buenos Aires. The meeting, which was hosted by the Confederation of Educational Workers of the Argentine Republic (CTERA), was held to coincide with the Ibero-American Summit in Bariloche. The teachers' objective was to voice their concern about the crushing problems they face and the uncertain future of education in the region.

They issued a declaration that criticizes the short-sightedness of neoliberal educational reforms, and declares that education should be considered a strategic investment in the future. The document emphasizes that only the long-term policies of democratic governments, hammered out with broad-based civic participation, will guarantee quality education. The teachers also called for overcoming the false contradiction between public education and modernization. They did so by affirming the four educational principles that underline democratic modernization: education should be non-sectarian, free, obligatory, and integrating. These principles, which have not been sufficiently adhered to by modern education systems, are now under attack by neoliberal policy makers.

According to the document, teachers want an education system which:

- is governed and managed with the participation of teachers, and not left entirely in the hands of bureaucrats and politicians.
- guarantees fair salaries and ongoing professional training.
- answers the demands of all sectors of the population and broadens economic investment.
- is multicultural and does not discriminate against minorities.
- keeps study plans up-to-date and regularly revises the curricula.
- responds to the infrastructural needs of public schools.

The teachers agreed that these educational reforms will not be possible without the participation of the unions and associations that represent educational workers. They demanded that collective bargaining be respected and that their unions be given a role in the discussion of education policies. They criticized the coercive measures that have been used to repress union activity, and government interference intended to weaken and atomize the union movement.

lunches and transportation for students and teachers have been eliminated. The Nicaraguan teachers' union has also criticized the closing of rural schools and the handing over of school buildings to private interests (6).

The push for privatization reflects the Bank's belief that national governments should not have to provide permanent support for education. The Bank does not take into account, however, the relative weakness of the private sector in Latin America. Private groups are not able or willing to take on the task of providing primary education to millions of children. Such an initiative would entail paying the salaries of thousands of teachers as well as providing proper equipment to the schools. Not even the Catholic Church, which has traditionally been the largest supplier of private education, could take on more than a small portion of the total number of students in need of education.

As governments in countries such as Mexico, Argentina, Colombia, and Chile began to decentralize their school systems in the late 1980s and early 1990s, a private educational market did grow at first. It soon, however, began to flounder. Business lost interest in investing in education, as shrinking real wages caused the pool of potential private-school pupils to diminish (7). In 1995, for example, a hundred private schools closed in Buenos Aires alone. This year (1996), the demand for public elementary education in Argentina has mushroomed as many middle-class parents are no longer able to afford private-school tuition fees. Quite a few children will likely be left without schools to attend, or be stuck in overcrowded classrooms (8).

For decentralization to flourish, there have to be social groupings able to take advantage of the new opportunities and responsibilities. But Latin American civil society, which is weak to begin with, has been hit hard by the recent economic crisis. The Bank argues that "decentralization of education and support to community and private schools will generate additional resources for education from families and other local sources" (2, p. 43). Since regional economies are bankrupt, people cannot pay higher local taxes or make the direct contributions needed to keep these transferred schools afloat. Nor do people struggling to make ends meet have the time or energy to run schools.

The debate about whether Latin America's school systems should be decentralized or centralized is not a new one. In fact, that discussion, which has never been definitively resolved, began at the end of the nineteenth century. Not surprisingly, the debate over decentralization is intimately linked to the issue of nation building. Despite all their problems, public school systems are the most important public arena in which a unified national culture can be constructed and passed from generation to generation.

Since the independence era, Latin American democrats have linked decentralization with participation. They envision unified national school systems which are nonetheless sensitive to local demands and proposals. They argue that members of local school boards should be democratically elected. Finally, they believe that responsibility for financing education rests primarily on governments, though state resources can be complemented by private contributions. They favor state-financed education because it guarantees the continuity of education programs, is much more stable than private support, and has universal reach.

Decentralization is not good in and of itself, or under any circumstances. It needs to occur as part of broader development initiatives that have widespread popular support. To be effective, decentralization should take place during moments of regional economic growth when money as well as responsibility can be passed to the local level. The public should also play a role in shaping the process. As one Bank report declares, "If secondary education is to be decentralized, all parties agree that it should be done with prior consultation between the parties involved" (9). Nevertheless, in practice, the World Bank has allowed countries to carry out decentralization without consulting the people affected.

Neoliberal economists insist that their reforms will increase the efficiency and quality of education (10). The indicators they use, however, are often far removed from issues of pedagogical practice (11). For example, economists measure the efficiency of a school's staff by comparing the hours worked to the number of teachers on salary. For secondary, university, and technical education, efficiency is measured by the number of graduates who find jobs. Following this logic, Minister of Economics Domingo Cavallo blamed Argentina's 20 percent unemployment rate on the poor quality of the education system.

Whatever the criteria used—whether economic indicators, test scores, or people's right to education—Latin America's school systems score poorly. In the 1990s—the era of neoliberalism—education levels across the region have declined. Illiteracy is making a comeback in countries such as Argentina and Uruguay whose literacy rates were traditionally as high as those of developed countries. The Argentine government will not release complete statistics, but several sources suggest that illiteracy is now 14 percent among Argentines over 15 years old, compared with 7.4 percent in 1970 and 6.1 percent in 1980. The drop-out rate in primary school currently averages 35 percent nationwide, although it approaches 70 percent in certain provinces. Nearly 20 percent of all secondary-school students in Argentina had to repeat their grade level in 1995 (12–16).

National exam results in many countries have declined significantly since the application of neoliberal policies. In Costa Rica, studies show that since structural adjustment measures were implemented in the 1980s, scholastic achievement levels have fallen in primary and secondary schools, and more students are failing grades in high school. Between 1988 and 1990, over 40 percent of students flunked national exams in math, 13 percent flunked Spanish, 19 percent social studies, and 17 percent foreign languages and science (17, p. 45).

In order to improve those results—but never straying from the neoliberal mindset—the Bank is encouraging countries to establish common mandatory basic curricula in all public and private schools, as well as standard programs to evaluate teacher and student performance. With these instruments, the neoliberal model is complete: the state pulls out of education entirely and the market takes its place; after relaxing economic controls, ideological controls are strengthened. Market liberalism meets ideological conservatism.

Professors' activities have become subject to rigid discipline. Compensation is now often tied to particular performance indicators. For example, in Mexico, half of researchers' salaries is paid according to efficiency indexes. These indexes force them to interrupt their research in order to pursue topics which will produce immediately applicable results that will provide universities with additional income. Teaching is discouraged as well since it is given less point value than research. Merit pay often amounts to two or three times the base salary of professors. In Argentina, the monthly base salary of a full professor with 20 years seniority is U.S.$ 1,500. The professor can receive another $1,000 in incentive pay depending on how his or her work fits within the norms of efficiency. This kind of control over professors' time and activities has led to disinterest, apathy, and deterioration in the quality of their work (18).

The poor test scores have also been used as an excuse to cut back on the number of teachers and their working conditions. Salaries remain the biggest chunk of education budgets, even though teachers have been underpaid. Primary school teachers in Latin America earn between $100 and $400 a month in countries where the minimum wage is between $80 and $120. In nearly all countries, teachers earn only about as much as unskilled workers. Neoliberal economists do not address this problem because fair wages for teachers would require permanent increases in school budgets. Instead, the Bank recommends paring down teachers' already measly salaries. In Costa Rica, for example, salaries have been cut back, and teacher training has deteriorated significantly (17, p. 41).

In Argentina, a national evaluation survey was carried out in 1994, five years after Carlos Menem took office and began to institute sweeping neoliberal reforms. Elementary-school students scored an average of 5.50 out of 10. The publication of these results in the media provoked a national scandal. Menem denied that his education policies were to blame. Instead he pointed the finger at teachers. Taking advantage of the uproar, he curried public support for more "flexibility" in teachers' contracts—which has translated into fewer posts, less job security, and deteriorating salaries and working conditions (19).

The large teachers' unions have also come under attack. These unions have been fundamental players in the struggle to maintain unity in public education systems. For example, the National Education Workers Union (SNTE) in Mexico, despite its links to the ruling Institutional Revolutionary Party (PRI), has been an important bulwark for defending the Mexican education system. Teachers' unions have also played a broader political role in many Latin American countries. The National Association of Salvadoran Educators (ANDES) was one of the sources of activists for the Farabundo Marti National Liberation Front (FMLN). The

Confederation of Educational Workers of the Argentine Republic (CTERA) leads the unions opposed to the Menem government. And the teachers' union in Brazil is one of the main unions affiliated with the Workers' Party (PT).

The type of decentralization that has been carried out under the tutelage of the World Bank has dispersed teachers' demands, eliminated collective bargaining agreements, and de-linked union activism and politics. Teachers' unions have always worked in defense of democratic educational principles and national public education systems. Today, they have moved to the forefront of opposition to the education reforms tailored by the World Bank because they believe the very survival of the teaching profession and the public education system is at stake.

Note — This chapter is adapted from an article published in *NACLA: Report on the Americas* XXIX(6), May/June 1996.

REFERENCES

1. Roffo, A. La escuela prepara para el trabajo? Entrevista a Silvia Montoya. *Clarín,* Buenos Aires, January 28, 1996.
2. World Bank. *El financiamiento de la educación en los países en desarrollo.* Washington, D.C., 1986.
3. World Bank. *Priorities and Strategies for Education: A World Bank Review.* Washington, D.C., 1995.
4. Coraggio, J. L. Economía y Educación en América Latina. Grupo de Trabajo de Economía y Educación de CEPAL, Chile, 1992.
5. Ley de participación comunal en la Gestión y Administración Educativas; Ley de Financiamiento Educativo; Ley de Mejoramiento de la Calidad y Ampliación de la Cobertura de la Educación Peruana. *El Peruano,* Lima, December 27, 1992, pp. 111471–111486.
6. National Association of Educators of Nicaragua (ANDEN). Privatización y defensa del servicio público de la educación en América Latina. First Latin American Conference on Education in Managua, Managua, Nicaragua, October 1992.
7. CEPAL-UNESCO. *Educación y Conocimiento: Eje de la Transformación Productiva con Equidad,* pp. 26–27. Centro Nacional de Información Educativa, Santiago de Chile, 1992.
8. Statistics from Pedagogical Alternatives and Educational Prospects in Latin America (APPEAL) of the Faculty of Philosophy and Arts, University of Buenos Aires, Argentina, 1996.
9. Kugler, B. *Argentina: Reallocating Resources for the Improvement of Education: A World Bank Study.* The International Bank for Reconstruction and Development, Washington, D.C., 1989.
10. Castro Silva, E. Riesgos y promesas del currículum de colaboración en contextos de descentralización administrativa. In *Revista Iberoamericana de Educación,* No. 3, pp. 63–89. Spain, September–December 1993.
11. Díaz Barriga, A. *Empleadores de Universitarios: un estudio de sus opiniones.* Centro de Estudios sobre la Universidad, Universidad Autónoma de México, Mexico, 1995.
12. CEPAL. *Anuario Estadístico de América Latina y el Caribe.* Santiago de Chile, 1993.
13. Instituto Nacional de Estadísticas y Censos (INDEC). *Encuesta permanente de hogares.* Buenos Aires, 1993.

14. Casi el 18% de los estudiantes secundarios repitieron el año. *Clarín,* Buenos Aires, February 24, 1996.
15. Torrado, S. *Estructura social en la Argentina (1945–1983).* Ediciones de la Flor, Buenos Aires, 1992.
16. Gallart, A. *The Diversification of the Education Field.* International Institute for Educational Planning, Paris, 1993.
17. Carnoy, M., and Torres, C. A. *Educational Change and Structural Adjustment: A Case Study of Costa Rica.* UNESCO, Bureau for Coordination of Operational Activities, Paris, 1992.
18. Díaz Barriga, A. (coordinator). *Los académicos ante los programas de Merit Pay, estudio sobre los estímulos en la UNAM y en la carrera magisterial, Informe Preliminar.* Centro de Estudios sobre la Universidad, UNAM, Mexico, 1995.
19. Puiggrós, A. *Volver a Educar: el desafío de la enseñanza argentina a finales del siglo XX.* Ariel, Buenos Aires, 1995.

CHAPTER 7

MARKET COMMODITIES AND POOR RELIEF: THE WORLD BANK PROPOSAL FOR HEALTH

Asa Cristina Laurell and Oliva López Arellano

During recent years, the health policy debate has been spurred by the negative impact of the crisis and of structural adjustment on health institutions. The *1993 World Development Report: Investing in Health* (1) published by the World Bank is central to this debate because it outlines an agenda for a new health policy designed especially for low- to middle-income and formerly socialist countries. This document is of particular importance for Latin America because it provides a blueprint for health reforms now in progress or soon to be launched in countries throughout the region. Thus, *Investing in Health* represents a systematic explanation and justification of the World Bank's existing programs as well as its future agenda.

This World Bank Report is therefore much more than simply one more document prepared by a national or international agency; it represents the programmatic proposal of an institution that has become a major policymaker through its imposition of structural adjustment programs (SAPs) during the last decade. Formerly, the World Bank was concerned primarily with economic policy, but with its *1990 Report on Poverty* (2), it began to intervene in the formulation of social policy.

The World Bank's powerful influence over national policy is largely due to the fact that neoliberal governments fundamentally agree with its basic theses. However, the Bank also has important financial instruments at its disposal, which it can use to impose its health policies on a country when necessary. In this sense, the Report states that loans and aid should be conditional on government compliance with reforms proposed by the Bank (1, p. 173). The significance of this requirement becomes obvious when one considers the quantity of financial resources managed by the Bank. In 1992, it provided $1.151 billion (U.S. dollars) in loans to health programs (1, p. 174), and it has recently begun to administer a growing proportion of bilateral aid.

In *Investing in Health*, the World Bank considers health to be linked to development, and it recognizes the dual nature of health: as an end in itself and as a means to foster development. However, throughout the text, health as a goal is progressively subordinated to health as a means (1, p. 18), and health service financing and provision are increasingly considered as relevant economic activities (1, p. 53). The idea that permeates the Bank's recommendations is that investment in health can be justified for strictly pragmatic economic reasons.

Thus the World Bank proposal is based on two primary strategies: the introduction of market forces into the health care sector, and the allocation of public resources according to criteria of technical and instrumental efficiency (1, pp. 14–17). The purpose of governmental intervention in health care should be to promote diversity and competition by facilitating private sector involvement. Public investment should be restricted to low-cost actions, targeting the poor, that render a high score in terms of disability-adjusted life years (1, p. 7).

OBJECTIVES AND PREMISES

The health policy proposed in *Investing in Health* has several basic objectives. One is to bring health policy into line with the neoliberal canon that ascribes health mainly to the private domain, accepting it as a public responsibility only under certain circumstances. Another is to adapt health policy to the priorities of fiscal adjustment, which requires reducing and restructuring public social spending, including spending on health. These two objectives guided the first World Bank proposal for health policy in *Financing Health Services in Developing Countries: An Agenda for Reform* (3). That publication provoked serious objections (4) because of its neoliberal orthodoxy and its indifference to the social deterioration and political conflicts that have accompanied structural adjustment processes.

Although *Investing in Health* is founded on the same basic conceptions, in this case the World Bank has clearly adopted a second set of objectives. The most outstanding of these are to develop consensus around its proposal, to tone down some of the most criticized aspects of the former document, and to include in its proposal policies devised to soften the political and social costs of the SAPs. In terms of the Bank's search to build consensus, it is worth noting that the 1993 Report is subscribed to by major international organizations and aid agencies (1, p. iv). The same concern about building consensus can be found in the attention given to two increasingly important social actors: women's organizations and nongovernmental organizations (NGOs).

On the other hand, there is a continued effort to develop the social discourse centered on the "war on poverty," initiated in the World Bank's 1990 Report (2). This objective conforms to the adoption of the UNICEF-generated slogan "Adjustment with a Human Face" (5) as well as the recommendations by the 39th

World Health Assembly in 1986 that SAPs should take health and nutrition into consideration (6).

However, a simple discourse is hardly sufficient to neutralize the social devastation and political conflicts caused by the neoliberal model, problems that are threatening to make it inviable. The basic contradiction of the modern state—namely, the need to actively promote the expansion of capital while regulating class conflict (7)—has restricted the Bank. This concern has apparently led the World Bank to modify its radical anti-statism and propose a model of state intervention that neither nullifies the neoliberal project nor destroys the legitimacy of the state.

In terms of health, this intervention is based on two complementary strategies (1, pp. 53–73). One is to promote the transfer of potentially lucrative health service provision and financing to the private sector; the other is to concentrate direct state action on selective low-cost programs that simplify service provision and redefine target populations to include only those living in critical poverty. This policy recreates a modern version of 19th century charity (8): the state intervenes in response to popular demands but the benefits provided are regarded as concessions rather than rights (9). This policy is consistent with the basic premise of neoliberalism that social welfare is the responsibility of the private domain and governments should only intervene when the private sector will not or cannot respond (10).

A second premise of the World Bank proposal is that the public sector is inefficient and frequently inequitable (due to the varying degrees of power wielded by different groups seeking to pressure the government), while the private sector is efficient and more equitable since it must necessarily comply with the market dynamics of free choice and competition. The third premise, presented as a realistic and pragmatic insight, is that public health resources are scarce and will continue to be so. The veracity of these premises, which are central to the World Bank proposal, is not proven anywhere within the document, and therefore they are essentially ideological judgments.

Based on these premises, the document recommends a new distribution of health care responsibilities between the public and the private spheres. This proposal defines four grounds for legitimate government intervention in health (1, pp. 55–60): (*a*) the provision of narrowly defined "public goods"; (*b*) certain activities directed toward the individual but implying large externalities, that is, activities whose collective benefits would extend beyond the person attended; (*c*) regulation and information to compensate for market failures; and (*d*) certain cost-effective health services as a means of poverty alleviation. These responsibilities correspond exactly with what would be considered justified according to the neoliberal model, since they represent tasks that the private sector cannot or does not wish to fulfill (11). Thus the definition of a "public good" is based on the criteria of nonrivalry (its consumption by one individual does not impede its consumption by another) and of nonexclusion (nonpaying consumers cannot be excluded). This narrow definition limits possible measures to those involving vector and pollution control, the provision of certain information, and so forth. The rationale for government intervention, then, is the private sector's lack of interest in providing these goods and services since they generally cannot become market commodities.

We should stress that this conception of "public" is one that has been depleted of all historical, valuative, and ethical significance; it disregards the fact that in the real world the public character of a good or an action is determined by the society's considering it valuable and/or a social priority and thus deciding to take it on and finance it collectively (12). For this reason, a majority of Latin American societies recognize health care for their members as a public concern and thus have established health care as a social right.

According to the World Bank agenda, government intervention measures involving large externalities, such as immunizations or the treatment of highly contagious diseases, are justified because they approximate "public goods." In the Bank's view, regulation and information are justifiable if they do not limit market freedom and if they are aimed at compensating some of the market's well-known failures.

Investment in health care for the poor through cost-effective actions is justified because it increases their human capital and productivity and does not provoke political resistance by powerful economic groups (1, p. 56). It is thus seen to be an economically efficient and socially acceptable strategy to reduce poverty and alleviate its consequences. However, measures should be taken to ensure that subsidized health services are offered only to those who are too poor to buy them in the market and therefore are not of interest to private providers (1, p. 56). These are the circumstances under which public resources should be dedicated to poverty relief.

THE NEO-CHARITY APPROACH TO ESSENTIAL HEALTH SERVICES

The practical outcome of this orthodox neoliberal logic is an agenda for health care reorganization that implies state withdrawal from the financing and provision of health services and a reorientation of public institutions toward selective assistance, in a scheme reminiscent of antiquated models of charity for the poor.

The proposal to lower costs and maximize impact through selective and limited forms of intervention is not new. One need only recall the drift from an integral concept of primary health care (13) to a selective one (14) to the short-term, limited proposals exemplified by *GOBI-FFF* (15–17). The World Bank carries this approach to its logical extreme by proposing that public resources be totally redirected toward low-cost interventions that could dramatically reduce the burden of disease (1, p. 8).

The technical basis for the Bank's proposal is the evaluation of health conditions in terms of the *Global Burden of Disease* (GBD) measured in *Disability-Adjusted Life Years* (DALY) (1, pp. 26–27). The GBD concept allows for a more integral evaluation of damage to health since it considers both disability and premature death. Furthermore, since its measurements are in terms of time, this indicator provides a common unit with which to calculate the impact of different forms of intervention on the GBD, as well as their cost (1, pp. 219–231).

However, in its present form this method suffers from some very serious conceptual and technical shortcomings, which shed doubts on whether it could serve as an adequate tool for decision-making. Furthermore, this linear, technical method for defining health needs and choosing forms of intervention disregards the political, ethical, cultural, and symbolic aspects of health care and reduces issues of collective health and death to simple problems of social engineering. The technocratic application of GBD and DALY is used to select public health and clinical interventions as part of an essential health package, since it provides a basis for defining low-cost (under $100), short-term actions with high DALY dividends (1, pp. 228–229).

The basic forms of public health care intervention recommended by the World Bank are limited to five clusters. The first involves an expanded program of immunization against measles, poliomyelitis, tuberculosis, diphtheria, tetanus, whooping cough, yellow fever, and hepatitis B. A second form of intervention involves the use of low-cost drugs to combat intestinal worms, to be distributed through the schools by nonmedical personnel (1, p. 76). Third is the tobacco and alcohol program, based on promoting healthy behavior through information provision and health education complemented by legal and fiscal measures to regulate consumption and marketing (1, pp. 89–91). Fourth is an AIDS-prevention educational program targeting high-risk groups; this also includes the regulation and control of sources of blood transmission as well as community treatment of the sick through low-cost protocols (1, pp. 106–107).

In addition to these four programs, the World Bank suggests a series of further public health intervention measures considered legitimate areas for government action, which could also serve to reduce the GBD at a reasonable cost. One is directed toward reducing malnutrition resulting from insufficient consumption of calories, proteins, and micronutrients (vitamin A, iodine, and iron) (1, p. 80). The actions recommended are nutritional education and micronutrient supplementation. The Report warns against any government intervention in the food market except in cases of outright famine, arguing that such forms of intervention are destructive because they obstruct market forces (1, pp. 83–84).

Among actions designed to promote a healthy environment, there is a special emphasis on the situation of families living in crowded and polluted dwellings without basic utilities and services. However, the World Bank insists that the government's role is to strengthen private initiative. According to the Bank, the government should establish and enforce environmental norms and define a legal framework that would facilitate a flexible and efficient system for private sector provision of the basic services (potable water and sanitation) needed by the population and for which people are willing to pay. Within this logic, governments should not provide or subsidize these services since they are privately appropriated and do not truly represent public goods (1, pp. 93–95). In contrast, government intervention is considered justified in the case of sewage treatment and pollution and vector control, since families do not sufficiently value these services and are less willing to pay for them. Furthermore, such forms of intervention are considered public goods since they benefit the entire community (1, pp. 95–96).

Finally, the Report recommends that public resources be assigned to certain public health programs that are closely linked to clinical services. One such program is community-based family planning programs targeting poor urban and rural women, particularly young, low-income women (1, pp. 86–89). This program would be justified because family planning is considered a low-cost measure that is highly effective in avoiding many of the risks associated with pregnancy, as well as one of the most efficient measures for improving child and maternal health. Another useful procedure for diminishing the GBD at a reasonable cost involves systematic screening and referral for common diseases (such as breast and cervicouterine cancer) that can be cured through early, low-cost treatment (1, pp. 76–77).

In the World Bank proposal, the particular package of essential, highly effective, low-cost clinical services to be provided by public institutions would vary from country to country according to health needs and income levels. However, it recommends a minimum of six groups of intervention measures. One involves prenatal care and delivery. An 80 percent coverage of these services throughout the world would reduce by about 40 percent the disease burden provoked by dangerous deliveries, at a cost of $4 to $9 per capita (1, p. 116). A second group, which overlaps with the public health package, is community-based family planning targeting rural areas and women and children from poor families, to be financed with public resources (1, pp. 84–89). The third program involves the short-term outpatient treatment of tuberculosis, this disease being the main cause of disability and death among the world's adult population (1, p. 119). The fourth program would combat common sexually transmitted diseases, whose most serious consequences are suffered mainly by women (1, p. 118). The fifth group of intervention measures involves community-based programs to treat widespread serious diseases affecting children (diarrhea, acute respiratory disease, measles, malaria, and severe malnutrition) (1, p. 117).

Finally, certain limited measures to provide care for adults are proposed, including pain control, the treatment of infections and minor traumas, and advice on how to reduce the incidence of chronic diseases. If additional resources are available, low-cost treatments for common chronic diseases could be included, such as aspirin for coronary disease, drugs for hypertension and certain types of psychosis, cataract removal, and low-cost rehabilitation (1, p. 10).

A public expenditure of $22 per person in middle-income countries would provide the package of these highly efficient, low-cost, essential services, if resources were redistributed in favor of primary care and regressive subsidies were eliminated. This would imply a drastic redefinition of the public-private mix, recovering for the market everything for which the population is willing to pay (1, pp. 95–112). In Latin America, this new "mix" would signify the liberation of about $83 per person, or a total of $35 billion for capture by the private sector, since at present the per person expenditure is $105 (1, p. 53).

A basic problem with the essential package proposal is one of ethics, since health is no longer considered a basic human need, and health care is considered a private good rather than an inalienable right. Thus the state abdicates its former obligation to guarantee the right of all citizens to health care and limits its public activities to those targeting the poor. This results in two polarized but complementary strategies: selective relief, a modern version of the poor law, in which one part of the population receives care because it is destitute; and selective privatization, in which another part of the population has access to care as "clients," according to their purchasing power (8). As a result, both groups actually lose their social citizenship, services are fragmented, and the provision of integral health care is impeded.

The crude technical approach used to select population groups and intervention measures neglects the ethical and political aspects of health care and gives technocrats the last say over issues of life and death. The economic rationale behind using cost-effectiveness calculations to select the contents of the essential health package for optimal use of resources might seem impeccable. However, in addition to technical difficulties, it also evades basic ethical issues (18).

The selective approach of the World Bank not only restricts public action to the poor, but it insists on a further targeting within the population thus labeled. Training and information programs for poor women (1, p. 43), programs to promote schooling for poor girls (1, p. 49), and the treatment of common serious diseases in poor children (1, p. 117) all illustrate the logic of this double targeting.

The reduction of state responsibilities to a minimal cluster of cost-effective interventions fragments public action and makes it possible to use special funds to structure vertical and limited interventions outside the realm of public institutions (19). Given the increasing power of supranational institutions such as the World Bank and medical corporations, such institutional by-passing serves to rapidly undermine public institutions (20). Under these conditions, limited short-term forms of intervention are extremely vulnerable to adverse circumstances and thus are easily dismantled. Their immediate relative success contrasts with their instability, particularly in a period when public health care is being fragmented and deinstitutionalized. On the other hand, these restricted forms of intervention reduce the possibility of developing integral action at different levels of the health care system and thereby favoring synergy between them (21).

False dilemmas, such as selectivity versus universality or effectiveness versus equity, should be recognized as such, and the complementary functions of different kinds of actions should be emphasized. A universal and integral health care system may, under certain circumstances, target some forms of intervention and select specific groups in order to ensure both equity and efficiency. The best way to ensure the long-term sustainability of targeted actions is by maintaining a strong public institution capable of developing a global policy of integral health care. Only under such conditions can targeted programs complement global structural change and obey a rationale of compensation for the disadvantaged instead of poverty relief for those excluded from the market.

HEALTH AS A PRIVATE RESPONSIBILITY

In line with its assertion that health is a private matter and health care a private good (3), the World Bank proposal focuses primarily on the private realm. However, in doing so it mingles three actors of a very different nature: the individual and the family, nonprofit organizations, and entities operating in the market in pursuit of profit.

True to its individualistic creed, the World Bank maintains that "what individuals do with their own lives and those of their children is much more important than anything that governments could do" (1, p. 38). In saying this, it overlooks all economic and social determinants of the realities within which individuals live and act. The person and the family, then, should bear the main responsibility for health and should adopt healthy behavior and resolve their health problems by purchasing necessary medical services in the market. The Report stresses the importance of women as caretakers and health promoters within the family, and several of its proposals are addressed to them (1, pp. 38–52). The essential purpose of these proposals is to strengthen the ability of the family, especially among the poor, to replace the former role of public health institutions, thereby facilitating cutbacks in spending and services. Contrary to the World Bank's claims (1, p. 162), this approach does not imply greater rights for women but rather greater obligations (22).

Private nonprofit organizations are also assigned a role in relation to the needs of those who are too poor to resolve their health needs in the market. There is a special focus on NGOs, and it is suggested that they should get public financial support to perform some tasks formerly handled by the government. The supposed justification for this proposal is that NGOs are generally considered to be more efficient than public institutions. However, there is an unmistakable spirit of privatization and institutional by-passing behind this proposal.

Although the Report dedicates considerable space to the role of individuals and nonprofit organizations, its main concern is with expanding the health market. The division of clinical services into "essential" and "discretionary" is crucial to this quest, since the latter, according to the World Bank, are private goods that should be provided as commodities in the market (1, pp. 60–73). The Bank recognizes that this would require the creation of financial instruments to ensure consumer purchasing power, that is, an effective demand and a stable market (1, pp. 111–129). This acknowledgment allows the Bank to introduce the insurance companies, together with private medical care providers, as prominent agents in the health field. The Report discusses at length various forms of articulating private financing and service provision to facilitate private sector involvement and to promote diversity and competition.

The three arguments used to justify the shifting of financial and/or clinical service provision from the public to the private sector are (*a*) the poverty of the state, (*b*) the inefficiency of the public sector, and (*c*) inequity in access to services. The first argument considers the present and future scarcity of governmental health resources as a natural and immutable fact. No mention is made that this assertion assumes that orthodox adjustment policies will be maintained. Consequently, no analysis is made of how public funds are distributed within government budgets or of how they have been restructured because of adjustment policies.

Such an analysis would reveal at least two important facts. First, public financial resources have been rechanneled in order to pay debt service at the expense of social spending (23), in a process that represents one of the most dramatic transferals of public resources from the "poor" to the "rich" in the last 50 years (24). Second, a majority of middle-income countries dedicate a relatively small percentage of their gross national product to public social spending, while a significant proportion of those resources classified as public spending actually correspond to social security funds paid by workers and employers, not to tax monies, meaning that fiscal social spending is even lower than reported (25).

The second argument in favor of the privatization of clinical care—the inefficiency of the public sector—represents a supposition that has yet to be proven[1] and one posed totally out of context. Nowhere does the Report mention that the rapid deterioration of public institutions is directly related to adjustment policies that have provoked both the severe underfunding of their services and the implementation of a conservative form of "modernization" (21).

Similarly, the argument concerning the inequity of public services is also posed without regard for context. For instance, it is claimed that those covered by social insurance are taking advantage of state subsidies at the expense of the poor. Such an assertion omits two crucial facts. First, the large majority of those covered by

[1] The Report states: "Those inefficiencies have been so clearly criticized and during such a long period that they evidently can only be overcome through . . . radical reforms" (1, p. 67).

social insurance are themselves poor or impoverished workers,[2] and second, the universalization of social insurance coverage would resolve this alleged injustice. Furthermore, no analysis is made of the inefficiency and inequity of the private sector in comparison with the public sector. The well-known and extensively documented chronic crisis of health care cost and coverage afflicting the United States (26), the country considered the most notable example of private health care, speaks eloquently of the inefficiency and inequity to be found within the private sector.

The inconsistent reasoning in favor of privatizing "discretionary" clinical services can only be understood by taking into account the World Bank's conception of clinical services. They are considered a private good because they are appropriated in variable amounts and are consumed by individuals. Thus, the argument goes, it is unjust for health care to be financed by public funds; instead, each person should pay for the services he or she consumes. This requires that a price be determined for these services, that is, that they be turned into market commodities.

The flaw in this argument is that the private, individual consumption of a good or a service does not prevent it from being considered a public good to be granted by society to all its members. Moreover, citizens' rights, themselves a founding principle of modern society, pertain to the public realm, even when they are exercised or enjoyed individually, because they represent shared ethical or social values and democratically established social priorities (27).

Furthermore, it could be argued that health is an absolute human need since it is directly related to the preservation of life and the development of human capacities (28). All human beings should then have a right to the optimal satisfaction of this need, and this right can only be granted through public measures. This is especially so in societies suffering from profound inequalities, such as those of Latin America. If this argument is accepted, it is both cynical and false to consider most medical services "discretionary," the mere option or whim of an individual. Likewise, it would be wrong to equate them with any other commodity, when access to these services may mean the difference between life and death, or the difference between serious biological or mental harm and the development of human capacities.

The World Bank proposal also claims that the economic rationale of cost-effectiveness should determine the contents of the public health package and should guide the choices of individuals in the market. The Bank thus pretends to exorcise all the historical, cultural, symbolic, and emotional significance to be found in issues related to health, life, and death. Such meanings are to be found even in the most highly commodified societies. They are extensively documented

[2] For instance, 80 percent of the insured in Mexico earn three times the minimum wage ($250 per month) or less, which is approximately equivalent to the cost of a basic food basket for a family of five.

in the scientific literature and serve as a central theme of all arts. The appeal to *Homo economicus* in the marketplace presages the failure of the World Bank to legitimize its health policy since it violates basic and widely held humanitarian values.

At this point, someone who has read *Investing in Health* might object that the present critique is not providing a fair treatment of the document's content. This is partly true because the Report is a pragmatic document aimed at achieving the consensus of a large number of agencies and organizations. Therefore, most positions that have been expressed within the health debate over the last decade are reflected in this document, and most of its participants could identify with one part or another of the document. This has meant that the Report simultaneously develops a variety of discourses and arguments, which frequently enter into contradiction. However, the conception that provides overall coherence to the proposal and which can be deduced from the agenda for action is unmistakably neoliberal in nature.

As mentioned earlier, one of the main proposals of the World Bank is to promote diversity and competition in the health market. This implies specific state intervention measures to encourage private service provision and financing. A series of contradictions arise as the proposal attempts to reconcile public spending restrictions with the promotion of private sector participation, given that the former precludes the use of subsidies. Although the document makes a stand against subsidies, it nevertheless recommends measures that, in practice, have led to indirect or hidden private sector subsidies. This is the case both with the Bank's recommendation of compulsory health insurance allowing for a choice between private and public systems, as well as its recommendation that public services be contracted out to private companies (29).

Another major World Bank proposal is that discretionary services should be paid for through a fee-for-service system. However, it is also recognized that fees constitute an obstacle to access and that flexible payment schemes in public institutions are also necessary (1, p. 160).

Given the high cost of clinical services in the market, the World Bank recommends the establishment of public and private health insurance schemes. It describes the possible forms of abuse that can arise in relation to private insurance, such as "skimming" or adverse selection, and the "moral hazards" of providers and clients (1, pp. 56–57). However, such negative and extensive practices do not discourage the Bank from endorsing state promotion of private insurance (1, p. 112).

So strong is the Bank's conviction of the blessings of the market (or so firm its decision to transfer health care funds to private financial groups) that it proposes a number of measures to regulate, reduce, or compensate abuse, but scarcely explores possible means for achieving public financing. Amazingly, all these measures have been taken from the U.S. experience, where none has yet proven successful (30). Nor does the evidence presented in the Report demonstrate the superiority of the private insurance systems that it endorses.

Let us give a few examples. Although it is claimed that universality has failed (1, p. 65), the universal social security systems of Costa Rica and Korea are recognized for their high level of equality and their ability to channel resources to the poor (1, p. 71). Inversely, although the Chilean health reform is proposed as a model because of its radical privatization, the Report recognizes that it has led to serious adverse selection and the impoverishment of the public social security system (1, p. 167). In an evaluation of cost and satisfaction in ten OECD countries, the predominantly private health system of the United States was found to have the poorest showing because of its high costs and low satisfaction (1, p. 72). The Report even states that while theoretically it should be possible to eliminate both inequities in access and "skimming" from a private system, in reality only those health systems financed through public or para-public collective funds have actually provided universal and equal access to health services (1, pp. 123–125).

As mentioned earlier, the central proposal for medical care provision involves stimulating diversity and competition between providers in order to improve quality and efficiency (1, p. 7). Nevertheless, the Report later acknowledges that the ability of competition to enhance quality and efficiency has not been clearly proven (1, p. 135). In addition, the Report admits that the objective and subjective conditions that would allow the "client" to make a rational choice between providers and therapies frequently do not exist, and this constitutes an unfortunate market failure.

Although it is widely accepted that the profit motive explains, to a great degree, health care inefficiency and the application of inadequate diagnostic and therapeutic methods, the Bank insists on encouraging private providers to take charge of discretionary services. Thus it does not seek ways to strengthen and improve existing public institutions, but rather claims that quality and efficiency can only be achieved through such means as regulation, adequate forms of payment (such as capitation) that do not induce utilization of expensive services, and provision of information to "clients" (1, p. 136).

The table that synthesizes the policies proposed to improve health care and their impact on distributive and technical efficiency and on accessibility for the poor (1, p. 130), provides revealing insights on the Report's internal contradictions. According to this table, public policies have the greatest impact while private sector policies hardly affect the three parameters considered to be relevant.

THE PRIVATIZATION GAMBLE

The decision to apply the basic proposals presented in *Investing in Health* would mean, in most Latin American countries, submitting a country's health care system to large-scale experimentation on very uncertain grounds. This is because there is no convincing evidence, as the Report itself shows, that the policies recommended will resolve the problems described. One could, of course, argue that governments are free to adopt these policies or not. However, the Bank's ability to exert coercion over underdeveloped countries in acute need of foreign exchange by making loans and other international aid conditional upon the application of its policies should not be underestimated.

Public institutions are most liable to suffer from the World Bank experiment, since far from being strengthened, they would be partially dismantled, programs would be eliminated, and dissociation between levels of care would result. In this context it should be stressed that, in spite of their rapid deterioration during the last decade, public systems continue to represent the only health care alternative available to the majority of Latin Americans. If their services are replaced with noninstitutional ones, such as those provided by NGOs or the private sector, secure and permanent access to health care will inevitably be diminished.

The World Bank's proposals represent an attempt to induce economic and social engineering, with questionable mid- and long-term sustainability, in countries having few resources with which to rebuild their dismantled public institutions if the experiment goes wrong. This implies a great responsibility, since the World Bank is triggering irreversible processes that will affect the very population that it claims to favor—the poor.

Furthermore, the social consequences of health policy reform are not contemplated, nor are the problems of legitimacy that will emerge when "discretionary" services are excluded from the care provided and granted by public institutions. The World Bank proposal also puts serious ethical questions on the agenda. For instance, it might seem rational to use proposed cost-efficiency calculations to determine which services should be included in (and excluded from) the public health package. However, what is really at stake is the determination of whose health is profitable for investment and, eventually, the power of decision over who should live and who should die.

Most modern societies resolve ethical and value questions relative to all their members through democratic means: through confrontation and subsequent agreements, social priorities are determined and recognized as rights with their corresponding obligations. The guarantee of the fulfillment of those rights is usually deposited in the state, which implements enforcement through public rules and institutions.

It is noteworthy that the Report disregards the use of democratic procedure for the resolution of ethical dilemmas, because of another argument put forth by neoliberal theorists (11). This argument asserts that the capacity of some groups, such as urban sectors and trade unions, to pursue their interests by exerting pressure on the government has perverted state activity (1, p. 130), and it is therefore illusory to believe that governments and parliaments can make fair decisions about health care. Hence, the problem is divided into two parts. On the one hand, decisions on the use of discretionary clinical services should be transferred to individuals in the market (31); on the other, government decisions on the essential health package for the poor are made "objective" through the application of cost-effectiveness calculations.

Such proposals not only serve as a way of justifying cutbacks in public health budgets in order to comply with fiscal adjustment, they also covertly seek to destroy the very concept or idea of social rights, a critical condition for the privatization and commodification of health financing and provision. Strictly speaking, it is meaningless to recognize social rights unless the corresponding social and public obligations are simultaneously specified (32). It is absurd to acknowledge the right to health while defining health care as a private good and dividing the population into two categories: the "poor," who are eligible for essential health services, and the "clients," who are consumers of discretionary services in the market. The abolition of the right to health and of egalitarian means of access is thus a necessary condition for the World Bank's proposed health reform. This is so because shifting the profitable aspects of health financing and provision to the private sector requires mechanisms of exclusion/inclusion. These are incompatible with the concept of the *right to health*, which, by definition, is universal.

Although the World Bank proposal can be interpreted as a neoliberal ideological campaign, it is not restricted to the terrain of ideas but is firmly rooted in the material world of economic interests. It seeks to legitimize the conversion of health finance and health care into private economic activities, thus recovering them as territory for direct capital accumulation. The hidden agenda behind the "agenda for action" is the attempt to invest in health for profit in the strictest meaning of the word.

This forms part of the drive to recommodify social services that underlies the attack on the welfare state all over the world (33, 34). These services, particularly those related to health care, currently represent very important economic activities. The other side of the argument that health care is too expensive to be paid for by the state, an assertion repeated throughout the Report, is that an activity involving so much money should not be controlled by the public sector but should be managed by the private sector for profit. As was mentioned earlier, in Latin America, the implementation of the World Bank proposal would liberate $38 billion for the private sector.

This means that the privatization of health care will only be pursued to the extent that it can become a realm for capital accumulation (35). One could argue that this is not the case in underdeveloped countries and therefore does not form part of the World Bank's hidden agenda. However, empirical evidence shows that the erosion of public institutions has spurred the growth of both medical corporations and private insurance companies in middle-income countries (36, 37). The specific characteristic of privatization in those countries is that it must be selective in order to be profitable, which explains the proposal to assign an essential health package to the public sector and reserve discretionary commodified services for the private sector.

An equally important condition is that an effective demand be generated for discretionary services. This requires restructuring health care funds so as to grant payments to private providers, a problem that is addressed extensively in *Investing in Health* as an argument in favor of promoting health insurance. The third condition for successful selective privatization is to establish criteria and mechanisms that would serve to separate the profitable from the unprofitable.

Health funds are the central issue in the current process of privatization. This is true not only because they are a condition for the expansion of private care but because they represent huge financial resources. The administration and control of these funds is more important even than the provision of services. This explains the increasing inroad of financial capital—the insurance companies—into the health sector, a tendency that is developing worldwide and is distinctively characteristic of the new wave of privatizations (38).

In this respect, the World Bank reform recommended for middle-income countries is that they increase health insurance coverage and give the consumer a choice between public and private insurance (1, p. 164). In practical terms, this means a shift from collective solidarity insurance to individual compulsory insurance which, in Latin America, corresponds to the Chilean model (39). The advantage of this model is that it resolves two of the crucial problems faced by privatization. On the one hand, it turns health insurance into a form of compulsory savings which ensures the collection of funds transferable to private sector administration. On the other, it furnishes a criterion, the amount paid in premiums, which can be used to segregate those who are profitable from those who are not. This scheme does not necessarily involve increasing the total amount of health funds available, but it does serve to redistribute funds from the public to the private sector. This means that funds are not distributed according to need, as in the case of collective funds, but rather according to individual premiums, thus separating out the higher payers for the private sector.

Although the rise of insurance capital is the major outstanding feature of the modern health industry, technological change in medical practice (40) has also played an important role in reshaping the landscape, by propelling the growth of hospital corporations. This means that the central economic dynamic of private medicine has shifted from the enrichment of physicians to capital accumulation by hospital corporations. In the context of structural adjustment, which in Latin America implies serious cutbacks in state health expenditure, private health funds are the necessary complement of hospital corporations since public funds are insufficient to cover the cost of private services. The promotion of private insurance is thus crucial to the consolidation of a private system of health provision and insurance parallel to the public system. Through this mechanism, the private system concentrates a major portion of health resources on covering the needs of a minority of the population, thus reducing the resources of the public system that is responsible for the majority. For instance, in Chile the private system covers 20 percent of the population and concentrates over 40 percent of all resources

(41). While the Bank certainly warns against adverse selection or "skimming," it is unable to prove that such can be avoided within the logic of the market, since the purpose of commercial firms is to maximize profit and not to satisfy social needs. An inevitable consequence of inducing the growth of private insurance and medical corporations is that they become powerful actors in the health field. Judging from the U.S. experience (42), we can expect that their capacity to influence health policy will greatly surpass that of any of the pressure groups that currently obsess the World Bank.

It is important to underline that major capital's inroads into the health sector do not necessarily imply the withdrawal of the state. To the contrary, this process requires two types of state intervention. On the one hand, the government must develop policies to promote and facilitate the expansion of the private sector; on the other, it must provide at least a minimal package of health services for a major portion of the population in order to conserve legitimacy.

According to the criteria set by the Bank in its Report, a health policy is satisfactory if it improves health conditions, user satisfaction, and equity while simultaneously reducing costs (1, p. 55). It is difficult to imagine how a policy that promotes selective privatization and neo-charity could satisfy any of these criteria from the perspective of common people. The exclusion of one part of the population from many discretionary services will not improve their health and certainly not their satisfaction with medical care. Nor is there any solid evidence to prove that the private financing and provision of services reduces costs, a fact that even the Bank recognizes on several occasions. And finally, far from improving equity, the polarization of the health sector between private affluence for a minority and public scarcity for a majority reveals a sharp increase in inequity, if equity in health care is defined as equal access to available care for equal need, equal utilization for equal need, and equal quality of care for all (6, p. 434). In its efforts to hide this fact, the Bank resorts to a very partial definition of equity, using it to refer only to the public domain, making it possible to overlook market-produced inequities. It is doubtful that this gimmick will convince people that the discriminatory and regressive policies defended and promoted by the World Bank are in their best interests, or that these policies will eventually accomplish equity, which is to say, justice.

REFERENCES

1. World Bank. *Informe sobre el Desarrollo Mundial 1993. Invertir en Salud.* Washington, D.C., 1993.
2. World Bank. *Informe sobre el Desarrollo Mundial 1990. La Pobreza.* Washington, D.C., 1990.
3. Akin, J. *Financing Health Services in Developing Countries: An Agenda for Reform.* World Bank, Washington, D.C., 1987.
4. Organización Panamericana de la Salud. *Economía de la Salud.* Washington, D.C., 1989.

5. Comia, G., Jolly, J., and Stewart, F. *Adjustment with a Human Face*. Clarendon Press, Oxford, 1987.
6. Whitehead, M. The concepts and principles of equity and health. *Int. J. Health Serv.* 22(3): 429–445, 1992.
7. Offe, C. *Contradicciones del Estado de Bienestar*. Alianza Editorial, Madrid, 1990.
8. López, O. La política de salud en México. ¿Un ejemplo de liberalismo social? In *Estado y Políticas Sociales en el Neoliberalismo*, edited by A. C. Laurell, pp. 165–183. Fundación Friedrich Ebert, Mexico, 1992.
9. Cohn, A., et al. *A Saúde como Direito e como Serviçio*. Cortez Editora, CEDEC, Sao Paulo, Brazil, 1991.
10. Laurell, A. C. *La Política Social en la Crisis: una alternativa para el sector salud*, pp. 9–15. Fundación Friedrich Ebert, Mexico, 1991.
11. George, V., and Wilding, P. *Ideology and Social Welfare*, pp. 19–43. Routledge and Kegan Paul, London, 1985.
12. Donahue, J. D. *La Decisión de Privatizar: Fines Públicos, Medios Privados*, pp. 31–60. Paidos, Buenos Aires, 1991.
13. Organización Mundial de la Salud. *Declaración de Alma Ata: Reporte de la Conferencia Internacional sobre Atención Primaria a la Salud*. Geneva, 1978.
14. Walsh, J., and Warren, K. Selective primary health care: An interim strategy for disease control in developing countries. *N. Engl. J. Med.* 301: 967–974, 1979.
15. Berman, P. Selective primary health care: Is efficient sufficient? *Soc. Sci. Med.* 16: 1054–1094, 1982.
16. Gish, O. Selective primary health care: Old wine in new bottles. *Soc. Sci. Med.* 16: 1054–1094, 1982.
17. Unger, P., and Killingsworth, J. Selective primary health care: A critical review of methods and results. *Soc. Sci. Med.* 22(10): 1001–1013, 1988.
18. Blanco, J., and Rivera, J. A. La Carga Global de Morbilidad: justificación para invertir en salud. In *Nuevas Tendencias y Alternativas en el Sector Salud*, edited by A. C. Laurell, pp. 111–128. Fundación Friedrich Ebert/UAM-X, Mexico, 1994.
19. Grodros, D., and Béthuna, X. Las intervenciones sanitarias selectivas: una trampa para la política de salud del tercer mundo. *Cuadernos Médico-Sociales* 60: 71–85, 1988.
20. Torres, C. Las políticas de salud de la región de las Américas para los 90. Paper presented at the XVIII International Congress of Latin American Studies Association, Atlanta, March 10–12, 1994.
21. Lopez, O., and Blanco, J. *La modernización neoliberal en salud. México en los ochenta*. Col. Ensayos, Universidad Autónoma Metropolitana-Xochimilco, Mexico, 1993.
22. Garduño, M. A., and Peña, F. Unidades familiares, mujeres y salud en el desarrollo. In *Nuevas tendencias y alternativas en el sector salud*, edited by A. C. Laurell, pp. 61–88. Fundación Friedrich Ebert/UAM-X, Mexico, 1994.
23. Zepeda, E. El gasto social en México, de la estabilización ortodoxa al liberalismo social. *Frontera Norte* 6(1): 171–196, 1994.
24. Laurell, A. C. Crisis, neoliberal health policy and political processes in Mexico. *Int. J. Health Serv.* 21(3): 457–470, 1991.
25. Laurell, A. C. Financing Health Services in Mexico. Paper presented at the International Conference on Health System Financing, Berlin, August 30–September 3, 1993.
26. Navarro, V. (ed.). *Why the United States Does Not Have a National Health Program*. Baywood, Amityville, N.Y., 1992.
27. Gurza, L. A. Contracrítica de lo público. Por una utopía al alcance de la mano. *Coyuntura* 37: 32–39, 1993.
28. Doyle, L., and Gough, I. *A Theory of Human Need*. MacMillan, London, 1991.

29. Requena, M. El financiamiento del sistema chileno de salud necesita ser reestructurado. *Salud y Cambio* 3(7): 12–19, 1992.
30. Bodenheimer, T. Should we abolish the private health insurance industry? *Int. J. Health Serv.* 20(2): 199, 1990.
31. Pierson, C. *Beyond the Welfare State?*, pp. 45–48. Polity Press, Cambridge, 1991.
32. Da Vita, A. O Lugar dos dereitos na moralidade política. *Lua Nova* 30: 5–34, 1993.
33. Navarro, V. The welfare state: Part of the problem or part of the solution? *Sistema*, Madrid, 1990.
34. Esping-Andersen, G. *The Three Worlds of Welfare Capitalism.* Polity Press, Cambridge, 1990.
35. Laurell, A. C. Privatización y la emergencia del capital financiero en salud. *Salud y Cambio* 4(13): 6–12, 1993.
36. Fleury, S. (ed.). *Estado y Políticas Sociales en América Latina.* FIOCRUZ-UAM, Mexico, 1992.
37. Price, M. The consequences of health services privatization for equality and equity and health care in South Africa. *Soc. Sci. Med.* 27(7): 703–716, 1988.
38. Himmelstein, D., and Woolhandler, S. The corporate compromise: A Marxist view of health policy. *Monthly Rev.*, May 1990, pp. 14–29.
39. Piñera, J. *El Cascabel al Gato. La Batalla por la Reforma Previsional en Chile.* Zig-Zag, Santiago, 1992.
40. Passos, N. R. El proceso de producción de los servicios de salud. *Educ. Med. Salud* 25: 15–27, 1991.
41. Tetelboin, C. Chile, políticas neoliberales y salud. In *Estado y Políticas Sociales en el Neoliberalismo*, edited by A. C. Laurell, pp. 145–164. Fundación Friedrich Ebert, Mexico, 1992.
42. Kemper, V., and Novak, V. What's blocking health care reform? *Int. J. Health Serv.* 23(1): 69–79, 1993.

CHAPTER 8

NEOLIBERALISM REVISED? A CRITICAL ACCOUNT OF WORLD BANK CONCEPTIONS OF GOOD GOVERNANCE AND MARKET FRIENDLY INTERVENTION

Ray Kiely

This chapter investigates recent attempts by the World Bank to revise its commitment to neoliberal ideas. The concepts of market friendly intervention and good governance are examined. Both concepts are rejected on the basis of their continued commitment to a flawed neoliberal paradigm, which wrongly sees states as inherently inefficient economic actors and reduces development to a simple process of technical policy-making. The chapter therefore also contends that the World Bank's optimism concerning the prospects for structural adjustment is misplaced, and some evidence is considered to back up this claim. Finally, I briefly suggest an alternative account, focusing on social structures within localities and the relationship between national economies and the global economy, which shows the continued relevance of state economic intervention for sustained capitalist development.

These issues are discussed in four sections. First, the "classical" neoliberal approach to development is briefly reviewed, along with the reasons why this view has been undermined. Second, the revised neoliberal view is outlined in some detail, and it is here that the ideas of market friendly intervention and good governance are introduced. The third section critically discusses these ideas, along with some consideration of their implications for adjustment policies. The fourth section briefly outlines the basis for an alternative approach to understanding the rise of the East Asian newly industrializing countries (NICs), and I then conclude by showing how this approach can be used to examine the prospects for late developers in the current global context.

NEOLIBERALISM AND DEVELOPMENT

The onset of the "debt crisis" in 1982 led to a serious challenge to "orthodox" development economics. Import-substituting nation-states faced a heavy debt-burden as the import of consumer goods replaced the import of capital goods, and state protection to domestic industry led to inefficiency and corruption. This scenario was in sharp contrast to the outward looking, export-oriented policies of the East Asian NICs. Although these too suffered from recession in the early 1980s, and South Korea was a large debtor nation in 1982, recovery was rapid and Korea continually managed to meet its interest repayments without the devastation that was witnessed in much of Africa, Latin America, and the Indian subcontinent.

It was in this context of unsuccessful import-substituting countries, and successful export-oriented countries, that the neoliberal "counter-revolution" (1) in development economics emerged. Neoliberals argued that the NICs were not "exceptions" to the rule of a North-South divide, but they in fact constituted a "model" for the rest of the developing world to follow. Success "was achieved not by economic tricks, but by sensible policies based on sound neo-classical principles" (2, p. 329).

Although some neoliberals pay lip service to the specificity of East Asian culture, other writers clearly regard the East Asian experience as something which can (or should) more or less be replicated by the rest of the world (3, pp. 100–108; 4). It is for this reason that the neoliberal counter-revolution can be described as a new version of modernization theory—the "western model" of Rostowian theory is replaced by the "East Asian model" of neoliberal theory.

Neoliberals argue that the success of the East Asian NICs can be attributed to three basic policies. These are:

1. limited government intervention in the economy;
2. a low level of price distortion in the economy;
3. an outward-oriented strategy of export promotion (5).

These principles formed the basis of structural adjustment and stabilization programs in the developing world in the 1980s and 1990s. Structural adjustment can be defined as a set of policies designed to promote economic growth through the opening up of economies to "competitive market forces." Stabilization policies, more closely associated with the International Monetary Fund (IMF), are designed to alleviate short-term balance of payments deficits. In practice the two are often hard to distinguish. Policies include the removal of obstacles such as state subsidies to industry, minimum wages, and price controls. Combined with a competitive exchange rate, prices are said to reflect the laws of supply and demand, and so investors and consumers can respond to the correct price signals, which in turn facilitates high levels of economic growth. The World Bank therefore places a premium on the close correlation between a low level of price distortion and rapid economic development (6, pp. 60–63). Policies of limited government intervention in the economy and an outward-oriented trade strategy are said to lead to a low level of price distortion, which thereby promotes efficiency. Prices should be set by the "natural" laws of supply and demand, unhindered by the distorting effects of government subsidies, minimum wages, or price controls. In a study of the performance of 31 developing economies in the 1970s (6), it was claimed that those with low rates of price distortion and an outward orientation to the world economy tended to perform far more effectively than medium- or high-distortion countries. The standard neoliberal conclusion was reached that "countries applying outward-oriented development strategies had a superior performance in terms of export, economic growth, and employment" (7, p. 16).

This version of the neoliberal perspective was undermined in two ways. First, the evidence that there was a strong correlation between low levels of price distortion and high economic growth was challenged. As the Bank's evidence itself makes clear, price distortions can only explain about one-third of the differences in growth rates between different countries (8, p. 193), while some of the classifications (such as free-market Chile having a high level of price distortion) are questionable. Perhaps most importantly, the evidence itself does not confirm the proposition that trade policy in itself is a major determinant of economic growth. The relationship between price distortion, outward orientation, and economic growth may be the result of a third factor, such as structural problems which slow down economic growth (8, p. 194). Thus, the strong inward orientation of many of the poorest economies in the world may be a *reflection*, rather than a *cause*, of slow rates of economic growth (9).

Second, East Asian industrialization processes had strongly interventionist states. A wide body of literature has convincingly challenged the crude neoliberal argument that East Asia is simply a model of development based on market forces, and has shown that in fact the state intervened heavily in all the NICs (10–12). After a period of import-substitution industrialization in the 1950s, South Korea moved to a policy of export promotion from 1961 onward. However, this policy did not mean that import substitution was abandoned as industries continued to be subsidized, and the state planned industrial output through institutions such as the Economic Planning Board and the Ministry of Trade and Industry. Moreover, banking was nationalized in 1961, and state control was thus used to target specific industries through access to credit. In the 1970s heavy industries such as iron and steel benefited from such preferential treatment. The most successful firms in terms of meeting export targets were also rewarded by the state by being granted access to restricted imports, and were allowed to recover losses made on the world market through sales in the lucrative protected domestic market. In Taiwan the state's control of credit led to a similar policy, while in Singapore and Hong Kong the state has played a key role in subsidizing food and public housing and (in the case of Singapore) in direct investment financed through the compulsory insurance scheme known as the Central Provident Fund (12–14).

THE REVISED NEOLIBERAL MODEL

The concern of this section is to examine a more subtle version of the neoliberal argument, based on the notion that interventions have been more market friendly in East Asia than elsewhere, and that this explains the success of the former and failure of the latter. This will be done through an examination of the notions of "market friendly intervention" and "good governance" (15–18).

Market Friendly Intervention

The basic contention of the World Bank's report *The East Asian Miracle* (18, p. 5) is that the East Asian miracle economies "achieved high growth by getting the basics right." This statement represents an important qualification to the older argument (6, pp. 60–63) that East Asian success was due to a low level of price distortion in the economy—in other words, high growth was a result of "getting prices right." The Bank accepts that intervention did occur in the East Asian economies—the 1993 Report lists a number of factors including targeting industries, subsidies, protecting domestic import substitutes, state banking, state-led research and development, and close consultation between the public and private sectors (18, pp. 5–6). However, the Report argues that these interventions meet the criteria of market friendly, as opposed to market distorting, intervention. In this development strategy, "the appropriate role of government is to ensure adequate investments in people, provide a competitive climate for private enterprise, keep the economy open to international trade, and maintain a stable macroeconomy" (18, p. 10). Market friendly intervention can take one of three forms (16, p. 5):

1. States intervene reluctantly, preferring to "let markets work."
2. States apply checks and balances, subjecting interventions "to the discipline of international and domestic markets."
3. States intervene openly, and are "subject to rules rather than to official discretion."

According to the World Bank, the interventions in East Asia conformed to these basic principles. The key to the high growth (and equitable development) can be found (18, p. 325):

> in fundamentally sound, market-oriented policies. Labor markets were allowed to work. Financial markets, although subject to more selective interventions to allocate credit, generally had low distortions and limited subsidies compared with other developing economies. Import substitution . . . was quickly accompanied by the promotion of exports and duty-free admission of imports for exporters. The result was limited differences between international relative prices and domestic relative prices. . . . Market forces and competitive pressures guided resources into activities that were consistent with comparative advantage and, in the case of labor-intensive exports, laid the foundation for learning international best practice and subsequent industrial upgrading.

Good Governance

The Bank has recognized that an excessive focus on economics is one-sided, and that there is also a need to emphasize the institutional context within which adjustment policies take place. Adjusting countries need to conform to the notion of "good governance" (15, 17). Although there has been some reluctance to provide a comprehensive definition of this concept, it appears to include an emphasis on political pluralism, accountability, and the rule of law (15, pp. 60–61, 192). The Bank has been cautious about arguing that these entail democratization, for fear of intervening in the political affairs of sovereign countries.

Most important, however, is that the Bank sees good governance as a means to an end; it is "synonymous with sound development management" (17, p. 1). Such management requires "not just less government but better government—government that concentrates its efforts less on direct interventions and more on enabling others to be productive" (15, p. 5). This argument, taken from the Bank's first work on the concept of good governance, repeats the classical neoliberal argument that state spending is unproductive and that it crowds out the wealth-creating activity of rational, individual entrepreneurs. The role of the state is to enable the private sector to lead economic activity—state activity, in other words, should be market friendly. As Schmitz argues (19, p. 69):

> The key thing to ask of developing countries was *not* whether they were democracies or autocracies . . . but whether they had the governing will and wherewithal to create the 'appropriate policy framework' required to achieve efficient markets and the successful implementation of donor and creditor-mandated economic liberalization programs.

In this way, the good governance argument complements the market friendly one. The East African miracle economies were models of good governance as interventions in the economy were either irrelevant or they canceled each other out. The rest of the developing world, particularly sub-Saharan Africa and including eastern Europe, should learn from their example. Good governance may refer to efficient civil servants, the rule of law, and so on, but the key point is that these institutions allow limited government to operate. In a 1994 report the Bank was quite explicit about this (20, pp. 2, 10):

> there is hope that Africa, like East Asia thirty years ago, will move onto a faster development track. For that to happen, more progress will be required in macroeconomic reform—to provide a stable environment in which economic activity can flourish. Good macroeconomic policies have paid off in East Asia, and they will pay off in Africa.

Such policies are said to include less taxation of agriculture, putting exporters first, liberalizing imports, privatization, and fiscal reform (20, pp. 10–14).

So, to summarize: the earlier neoliberal view (5) that East Asian success was a product of sound policies of limited government has been altered so that proper recognition is given to the fact that the state was interventionist. The new view accepts the reality of state intervention, but argues that this did not fundamentally alter a policy of industrial development through market forces. State regulations did not hinder the development of an industrial structure that would have emerged through market forces anyway. This argument is similar to that proposed by Berger who argued that (21, p. 64):

> the crux of the Korean example is that the active interventionist attitude of the state has been aimed at applying moderate incentives which are very close to the relative prices of products and factors that would prevail in a situation of free trade. . . . It is as though the government were 'simulating' a free market.

Such interventions are contrasted with the distorting activities of states in much of the developing world (18, p. 351). Good governance includes a number of institutional factors, which are considered important insofar as they will allow market friendly intervention to occur.

ASSESSING THE REVISED MODEL

This section examines the revised neoliberal model through an assessment of (*a*) the idea of market friendly intervention, (*b*) the idea of good governance, and (*c*) the implications for structural adjustment.

Market Friendly Intervention

The main problem with the World Bank's report is its tendency to isolate specific examples of state intervention, and to then show how these were counter-balanced by further interventions. For example, in South Korea and Taiwan the potentially damaging policy of import substitution was said to be canceled out by policies of export promotion, with the result that a market-conforming structure emerged despite the interventions (18, pp. 292–316). However, the effects of intervention cannot be adequately assessed in this way; they must be analyzed through their impact *on the economy as a whole.* Thus for example, industrial policy affects a country's balance of payments through the spin-off effects into other industries (22, p. 17). Furthermore, the Bank's argument (18, p. 316) rests on the mistaken assumption that the textiles industry was not protected by the state. In fact, despite the labor-intensive nature of this particular industry, it was heavily protected from foreign competition. It was specifically promoted by the state from the early 1960s, receiving preferential loans and tax and tariff exemptions (11, pp. 66–68). Therefore, the existence of a large textiles industry "is not proof that industrial policy did not work but in fact suggests that it worked really well, as this was one of the most heavily promoted sectors" (23, p. 214).

The argument that protectionism was largely irrelevant because it was counterbalanced by the setting of export targets is similarly problematic. This claim ignores how protectionism alleviated potential balance-of-payments constraints and helped to promote technical change and hence productivity growth through the linking of import controls to export targets (22, p. 20).

Similarly, the World Bank recognizes that South Korea and Taiwan were restrictive in their policies toward direct foreign investment, but argues that this was counteracted by a policy of openness to foreign technology acquisition (18, p. 21). However, as Lall argues (24, p. 651):

> There is no analysis in the study . . . of the effects of different modes of technology import on the industrial development: different forms of openness were perceived by these countries to have different implications for the development of their own innovative capabilities, and this formed a crucial element of their industrial strategies.

In particular, in Korea and Taiwan the state policy of guiding the market was achieved far more easily by a reliance on domestic rather than foreign firms, and it facilitated the growth of substantial research and development activities (22, pp. 21–22).[1] These developments were clearly crucial to the ability of Korea and Taiwan to "unpack," utilize, and build upon imported technologies, and in the long run to become internationally competitive and break into export markets (24, p. 651). This contrasts sharply with the alleged failures of import substituters in Latin America (though not India), which, in terms of its open-door policy to foreign investment, was if anything more "market friendly" than Korea and Taiwan (25).

[1] South Korea (1.9 percent of GNP in 1988) and Taiwan (1.2 percent) have far greater levels of investment in research and development activities than most of the more industrialized developing countries—for example Argentina (0.5 percent in 1988), India (0.9 percent in 1986), and Brazil (0.4 percent in 1985). This is lower than Japan (2.8 percent in 1987) and Germany (2.8 percent in 1987), but higher than Belgium (1.7 percent in 1987) and Italy (1.2 percent in 1987) (22, p. 22).

Some "market unfriendly" technological upgradings, such as Korea's heavy and chemical industry drive, are recognized by the Bank. In this case, however, the non-market-conforming interventions are criticized for their costs in terms of support for inefficient and expensive industries (18, p. 309). Closer empirical scrutiny of these costs shows that in fact the most targeted heavy industries (chemicals and machinery) accounted for a lower share of outstanding non-performing loans than outstanding total loans, and that 60 percent of all nonperforming loans were accounted for by the construction industry's over-investment in the Middle East (26). Furthermore, the drive can hardly be considered a disaster when one considers that by the early 1980s, heavy industries accounted for most of the country's export earnings (27, p. 631). It was in this period that the Korean economy was substantially liberalized, but only the most wishful of neoliberal thinkers would attempt to argue that it was this process (which only began in 1981) which led to the competitiveness of Korean heavy industry. The liberalization of trade did go hand in hand with the expansion of heavy industries in the 1980s, but the *causal* factors were those market unfriendly policies of state targeting and technical upgrading in the 1970s. Moreover, the Korean state has continued to protect high-technology sectors that would otherwise be undermined by foreign competition (28, pp. 206–210).

These examples show the inadequacies of the World Bank Report, and its stubborn refusal to make a bold move away from the neoliberal paradigm. The Report "is almost a textbook example of neoclassicists visibly confused but too proud to admit their failure—having been so quick to blame government for economic failures in the past, they are now reluctant to admit a positive role for government in a successful economy" (29, p. 635). Such confusion leads to faulty logic in places and a number of contradictory claims. For example, the Bank (18, p. 6) argues that one cannot establish statistical causal relationships between intervention and growth, as we cannot know what would have happened in the absence of such an intervention. However, this does not stop the Bank from using such a methodology in order to try to establish a causal link between growth and *non-intervention* (18, p. 325; 27, p. 628). Thus, in arguing that industrial policy created a market-conforming industrial structure, the Report concludes that industrial policy was ineffective. But: "As this test is formulated, industrial policy cannot win: if it fulfills neo-classical expectations, it is 'ineffective'; if it violates them, it is inefficient" (27, p. 629).

One final, and most important, point must be made about the market friendly approach. The basic argument is that interventions were largely irrelevant in East Asia because they were market-conforming, and therefore "relative price distortions were limited and indeed smaller than in most other developing countries" (18, p. 351). Of course, this assertion can be subject to exactly the same criticisms as that of the price distortion index in the 1983 *World Development Report*, discussed above. But even leaving that aside, the evidence in the 1993 Report can be used against the Bank's own arguments. This is because the Bank (18, p. 301) recognizes that the degree of high outward orientation and low price distortion varied between the Asian NICs—Hong Kong, Malaysia, Singapore, Indonesia, and Thailand have a low rate of price distortion, whereas Japan, Korea, Taiwan, and China do not do so well. In fact, these latter countries actually rank *below* supposedly inefficient import-substituting industrializers such as Brazil, India, Mexico, Pakistan, and Venezuela.

Interestingly, the Report only comments on the variations within the Asian NICs, rather than the fact that the Bank's evidence on prices implies that Brazil and India are more market friendly than Korea and Taiwan—*even though the Report is supposed to prove the opposite.*

Good Governance

Given that the Bank's idea of market friendly intervention is unconvincing, it is not surprising that the concept of good governance is too. The link between the two ideas is that East Asian miracle economies were models of market friendly intervention and good governance. My arguments above, however, suggest that these economies did not conform to the principles of market friendly intervention—which itself is an inconsistent concept—and so in this respect cannot be regarded as models of good governance. As regards the *source* of the model (East Asia), the Bank is mistaken, and so it follows that its applicability to other parts of the world is seriously undermined.

However, the concept of good governance needs further investigation in its own right. The idea that liberal democracy will promote economic growth is itself problematic (30, pp. 94–112). Certainly in this respect the East Asian economies, with their long tradition of authoritarian politics, cannot be regarded as models. This does not mean that authoritarianism is essential, but the long history of capitalist development does not give much room for optimism.

The relationship between adjustment and the observance of good human rights practices is similarly problematic. Certainly, much of sub-Saharan Africa (and elsewhere) has seen an improvement in human rights practices in the adjustment period. But there can be no convincing claim that there is a causal connection; in fact, "the only clear link between adjustment and human rights issues is that in some countries . . . organized opponents of adjustment have had their human rights infringed" (31, p. 23).

The underlying weakness of the concept of governance, however, relates to its excessively narrow view of politics. In focusing on *governance*, the Bank has reduced the *politics* of development to a purely technocratic issue. Wider social and political interests are largely ignored, and so the need for better governance linked to a "free enterprise" economy is reduced to rhetoric. There is no analysis of the vested interests, both within and outside the state, which may win or lose from structural adjustment. Moreover, the existence of such interests is a major factor in assessing the likelihood of adjustment programs being implemented in the first place (32, p. 266). Development "is not simply a managerial question, as the World Bank's literature on governance asserts, but a political one. For all processes of 'development' express crucially the central core of *politics*: conflict, negotiation and co-operation over the use, production and distribution of resources" (33, p. 620).

Thus, to return to the East Asian "model." The World Bank scenario of successful development in South Korea is based on the belief that a rational bureaucracy allowed market forces to operate, or at least only intervened in a market friendly way. But such a scenario simply flies in the face of South Korean history, which has included precisely the kind of political conflicts which the Bank ignores. In the case of both South Korea and Taiwan, radical land reforms were introduced by the state in response to serious conflict (in the latter case on the Chinese mainland) after the Second World War. These reforms laid the basis for (*a*) more equal income distributions compared to much of the world and (*b*) a transfer of resources from countryside to town without fully impoverishing the latter, and (*c*) broke the power of vested interests in the countryside, which may otherwise have influenced the state. The issue of land reform, and its results then, was one of *politics and not governance*.

The Bank's limited approach to politics can be traced back to its neoliberal conception of the state. It is not surprising that neoliberals argue that state intervention in East Asia was largely irrelevant, because the assumption that state intervention *must be inefficient* is built into their theoretical system. At the heart of the neoliberal critique of the state is the contention that state officials *always* act in a self-interested way. These officials are said to expand the activity of the state for their own good, rather than the interest of society. Such a viewpoint represents a clear attempt by neoliberals to explain politics, as well as economics, by sole reference to the self-interested, utility-maximizing individual. The best policy option is to secure the most effective context for such behavior to operate efficiently, and this is one in which competitive market forces are allowed to flourish by a "nightwatchman state" (34).

Clearly, there are many examples of unproductive rent-seeking activity throughout the world, but the neoliberal argument is far stronger than this. It is that the state acts in its own interest *irrespective of time and place* (35). Taken to its logical conclusion, such a view provides no justification for *any* state. As Evans argues: "How does such a state arise out of individual maximizers? It is hard to explain why, if office-holders are primarily interested in individual rents, they do not all 'free-lance' " (36, p. 25). The Bank echoes these inconsistencies in its approach to governance. The state is seen as the problem—it intervenes too heavily. It is also seen as the solution—it must reform itself in order to allow for wealth-creating activity. But if states are *purely* self-interested, then why should state officials carry out the necessary reforms? Again, *on its own terms*, the arguments of the Bank are full of inconsistencies.

The Implications for Structural Adjustment

Assessing structural adjustment policies in practice is extremely difficult. This is because there is considerable dispute over the extent to which policies have been implemented. Critical analysis of adjustment programs has often presented them as simple impositions by the World Bank or IMF onto supposedly sovereign nation-states, when in fact they are the outcome of complex negotiations between international institutions and national governments (37). Nevertheless, there is a certain "family resemblance" between adjustment policies, which often include exchange rate devaluations, the removal of import quotas, increased export incentives, revisions in agricultural pricing policies, and reform of the national budget (38, p. 29).

But even if we accept the above qualification, there are further difficulties, which relate to the reasons for the "successes" and "failures" in particular cases (38). Despite these difficulties, the World Bank (20) has recently claimed that there is a strong correlation between the strongest adjusting countries and economic growth. However, this report suffers from precisely the methodological weaknesses cited above; for instance, economic growth may be caused by favorable increases in terms of trade rather than specific economic policy. Moreover, even the Bank's own evidence suggests that there were as many policy differences among the six "good" policy performers and the 23 "others" (39, 40).

Gibbon's (41) alternative methodology is to examine "adjustment situations," which he defines as "a combination of actually implemented adjustment policies with other novel independent or semi-independent variables also of predominantly exogenous origin." The causal roles of adjustment policies may themselves be secondary, but this can only be determined by careful empirical analysis. In a long-term analysis of economic trends in sub-Saharan Africa (31), it was found that adjustment situations had made little positive difference to growth or poverty alleviation.

For example, using statistics collected by the Food and Agricultural Organization, it was found that growth rates in 37 adjusting African countries were not significantly different in the adjustment years of 1986–1993 than they had been in the previous seven-year period. Of the sampled countries, 24 percent had better growth rates, 22 percent had the same, and 52 percent had worse rates (31, p. 34).

These unimpressive results can be linked to the fallacious thinking of the World Bank on agriculture, which argues that by simply freeing producers from price controls production will soar (42). This assumes that producers can respond to price rises in a similar way, therefore ignoring rural differentiation, and ignores the all important role of infrastructure and transportation in what are often remote settings.

Similarly, industry has shown no marked increase in output, and no increase in investment (31, p. 42). Some industries are bound to suffer from devaluations as essential imports become more expensive, and trade liberalization can have disastrous consequences through the encouragement of cheaper imports. These comments apply even to Ghana, the African country that the World Bank upholds as a model of successful adjustment policy. Ghana's adjustment program since 1986 has included such market friendly policies as exchange rate devaluations, the removal of many import controls, privatization, and the liberalization of foreign investment regulations (43). Manufacturing grew in the adjustment period, but this was largely because imported inputs were made available to industries that had suffered from excess capacity. As liberalization spread and excess capacity was used up, the exposure to foreign competition led to a deceleration of industrial growth—from 5.6 percent in 1988, to 2.6 percent in 1991 and 1.1 percent in 1992. Employment in manufacturing fell from 78,000 in 1987 to 28,000 in 1993 (44, p. 2025). Industrial survivors and new entrants are largely in small enterprises making low-income products for localized markets, while success in attracting foreign investment has been minimal.

Similarly, the World Bank's hope that the informal sector can form the basis of a new, dynamic capitalist sector is misplaced. Thus (41, p. 769):

> Contrary to some proponents of adjustment, these constraints are not mainly of a regulative kind, for they are also found in sectors which were never regulated. Amongst the most important are the primitive technical level of the operations, shortages of skilled labour, and continuous competition for household and enterprise resources with other household income-generating activities.

The prospects for countries undergoing adjustment are not good, then. Indeed, even the Bank (20, p. 153) admits that investment rates have not increased in sub-Saharan Africa. Similar criticisms could be made of adjustment experiences in eastern Europe (45) and Latin America (46).

CLASS, STATE, AND GLOBAL ECONOMY IN LATE CAPITALIST DEVELOPMENT

In this section I put forward an alternative explanation for the rise of the East Asian NICs, and draw out some of the implications for understanding the prospects for capitalist development in the rest of the developing world. Most of my discussion will focus on South Korea, not in order to present this country as a model (neoliberal or Keynesian) for others to follow, but in part to emphasize the *particularity* of the South Korean experience. However, at the same time I will also argue that there are *specific lessons* to be learned from this experience, as opposed to a *general model*. In order to illustrate my alternative approach, I will examine South Korea in relation to the world economy, and the particular social structure within South Korean society.

It should be clear by now that the World Bank has a particularly optimistic account of the relationship between national economies and the global economy.

The Bank remains convinced of the neoliberal view that there is no need for protection to domestic producers because open competition on the world market will benefit all countries—that is, countries produce those goods in which they have a comparative advantage, and they can only establish what these goods are through open competition. In fact the "advanced" capitalist countries have often selectively applied this policy. Indeed, South Korea and Taiwan benefited from relatively open access to the U.S. market in the 1960s and 1970s, partly because they were favored allies in the Cold War. For similar reasons they were also major recipients of U.S. aid, especially in the 1950s. In the 1980s and 1990s, potential new Koreas and Taiwans have often faced far greater protectionism from the First World, particularly in labor-intensive sectors such as clothing, where the developing world could have a comparative advantage (14, Chapt. 5).

Moreover, even a consistent pro-free-market view ignores the inequalities inherent within capital accumulation (23, p. 215):

> that there are formidable entry barriers for developing countries attempting to move up the ladder of the international division of labour—because of cumulative causations in technical progress . . . imperfect domestic and international financial markets . . . a lack of marketing skills and infrastructure, and so on.

It was precisely for these reasons that state intervention in South Korea (and Taiwan) was market *un*friendly. Indeed, the South Korean state often deliberately "got prices wrong." In the 1960s, many firms exported at a loss, including those in labor-intensive sectors such as textiles (11, Chapt. 6). Losses were recovered through sales in the protected domestic market, but this reward was only granted to the most successful exporters—these sales were tied to performance standards set by the government. Hamilton (47, p. 83) claims that in fact the average deviation of production prices from actual prices increased from 7.8 percent in 1966 to 11.8 percent in 1978. Such figures suggest that state manipulation of prices was far from market friendly or irrelevant, and in fact was vital to Korea's export success. "Getting prices wrong" was therefore a major component of Korea's (and Taiwan's) transition to successful NIC status. The neoliberal critique is narrowly concerned with the (static) "allocative efficiency" of getting prices right, and therefore lacks an account of the *dynamics* of the process of changing comparative advantage. As Amsden points out, "it is quite possible that if the Bank had determined East Asia's overall growth strategy, the outcome might have been a lot worse—rather than as good as or better than—what did happen" (27, p. 629). For instance, the absence of capital controls may have led to massive capital flight, and the absence of import controls may have led to domestic industry being swallowed up by cheap foreign imports. In this situation Korea and Taiwan would still be exercising their "comparative advantages" in primary products, and thereby experiencing far lower rates of growth.

This suggests, then, that contrary to the neoliberal model, the state played a leading and effective role in capitalist development in South Korea. One possible implication that could be drawn is that it therefore represents a different model of development, based on rational state intervention. In other words, is there a different model of good governance, one in which the state plays an active role in the promotion of capitalism?

While such a scenario could potentially apply to certain countries, it cannot be used as an a priori model, applied independent of specific independent evidence. This is because such a model begs the question of why some states have actively promoted capitalist development, while others have hindered it. Thus (25, pp. 200–201):

> The question is not so much how to explain policy differences, but rather how to account for differences in the effectiveness of economic policy. . . . [This] implies that the failures in Latin America are not a consequence of incorrect policy choices, but of the way in which the state's lack of autonomy precluded certain policies from being pursued.

So it is not just a question of state policy per se (although this is important), but of the social context in which particular states operate. Both neoliberalism and neo-Keynesianism reify the state, measuring its policy effectiveness solely by reference to the degree of intervention within the economy. An alternative approach would be to recognize that both state and economy are constituent parts of the social relations of production, and to account for the development of capitalism on this basis (48, 49).

In the cases of South Korea and Taiwan, a key factor was the aforementioned land reforms implemented in the late 1940s and early 1950s. In Taiwan, fearing a repeat of the peasant revolts on the mainland (China), the nationalist Kuomintang introduced a radical land reform. The result was that "almost overnight the countryside in Taiwan ceased to be oppressed by a small class of large landlords and became characterized by a large number of owner-operators with extremely small holdings" (50, p. 85). Although reform in South Korea was not as far-reaching, it also led to the defeat of a powerful landlord class. These reforms acted as a kind of "punitive forced investment in industry" (51, p. 115), by turning the former landlords into peasants or workers through bankruptcy, or a nascent capitalist class strongly supervised by the state.

Thus, the development of a particular relationship between the state and civil society was conducive to rapid industrial capitalist development in South Korea (52). In other parts of the developing world, the continuing power of certain classes has hindered a similarly rapid development of industrial capitalism. For example, the continued power of unproductive landowning classes in parts of Latin America and Asia has meant that capitalist development has been far more uneven (53, 54). Similarly, the states in South Korea and Taiwan were able to discipline capital far more effectively than in Latin America, and so switch more effectively to an export-oriented development strategy from the 1960s. This policy was reinforced by the organizational weakness of labor in East Asia compared to Latin America (25, p. 208).

Clearly then, one reason that the optimism of adjustment policies is misplaced is its belief that a dynamic capitalism can be implemented without fundamental changes in the social relations of production. In many parts of the periphery, the emergence of a dynamic capitalism has been uneven or has hardly begun, and adjustment actually appears to *hold back* its further development.[2] In other words, adjustment policies can be seen as a failed attempt to introduce a more dynamic capitalism onto social relations which are not conducive to such development. In much of sub-Saharan Africa and Eastern Europe, adjustment policies have reinforced the existence of unfree forms of labor or merchant capital interests, which profit from the trade of goods produced by "non-capitalist" activity (55–57). In such cases, there is little compulsion for the owners of the means of production to rapidly develop the productive forces and thereby promote high levels of economic growth.

CONCLUSION: FUTURE PROSPECTS FOR CAPITALIST DEVELOPMENT IN THE PERIPHERY

The Bank's recent literature on market friendly intervention and good governance is unconvincing. It displays a continued reluctance to recognize the key role of the state in capitalist development, dismissing intervention as insignificant or irrelevant and reducing governance to purely technical questions of policy-making, such as "getting the basics right." Although technical policy-making is an important factor in promoting economic growth, in the case of the Bank's interpretation it is far too narrow and continues to focus one-sidedly on the question of "getting prices right." This abstracts from the inequalities inherent in capital accumulation and rigidly separates efficient "market forces" from inefficient "state intervention." Every case of capitalist development has had a strong state, and *the later the capitalist development, the greater the need for strong state "intervention" in the economy*. States can of course be inefficient and oppressive, in both socialist and capitalist contexts. However, states are not *necessarily* inefficient. Markets, on the other hand, are unequal, hierarchical, and incapable of working without the existence of states.

An alternative account recognizes the centrality of the state to capital accumulation, and in particular how late capitalist developers rely on the state precisely because of the way that markets work (see below). Socialists can learn some specific lessons from the East Asian experience for countries undergoing

[2] In this way, the Bank repeats the errors of "neo-Smithian Marxism" which argued that the origins of capitalism can be rooted in the extension of trading relations rather than a change in the social relations of production (48).

painful processes of adjustment in the developing world. In particular they should criticize the continued dogma that states hinder economic growth. In terms of technical policies, socialists can and should draw on the work of structuralist reformers such as Taylor (58), who propose the development of alternative adjustment policies on a case-by-case basis. The work of Sender and Smith (59, 60) and Mosley and Weeks (61) is particularly valuable in that it attempts to provide alternative policies on the basis of effective reality rather than wishful thinking. For example, Mosley and Weeks (61) suggest that, depending on specific circumstances, exchange rate devaluations may be of some value in promoting exports, while at the same time criticizing the World Bank's indiscriminate proposals for liberalizing trade and ending all protection to domestic producers. This strategy is in marked contrast to the ultra-left voluntarism of Cleaver (62) who proposes nothing less than the immediate closure of the IMF and the ending of development. Such a strategy says nothing about the strength of class forces in the world today, nor the immediate alternatives.

Having said that, socialists must recognize that there is no such thing as technical policy in itself. All such policies will affect class forces in the developing world, and they should in part be considered on this basis. Moreover—and this is the main lesson that can be drawn from the East Asian experience—capitalist development is not a purely technical issue but is the outcome of particular sociopolitical forces. In the long term, this is what has ultimately determined the path of capitalism in the region, and it is the contingent outcome of class forces elsewhere that will determine other paths of capitalist development. Capitalist development thus rests on the development of a particular *social structure of accumulation* (SSA). This refers to "the complex of institutions which support the process of capital accumulation. The central idea of the SSA approach is that a long period of relatively rapid and stable economic expansion requires an effective SSA" (63, p. 1).[3]

Finally, as dependency theory somewhat one-sidedly reminds us, successful capitalist development rests on contingent international factors too. The global economy comprised hierarchies of production which in turn mean that the world market is not the level playing field that neoliberals imagine. Late developers face enormous constraints, both in developing effective producers that can compete with foreign capital in their domestic economy, and in breaking into

[3] The approach in this chapter is not completely compatible with the SSA approach, however. SSA approaches can easily lead to functionalism. In focusing on appropriate foundations for capital accumulation, the SSA school can exaggerate the degree of integration of any SSA, and thereby downplay the reality of conflict within all capitalist societies. In this way, an appropriate SSA can be regarded as an appropriate structure which functions for the hegemony of capitalism, thereby ignoring the contradictions of *any* social structure of accumulation and the role of exploited classes as makers of their own history. My approach here suggests that SSAs are crucial to the "success" of capitalist development, as opposed to those technicist policies advocated by the World Bank, but also that such structures are contingent and based on historical processes as opposed to ahistorical models.

export markets and thereby competing in the world economy. These barriers are not completely insurmountable, however, and the East Asian NICs have enjoyed some considerable success on both fronts. Having said that, their success rested on favorable world market factors and the existence of a strong, effective state that disciplined capital as well as labor. Neoliberal dominance of international trade, financial, and development institutions hinders the prospects for successful capitalist development in the current period. On the other hand, a scenario of completely unregulated global market forces is unlikely to be implemented, and the world economy does offer opportunities for late developers as well as constraints. These opportunities include the prospect (with all the contradictions these entail) of foreign investment, of established overseas markets, and of acquiring advanced technology. The prospect for successful late capitalist development thus appears to rest on a policy of being "in and against the [world] market."[4] Successful late developers will be *in* the world market in that they attempt to draw on its opportunities, but will be *against* it in that the state will play a crucial role in removing its constraints. This, rather than a spurious concept of market friendly intervention, is the most important lesson that can be learned from the East Asian experience.[5]

Note — This chapter is adapted from an article published in *Capital and Class*, 64: 63–88, Spring 1998.

REFERENCES

1. Toye, J. *Dilemmas of Development.* Blackwell, Oxford, 1987.
2. Tsiang, S., and Wu, R. Foreign trade and investment as boosters of take off: The experience of the four Asian NICs. In *Foreign Trade and Investment*, edited by W. Galenson, pp. 320–343. University of Wisconsin Press, Madison, 1985.
3. Fukuyama, F. *The End of History and the Last Man.* Penguin, London, 1992.
4. Berger, P., and Tsaio, H.-H. *In Search of an East Asian Model of Development.* Transaction Books, New York, 1987.

[4] The idea of being "in and against" capitalism is derived from the work of the Conference of Socialist Economists on the state (64, 65). It is based on the recognition that important reforms (opportunities) can be gained from being *in* the capitalist state, but that these are always compromised (constrained) by the dominance of capitalist social relations and the role of the state in securing this dominance, and so there is a need to be simultaneously *against* the state.

[5] The recent downturn in economic growth in the East Asian region is fully compatible with the analysis offered in this chapter. Although the IMF and World Bank have argued that the recession has been caused by too much government intervention in the economy, in fact the roots of the recession in South-East Asia lie in the failure of the state to regulate unproductive economic activity, particularly speculation in finance and land. The recession in South Korea also shows the fallacy of neoliberal arguments, as it is rooted in the gradual deregulation of the economy over the last 15 years. In particular this has encouraged over-borrowing by the commercial banking sector and overcapacity in unplanned industrial sectors.

5. Balassa, B., et al. *Adjusting to Success: Balance of Payments Policy in the East Asian NICs*. Institute of International Economics, Washington, D.C., 1986.
6. World Bank. *World Development Report 1983*. Oxford University Press, Oxford, 1983.
7. Balassa, B. *The Newly Industrializing Countries and the World Economy*. Pergamon, New York, 1981.
8. Jenkins, R. (Re-)interpreting Brazil and South Korea. In *Industrialization and Development*, edited by T. Hewitt, H. Johnson, and D. Wield, pp. 167–198. Oxford University Press, Oxford, 1992.
9. Singer, H. The World Development Report 1987 on the blessings of outward orientation: A necessary correction. *J. Dev. Stud.* 24: 232–236, 1988.
10. White, G. *Developmental States in East Asia*. Macmillan, London, 1988.
11. Amsden, A. *Asia's Next Giant*. Oxford University Press, Oxford, 1989.
12. Rodan, G. *The Political Economy of Singapore's Industrialisation*. Macmillan, London, 1989.
13. Schiffer, J. State policy and economic growth: A note on the Hong Kong model. *IJURR* 15: 180–196, 1991.
14. Kiely, R. *Industrialisation and Development: A Comparative Analysis*. UCL Press, London, 1998.
15. World Bank. *Sub-Saharan Africa: From Crisis to Sustainable Growth*. Washington, D.C., 1989.
16. World Bank. *World Development Report 1991*. Oxford University Press, Oxford, 1991.
17. World Bank. *Governance and Development*. Washington, D.C., 1992.
18. World Bank. *The East Asian Miracle*. Oxford University Press, Oxford, 1993.
19. Schmitz, G. Democratization and demystification: Deconstructing 'governance' as development paradigm. In *Debating Development Discourse*, edited by D. Moore and G. Schmitz, pp. 54–90. Macmillan, London, 1995.
20. World Bank. *Adjustment in Africa*. Oxford University Press, Oxford, 1994.
21. Berger, F. Korea's experience with export-led development. In *Export Promotion Policies*, edited by B. De Vries, pp. 60–82. World Bank, Washington, D.C., 1979.
22. Singh, A. How did East Asia grow so fast? *UNCTAD Discussion Paper*, No. 97. UNCTAD, Geneva, 1994.
23. Chang, H.-J. Explaining 'flexible rigidities' in East Asia. In *The Flexible Economy*, edited by T. Killick, pp. 197–221. Routledge, London, 1995.
24. Lall, S. 'The East Asian miracle' study: Does the bell toll for industrial strategy? *World Dev.* 22: 645–654, 1994.
25. Jenkins, R. The political economy of industrialization: A comparison of Latin American and East Asian newly industrializing countries. *Dev. Change* 22: 197–231, 1991.
26. Amsden, A., and Euh, Y.-D. Republic of Korea's financial reform: What are the lessons? *UNCTAD Discussion Paper*, No. 30. UNCTAD, Geneva, 1990.
27. Amsden, A. Why isn't the whole world experimenting with the East Asian model to develop? Review of 'The East Asian Miracle.' *World Dev.* 22: 627–633, 1994.
28. Amsden, A. Trade policy and economic performance in South Korea. In *Trade and Growth*, edited by M. Agosin and D. Tussie, pp. 187–214. Macmillan, London, 1993.

29. Kwon, J. The East Asia challenge to neo-classical orthodoxy. *World Dev.* 22: 635–644, 1994.
30. Healey, J., and Robinson, M. *Democracy, Governance and Economic Policy.* Overseas Development Institute, London, 1992.
31. Engberg-Pedersen, P., et al. *Limits of Adjustment in Africa.* James Currey, London, 1996.
32. Uvin, P. *The International Organization of Hunger.* Routledge & Kegan Paul, London, 1994.
33. Leftwich, A. Governance, democracy and development in the third world. *Third World Q.* 14: 605–624, 1993.
34. Buchanan, J. *Liberty, Market and the State.* Wheatsheaf, Brighton, England, 1986.
35. Toye, J. Is there a new political economy of development? In *States or Markets,* edited by C. Colclough and J. Manor, pp. 321–338. Clarendon, Oxford, 1991.
36. Evans, P. *Embedded Autonomy.* Princeton University Press, Princeton, N.J., 1995.
37. Harrigan, J., Mosley, P., and Toye, J. *Aid and Power.* Routledge, London, 1991.
38. Toye, J. Structural adjustment. In *Structural Adjustment and Beyond in Africa,* edited by R. van der Hoeven and F. van der Kraaij, pp. 18–35. James Currey, London, 1994.
39. Mosley, P., Subasast, T., and Weeks, J. Assessing adjustment in Africa. *World Dev.* 23: 1459–1473, 1995.
40. White, H. Review article: Adjustment in Africa. *Dev. Change* 27: 785–815, 1996.
41. Gibbon, P. Structural adjustment and structural change in sub-Saharan Africa: Some provisional conclusions. *Dev. Change* 27: 751–784, 1996.
42. Schiff, M., and Valdes, A. *The Plundering of Agriculture in Developing Countries.* World Bank, Washington, D.C., 1992.
43. African Development Bank. *African Development Report 1994.* Abidjan, Ivory Coast, 1994.
44. Lall, S. Structural adjustment and African industry. *World Dev.* 23: 2019–2031, 1994.
45. Gowan, P. Neo-liberal theory and practice in Eastern Europe. *New Left Rev.* 213: 32–65, 1995.
46. Weeks, J. The manufacturing sector in Latin America and the new economic model. In *The New Economic Model in Latin America and Its Impact on Income Distribution and Poverty,* edited by V. Bulmer-Thomas, pp. 271–294. Macmillan, London, 1995.
47. Hamilton, C. *Capitalist Industrialization in Korea.* Westview, London, 1986.
48. Brenner, R. The origins of capitalist development: A critique of "neo-Smithian" Marxism. *New Left Rev.* 104: 25–92, 1977.
49. Kiely, R. *Sociology and Development: The Impasse and Beyond.* UCL Press, London, 1995.
50. Amsden, A. The state and Taiwan's economic development. In *Bringing the State Back In,* edited by P. Evans, D. Rueschmeyer, and T. Skocpol, pp. 78–106. Cambridge University Press, Cambridge, England, 1985.
51. Seldon, M. *The Political Economy of Chinese Socialism.* M. E. Sharpe, New York, 1988.
52. Seddon, D., and Belton-Jones, T. The political determinants of economic flexibility, with special reference to the East Asian NICs. In *The Flexible Economy,* edited by T. Killick, pp. 325–364. Routledge, London, 1995.

53. de Janvry, A. Peasants, capitalism and the state in Latin American culture. In *Peasants and Peasant Societies*, edited by T. Shanin, pp. 390–398. Blackwell, Oxford, 1987.
54. Hamilton, C. Can the rest of Asia emulate the NICs? *Third World Q.* 87: 1225–1256, 1987.
55. Watts, M. Peasants under contract: Agro-food complexes in the third world. In *The Food Question*, edited by H. Bernstein, pp. 69–79. Eartscan, London, 1990.
56. Raikes, P. *Modernizing Hunger*. James Currey, London, 1988.
57. Burawoy, M. The end of sovietology and the renaissance of modernisation theory. *Con. Sociol.* 21: 774–785, 1992.
58. Taylor, L. *The Rocky Road to Reform*. WIDER, Helsinki, 1993.
59. Sender, J., and Smith, S. What's right with the Berg Report and what's left of its critics. *Capital and Class* 24: 125–146, 1985.
60. Sender, J., and Smith, S. *The Development of Capitalism in Africa*. Methuen, London, 1986.
61. Mosley, P., and Weeks, J. Has recovery begun? Africa's adjustment in the 1980s revisited. *World Dev.* 21: 1583–1599, 1994.
62. Cleaver, H. Close the IMF, abolish debt and end development: A class analysis of the international debt crisis. *Capital and Class* 39: 17–39, 1989.
63. Kotz, D., McDonough, T., and Reich, M. *Social Structures of Accumulation*. Cambridge University Press, Cambridge, England, 1994.
64. Conference of Socialist Economists. *Struggles Against the State*. Pluto, London, 1979.
65. LEWRG. *In and Against the State*. Pluto, London, 1980.

CHAPTER 9

IN PURSUIT OF "GROWTH WITH EQUITY": THE LIMITS OF CHILE'S FREE-MARKET SOCIAL REFORMS

Pilar Vergara

The 1990 inauguration of President Patricio Aylwin, head of the *Concertación* of Parties for Democracy, a coalition of center and left-wing political parties, marked the end of 17 years of harsh military rule and the beginning of Chile's transition to democracy. The principal motto of the Aylwin administration was "growth with equity"—a notable counterpoint to the neoliberal model implemented by the previous military regime, which maintained that income redistribution could only come from economic growth. While the dictatorship had succeeded in achieving high economic growth rates—8 percent annually by the end of the 1980s—income inequalities actually worsened. The number of poor Chileans doubled during the Pinochet regime. By 1989, 44 percent of Chileans lived in poverty. The Aylwin government argued that economic growth was a necessary—but not sufficient—condition for achieving greater equality in Chile. This emphasis on equity was not based only on an ethical concern for social justice, however. The Aylwin administration also sensed that the equity issue was key to the consolidation of Chile's newborn democracy.

The government did not propose either a return to the populist practices of the past—a strategy that other Latin American governments presiding over new democratic regimes had tried, with disastrous results—or a continuation of the dominant neoliberal ideology of the military government. Its proposal was based on the premise that policies promoting economic growth and stability must continue, but that they should be complemented with social policies designed to promote greater equality. The Aylwin administration's approach to equity diverged from the neoliberal model in its emphasis on promoting greater equality among Chileans through social and labor policies directed at the poorest sectors of Chilean society. Nevertheless, it remained firmly within the framework of the free-market model inherited from the military. President Eduardo Frei, also from the *Concertación,* was elected to office in 1993. His administration continued the previous government's efforts to make economic growth compatible with achieving greater equity.

Over the past decade, the social reforms carried out by the Chilean military regime have been celebrated as a model for other Latin American countries anxious to overcome the endemic crises of their social security systems. The policies introduced by the Aylwin and Frei governments to reduce poverty levels within the free-market system, and the initial success of those efforts, reinforced the belief that Chile was a viable model for other countries engaging in social reform. Little attention has been paid, however, to the way the *Concertación* governments' redistributive efforts have been hampered by the new social institutions established during the Pinochet regime. An examination of the successes and limitations of Chile's social policy reveals how neoliberal social reforms have fundamentally restricted the scope and impact of the *Concertación's* attempts to achieve "growth with equity."

Social inequalities had reached unprecedented heights during the 17 years of military rule. The deterioration of basic public services due to constant cuts in social spending under Pinochet affected not only the poorest sectors of society, but also large segments of the middle class. Pent-up social problems had given rise to great expectations of reforms under a democratic government, raising the specter of an explosion of demands that could destabilize Chile's new democracy.

The Aylwin government's ability to implement redistributive policies, however, was seriously limited by other legacies of authoritarian rule. The military's neoliberal economic policies—including the steady lowering of tax rates and hence government revenue since 1984, the public debt contracted to rescue the financial system after the 1982–1983 crisis, and the end of revenue from the privatization of public enterprises, which were all sold off by 1989—imposed serious budget constraints on the new democratic regime. This impeded the Aylwin administration's ability to increase social spending without creating fiscal problems.

Within this context of sharp social tensions and budgetary constraints, the government devised an overarching plan to carry out its redistributive tasks. The plan consisted of three basic elements. First, the government implemented a tax reform to generate more funds to underwrite the state's social policy programs. Together with international grants and loans, this tax reform permitted the government in its first year to increase social spending by 17 percent without provoking macroeconomic imbalances. Resources devoted to social spending increased from year to year. By 1993, social spending had returned to its historic level of 15 percent of the gross domestic product (GDP), although it remained below 1970 values in per capita terms.

The second element of the Aylwin government's program was the targeting of social spending to reach the poorest sectors of the population. This strategy, the government believed, would help avoid the market distortions that other redistributive mechanisms, such as price controls, caused. New and innovative social programs were designed that focused on social groups such as female heads of household, youth, and indigenous communities. The government increased subsidies to low-income groups, and raised the minimum wage. Primary health care was expanded, and the government invested in new hospital equipment. A program was launched to improve the quality of basic education and to expand the school nutrition program. These programs were implemented in a decentralized manner, and emphasized the participation of the beneficiaries and the promotion of local self-help efforts. Overall, the government gave priority to social programs that represented an investment in human capital, which would promote long-term growth, as opposed to aid programs.

As part of this effort, the government established the Solidarity and Social Investment Fund (FOSIS), whose principal objective is to finance projects that promote productive employment for the poorest sectors. The FOSIS does not directly implement projects. Rather, it finances projects designed and administered directly by the social organizations of the poorest communities within each region, often in coordination with local non-governmental organizations (NGOs). The FOSIS has funded 52,000 projects in its four years of operation. These projects tend to be small and short-term. They are focused on marginalized sectors of society such as unemployed youth, campesinos, and small-enterprise workers. The FOSIS initially promised to work closely with existing government ministries, but in practice it often operated independently of them. While this permitted the FOSIS greater flexibility and helped avoid bureaucratic tangles, it also undermined the continuity of the projects.

Finally, the government proposed a labor reform law, which, after some modification, was accepted by labor, business, and the opposition parties, and approved by parliament in 1990. The new law reestablished a series of rights and guarantees that had been denied to workers under the military regime—including the rights to strike, to form a union, to collective bargaining within productive sectors, and to protection against arbitrary firing or lay-offs. Workers were thereby given the chance to negotiate how the benefits of growth were distributed. Chilean businesses are, however, still allowed to adjust salaries in times of economic downturns or macroeconomic changes in order to protect their ability to remain competitive with foreign companies.

This new set of policies registered quick and positive results in the context of strong economic growth. In the three years of Aylwin's administration, the minimum wage increased 24 percent in real terms, the purchasing power of Chilean families increased 70 percent, and average incomes grew almost 18 percent. These upward trends, coupled with the hundreds of new jobs that were created, led to a significant increase in the portion that household income represented within the GDP. Since 1993, these indicators have continued to improve, though at a slower rate than before. The crowning achievement of the Aylwin administration's new social policy was the reduction of poverty: the percentage of

Chileans living in poverty declined from 44.6 percent in 1989, to 33 percent in 1992 and 28 percent in 1994.

Not all of the Aylwin government's redistributive initiatives, however, enjoyed the same level of success. The limitations of these efforts became increasingly evident during the Frei administration. While the huge inequalities of income distribution that had congealed under the military regime were reduced (though only slightly) during the Aylwin administration, by 1995 they appeared to be increasing again. For example, while the average Chilean family augmented its per capita income by 5 percent between 1994 and 1995, the poorest 10 percent saw their income fall by 4.3 percent. The same concentration of wealth can be seen from a different angle. For the first time since the return to democracy, the annual growth of real incomes fell from 5 percent in 1994 to 4 percent in 1995, dropping below the increase of average economic productivity (7.1 percent). As a result, the income share of GDP fell (34.8 percent to 33.4 percent), while the share of capital profit increased (from 38 percent to 44 percent).

Although Frei has a more openly pro-business bent than his predecessor, he has also encountered a less auspicious environment for his redistributive policies. For example, the government's attempt to extend the 1990 tax reform, which was initially approved for a period of only four years, ran up against implacable resistance from the business owners' association as well as right-wing opposition parties. Consequently, the Frei administration was stripped of an essential tool to reduce social inequalities. The government's attempt to expand the labor reforms to include non-unionized workers, who represent nearly three-quarters of the labor force, has also run up against a brick wall. After nearly two years, the government has still not obtained parliament's approval for these modifications. As a result, the Frei government's social policy has been unable to go beyond Aylwin's initial achievements or to reverse the country's widening income gap.

State social spending has historically been the principal mechanism in Chile by which social inequalities were reduced and channels of social mobility opened. Despite the best intentions of the Aylwin and Frei administrations to overcome fiscal constraints on social spending, however, insufficient resources have been directed to social programs over the past few years, given the magnitude of the accumulated social needs. In 1990, for example, the government-mandated increase of family allowances and workers' minimum pension payments alone ate up half the total funds generated by the new tax reform.

An analysis of the overall impact on living standards of the government's economic and social policies highlights how ineffectual social policy has become as an instrument of redistribution. The reduction of poverty in the first year of the Aylwin administration can be largely attributed to economic growth, rather than the new social policy. It's important to remember that the expansion of employment, which began after 1989, took place as Chile was recovering from a severe economic recession. Growth in real wages during this period was facilitated by the 1990 labor reforms and government-mandated increases in the minimum wage as well as by the elimination of restrictions on union activity. Furthermore, the drop in inflation improved the overall purchasing power of the population. Once growth rates begin to stabilize and are sustained by increases in productivity rather than the use of idle labor capacity, the benefits to the poor will begin to taper off.

In addition, significant segments of society have been systematically marginalized from the benefits of economic growth, at least in part because they lack the skills and training to join the workforce. This "hard core of poverty"—subsistence farmers, rural migrants to the cities, the elderly, and women and youth who lack vocational training—will only be reduced with the help of specific social policies and programs. While the government has developed social programs directed at the poorest, the amount of resources directed to this sector remains meager. The FOSIS, for example, represents less than 1 percent of the government's social budget—far too small to have any enduring impact.

An important segment of Chile's middle class, which fell into poverty during the military regime, has also not benefited from economic growth or the government's new social policy. The impoverished middle class lacks the personal resources to pay for private services, but has also remained largely ineligible for state benefits. The hopes that this group in particular placed in Chile's new democratic governments have been dashed, giving rise to social protests, especially among teachers and health care professionals who work in the increasingly beleaguered public sector.

A more fundamental problem with Chile's social policy is rooted in the model of social welfare inherited from the dictatorship. Under the military, the state reduced social spending and retreated from the social sector by privatizing social services and creating new institutions guided by the laws of the market. A broad program of reforms, referred to as social "modernization," transferred to the market and the private sector the task of providing goods and social services previously offered by the state. As a result, the state's capacity to influence the living conditions of the population through traditional social policy measures was significantly reduced.

A brief look at the reforms of the social security system and the health care sector reveals the underlying principles that guided social reform under the military regime. As these social sectors were privatized, new institutions emerged that have fundamentally reshaped the provision of social welfare in Chile. While the state continued to provide limited benefits to the poorest, the social sector soon became dominated by powerful private institutions guided by the profit motive.

The old public social security system in Chile was based on combined contributions from workers, their employers, and the state that were distributed by the government once the worker retired. Reforms initiated in 1981 replaced the old system with a new one based solely on workers' individual contributions, which are administered by private, profit-making entities known as the Administrators of Pension Funds (AFPs). Workers who chose the new system were given "bonds of recognition" which permitted them to transfer their contributions to the old system into the AFPs. While the traditional social security system continued to be administered and guaranteed by the state, strong incentives—including a reduction of the payment rates from 23 to 13.5 percent—convinced most workers to switch to the new system. The state had to pay out the accumulated contributions of all those workers who switched to the new AFPs, resulting in the systematic transfer of state resources to the private sector. Every year, a quarter of the state's social budget goes toward these payouts. The impact on the old social security system was devastating: this crucial loss of resources generated a deficit of nearly 5 percent of GDP within the traditional social security system, which will last at least until the end of the decade.

Private medicine was also given a boost when the government authorized the establishment of Institutions of Provisional Health (ISAPRES). These profit-making enterprises, which resemble health maintenance organizations (HMOs) in the United States, offer medical services in exchange for an obligatory contribution of 7 percent of affiliated workers' salaries. Huge resources that once sustained the state-run clinics and hospitals were then transferred to the ISAPRES, resulting in a serious deterioration of the public health system and, consequently, of the health of the poorest who depend on that system. By the end of the 1980s, about half of the health care contributions of workers, as well as nearly 30 percent of state expenditures for the health sector, went to the ISAPRES, even though they provided health care services to only 12 percent of the population.

Because the ISAPRES are profit-making enterprises, they have excluded elderly people, the chronically infirm, those who suffer from preexisting maladies, and individuals with large families. These groups have been pushed into a public health sector that is increasingly underfinanced, understaffed, and underequipped. The majority of the ISAPRES affiliates cannot afford plans that include coverage for costly diseases or health problems. As a result, people suffering from illnesses that demand expensive treatments have little alternative but to turn to the public health system—even though many of them have paid into the ISAPRES system. The already inadequate public health system is thus further overloaded. In addition, the ISAPRES do not engage in educational activities to promote preventive health care, nor do they cover maternity care or workers' compensation.

The privatization of social services has had important implications for the process of capital accumulation. Coupled with neoliberal economic reforms, including the privatization of public enterprises, tax reductions, and lower overall state spending, this type of social sector reform has resulted in a transferal of most of the country's internal savings to the private sector. The AFPs alone have accumulated funds totaling nearly 25 percent of the GDP. By the end of the 1980s, they had become one of the principal investment institutions in the country.

The privatization of the social welfare system has been good for business, but it has seriously undermined the efficacy and scope of state social policy as a redistributive tool. In effect, privatization has created a dual welfare system, in which a private system with high-quality services for high-income groups coexists with an increasingly underfinanced state system for those who cannot afford private services.

As a consequence of privatization, overall state social spending has actually benefited the poorest the least. In 1993, for example, the wealthiest fifth of the population received nearly double the amount of social spending that the poorest fifth of the population received. This distribution of resources is due less to the inefficiencies of targeting strategies than to the high percentage of the government's social budget that is transferred directly or indirectly to the privatized social service sector.

Inefficiencies rooted in the persistence of centralization, bureaucratic inertia, and institutional fragmentation within state institutions present further barriers to an effective social policy. In fact, despite all the neoliberal hype, the archaic and inefficient state structures of the past have survived both the anti-statist revolution of the military government and the modernizing efforts of the post-dictatorship governments.

Decentralization, which was initiated during the authoritarian regime and pushed vigorously by the *Concertación* governments, has moved forward, as reflected in the new targeted social programs. In practice, however, social policy continues to be designed at the level of the central government. Moreover, the heavy centralist legacy seems to reproduce itself at the local level. The absence of well-trained functionaries in local communities has conspired against effective decentralization, and has reduced the efficacy of local initiatives. The task of restructuring the state social apparatus is admittedly formidable, given its complexity as well as the existence of entrenched interests that continue to resist change.

Despite these fiscal and institutional constraints, the state does retain some leverage. Pinochet's social reforms reduced the state's role in social policy, but they did not wipe it out completely. While the private sector is now largely responsible for financing and directly administering social programs, the state is still responsible for regulating private sector activities and setting standards. The state also retains the capacity to determine which elements of social policy should remain part of the public sphere and which should operate in conjunction with the market.

Yet, the *Concertación* governments have made little use of these powers. If the government had established stronger regulations governing private social service enterprises, many of their most egregious discriminatory and abusive practices might have been eliminated. For example, the high operating costs of the AFPs, which cut into the benefits paid to affiliates, could have been reduced by effective regulation. The state could have also imposed rules prohibiting the ISAPRES from refusing to treat high-risk patients and costly illnesses. Stricter controls over the transferal of state resources to social service enterprises in the private sector would have mitigated the imbalance that now exists in Chile between a well-funded private social service sector and a seriously deteriorated public one. Rules governing mergers and takeovers might have thwarted social service enterprises becoming virtual oligopolies. These harmful practices are extremely difficult to modify now that they have become entrenched—and more importantly, legally sanctioned.

The critical defect of the *Concertación* governments' social policy has been their reluctance to revamp the social sector reforms implemented under Pinochet. Neither the Aylwin nor the Frei administration proposed modifications in the newly privatized system of social services and the dualism that underlies it. This partly reflects the widespread belief that privatization helped resolve the fiscal crisis that had characterized the state social welfare system for decades. At the same time, the *Concertación* governments feared that given the social cost of these reforms, Chilean society would have bristled at the prospect of undergoing new structural changes.

This continuity with the social reform model inherited from the military regime undercuts the viability of government efforts to obtain real social equality. By subordinating social programs to the logic of the marketplace, the *Concertación* governments—despite their best intentions—are incapable of countering the widening chasm between rich and poor that the neoliberal economic model itself generates. In this model, the state assumes responsibility for ensuring the subsistence of the poorest by providing them with direct subsidies, but it renounces one of the principal social functions it once fulfilled—promoting a genuine redistribution of income.

Note — This chapter is adapted from an article published in *NACLA: Report on the Americas* XXIX(6), May/June 1996.

BIBLIOGRAPHY

Banco Central de Chile. *Informe Mensual.* Santiago, 1994 and 1995.

CEPAL. *Focalización y Pobreza.* Santiago, 1995.

Fondo de Solidad e Inversión Social (FOSIS). *Memoria FOSIS 1994.* Santiago, 1994.

Marcel, M. El financiamiento del gasto social. *Colección Estudios CIEPLAN* 31, March 1990.

Marcel, M., and Arenas, A. Reformas a la seguridad social en Chile. *Serie de Monografías,* No. 5. Banco Interamericano de Desarrollo (BID), Washington, D.C., 1991.

Ministerio de Planificación y Cooperación (MIDEPLAN), República de Chile. *Encuesta de Caracterización Socioeconómica.* Santiago, 1990, 1992, 1994, and 1996.

Ministerio de Planificación y Cooperación (MIDEPLAN), República de Chile. *Integración al Desarrollo, Balance de la Política Social: 1990, 1993.* Santiago, 1994.

Miranda, E. Descentralización y privatización del sistema de salud chileno. *Estudios Públicos* 39, Winter 1990.

Miranda, E. (ed.). *La salud en Chile: Evolución y perspectivas.* Centro de Estudios Públicos, Santiago, 1994.

Raczynski, D. Políticas sociales y programas de combate a la en Chile: Balance y desafíos. *Colección Estudios CIEPLAN* 39, June 1994.

United Nations. El gasto social en América latina: un examen cuantitativo y cualitativo. *Cuadernos de la CEPAL* 73, 1994.

Vergara, P. Ruptura y continuidad en la política social del gobierno democrático. *Revista Mexicana de Sociología (RMS)* 3, July–September 1993.

Vergara, P. Market economy, social welfare, and democratic consolidation in Chile. In *Democracy, Markets, and Structural Reform in Latin America,* edited by W. C. Smith, C. Acula, and E. A. Gamarra. North-South Center, University of Miami, and Transaction Publishers, Brunswick and London, 1994.

World Bank. *World Development Report.* New York, 1995.

CHAPTER 10

A FUNDAMENTAL SHIFT IN THE APPROACH TO INTERNATIONAL HEALTH BY WHO, UNICEF, AND THE WORLD BANK: INSTANCES OF THE PRACTICE OF "INTELLECTUAL FASCISM" AND TOTALITARIANISM IN SOME ASIAN COUNTRIES

Debabar Banerji

Giving a personal account of studies on class, health, and quality of life during 1965–1977 in the United States, Vicente Navarro (1) has brought back chilling memories of the dreaded McCarthyism which overshadowed almost every facet of intellectual life in that country (see Chapter 1). He has, very appropriately, used the term "intellectual fascism" to describe this phenomenon. The intellectual fascism that is being practiced by the rich countries of the world on the health services of the poor, dependent countries is of an even more malignant variety. There is an unholy nexus between the ruling classes of the rich and the poor countries in imposing health programs on the poor, because it serves their commercial and political interests. Even the most cogent, well-documented, and well-argued observations questioning the scientific validity of these programs are ignored. Making use of the market-generated information revolution, the rich have brainwashed the helpless masses of the poor to sell their programs. They have also ignored the fact that health policy formulation is a highly complex process, requiring optimization of very complex systems. The task becomes even more complicated when it has to be performed in the context of poor, non-Western countries. These considerations have received scant attention from the health policy experts hired by rich countries.

Asia is a huge continent, with extreme variations in geography, population, ethnic composition, and political commitments. In this chapter, only the countries that fall in the "median" positions will be taken into account. Among them, again, very brief references will be made to the cases of health service developments on the Indian subcontinent and in China to provide a setting for discussion. Together they account for more than two-fifths of the entire population of the world, and a much higher proportion of the world's poor.

The long experience of India in developing its health services has escaped the attention of scholars from the rich countries, of both the hired and the "progressive" varieties. It has been a most virulent form of intellectual fascism. These scholars were actively ahistorical, apolitical, and atheoretical. After Independence, India's ruling class, which had led the freedom struggle against the colonial rulers, was impelled by the working class to fulfill the promises it had made while mobilizing them for the struggle. This was the compelling motive force for its ushering in very ambitious health programs to cover the needs of the unserved and the underserved during the first two decades of independence, even though the country faced massive problems.

The situation in China is entirely different from that in India. Significantly, the two major ideas in public health that emanated from China—the barefoot doctor and the use of the traditional Chinese systems of medicine in their health services—are the outcomes of the revolutionary movement, particularly the Long March. Unfortunately, China also adopted the now well-discredited Soviet model, which failed to work. Deng Xiaoping's move to promote "market socialism" dealt an almost deadly blow to the village commune system, which sustained the barefoot doctors.

Other Asian countries such as Sri Lanka, Pakistan, Bangladesh, Malaysia, Indonesia, Thailand, and the Philippines have also made "progress" in developing their health services. The four last-named countries were among those specially favored by the world capital for stimulating rapid economic growth during the past two decades. Even at the peak of their growth phase, serious flaws have been observed in the health services in the form of rapid privatization leading to gross overcapacity in private hospitals and almost criminal neglect of the poor because of further decay of the already inadequate health services for poor people. One can well imagine the health and health service consequences of the severe financial crises that have overtaken these "Tiger" countries since 1997.

The ferment in the development of health services in Asia and elsewhere during the 1960s and 1970s triggered major changes in World Health Organization (WHO) policies. The Alma-Ata Declaration on Primary Health Care was the culmination of the chain reaction. Apparently for tactical reasons, all the rich countries of the world signed the Declaration. But their retribution for such a daredevil declaration by the poor was swift and sharp. As if from nowhere, they "invented" the concept of Selective Primary Health Care (SPHC). A large number of concerned scholars categorically questioned the scientific validity of the concept, but all failed to make any impression on the exponents of SPHC.

Two main issues stand out from the awesome manifestation of power by the rich countries in imposing their will on the poor. First, although they lay claim to being the inheritors of the European Enlightenment, which involves a deep commitment to the scientific method, they have shown contemptuous disregard for these principles whenever scientific data stood in the way of their commercial and political interests. Second, the bulk of public health scholars, who proclaim their allegiance to the scientific method and commitment to social justice, found it worthwhile to remain silent while such active desecration took place.

As a follow-up, the ruling classes of the countries of the world exercised their control over international organizations such as UNICEF, WHO, and the World Bank (WB) to get them started with formulating some selected programs as "global initiatives." These were bristling with inconsistencies, contradictions, and patent scientific infirmities. Even the main planks for the formulation of these initiatives were profoundly flawed. First, how can one have a "prefabricated" global initiative given the extreme variations among and often within poor countries? Second, selection of health problems for action conformed more to the special interests of the rich countries than the poor. Third, a technocentric approach to problem-solving was adopted. Fourth, there is an obvious contradiction in the scientific bases of the claim that the suggested globe-embracing programs are cost-effective given the profound variations among and within countries. Fifth, by their very nature, international initiatives cannot promote community self-reliance. Sixth, there is the key question of dependence and sustainability; "donors" have used their tremendous influence on the pliable ruling classes of the poor countries to ensure that the ill-conceived, ill-designed, and ill-managed global initiatives are given priority over the ongoing work of the health organizations. Finally, and above all, these programs are the very antitheses of the Alma-Ata Declaration.

It is grimly ironic that soon after the leadership given by WHO and UNICEF in writing one of the brightest chapters in the history of public health practice, in the form of acceptance of the Alma-Ata Declaration by all countries of the world in 1978, the ruling classes should have started the international initiatives that opened one of the darkest chapters. By the early 1980s, UNICEF let loose a barrage of global initiatives on the poor countries of the world. WHO and the World Bank lent the full weight of their considerable prestige and influence in strengthening this menacing trend in public health thinking and action.

The outbreak of the AIDS epidemic in 1982, which later took the form of a pandemic, legitimately thrust on WHO the onerous responsibility for action on a global scale. It developed the Global Programme for AIDS. Despite the bewildering variations in the epidemiological behavior of the disease—including its complex social and cultural dimensions, which required a very flexible approach to program formulation—the program conformed to a set pattern which was principally shaped in the United States.

WHO's declaration of the tuberculosis problem as a "Global Emergency" was a totally surprising move. The database to justify such a sweeping declaration was virtually nonexistent. Ironically, allocation of overriding priority to the international initiatives, all down the line, led to the neglect of other services provided at the peripheral or grassroots level. This included tuberculosis work. WHO had also launched two other global programs with considerable fanfare. One was the diarrheal disease control programme and the other was meant to deal with acute respiratory infections in infants and children. Mercifully, these programs failed right at the take-off stage. The World Bank had joined WHO to launch yet another international initiative called the Safe Motherhood Initiative. This too has a very long way to go.

Some high-profile research administrators got together to set up a global Commission on Health Research and Development in 1987. Practice of Essential National Health Research was the centerpiece of the report. Even the very scanty materials produced to document progress in its implementation leave little doubt that the initiatives taken could have little impact on the strengthening of health services in the countries of the world.

It should come as no surprise that virtually every global initiative taken by WHO, UNICEF, and the World Bank since the promotion of SPHC by the rich countries suffered from serious infirmities. Remarkably, even when these infirmities were pointed out to the organizations, they failed even to enter into discussion on the issues raised or take any corrective measures. It is not necessary here to make a comprehensive critique of all the programs. Only three of the major ones—on immunization, AIDS, and tuberculosis—will be taken up here, and these only very briefly.

Even a very broad analysis of the process of policy and program formulation and implementation of the immunization program (EPI/UPI) reveals that the apical organizations of international public health have shown scant regard for some of the fundamental principles of public health practice. They have dared to launch a global/universal immunization program without caring to have a reasonably reliable epidemiological baseline. They have tended to "homogenize" the situation; even the 100 or so poor countries have widely varying parameters. When there is no epidemiological baseline, how is it possible to assess the epidemiological impact of the program? Without paying any attention to these vital infirmities, the WHO/UNICEF/WB establishment has not hesitated to repeat in 1998 the wild claim that: "Today 80 percent of the world's children receive this form of protection against childhood diseases during their first year of life."

WHO and UNICEF had joined the Government of India to get the Indian program systematically evaluated in 1989. The results were published in the form of a book, which was widely circulated. The findings seriously questioned the claims by WHO/UNICEF/WB. Another all-India study conducted in 1992–1993 revealed that at the national level as few as 35.4 percent of eligible children were fully protected, with the coverage hovering around 9 to 22 percent among many of the highly populated states with the poorest records of infant mortality. If the situation is so bad in India, the conditions prevailing in the world's least developed countries, and many more, will certainly not be any better.

The same trend was followed when WHO, along with a large number of U.N. agencies, set out to design the Global Programme for AIDS (GPA), which was principally directed toward the poor countries. Despite the efforts by WHO/WB officials and their Indian camp followers to control information and extensively spread unsubstantiated information, it was possible, as early as in 1992, to bring out a monograph that called into question a number of critical assumptions in the formulation of the GPA in India. This too was disregarded.

The justification given by WHO/WB for launching the Global Programme for Tuberculosis (GPT) is even more fantastic and incredibly contradictory. Out of the blue, as it were, in the early 1990s, WHO/WB sounded a maximum-alert alarm bell to proclaim that tuberculosis had become a "Global Emergency" and the GPT was the way of tackling it. Once again, despite putting on a cloak of secrecy while selling the program in India, a comprehensive document was prepared pointing out major epidemiological, sociological, economic, and organizational and management flaws in the GPT. But this did not deter the authorities from pushing on with their doomed venture.

A very large area is covered in this report to demonstrate how the imposition of an enormous, high-priority, prefabricated health service agenda of the rich countries on the poor ones has virtually decimated the somewhat promising growth of people-oriented health services in a country such as India. The overriding priority assigned to a Malthusian family planning program for over four decades by the ruling classes, both national and international, has also had a devastating impact on the growth and development of the health services in India. As described later, Nicholas Demerath, Sr., has given a well-documented account of the various ways in which India's family planning program has been influenced by the U.S. government (U.S. AID) and other U.S. agencies.

In conclusion, let me list just a few of the major areas of distortion. First, the "public health" practiced by exponents of the international initiatives is starkly ahistorical. Second, the scientific term "epidemiology," which forms the foundation of public health practice, has been grossly misused by the new breed of experts. Third, suppression of information, use of doctored information, spread of misinformation and disinformation, and lack of effective evaluation/surveillance are expected outcomes. Fourth, directors-general of two top public health institutions in India extended their support to the GPT, even though serious flaws in the program were repeatedly brought to their attention. After they endorsed the WHO/WB program, they found highly lucrative positions in WHO. This and many other such instances mark the rock-bottom of the moral and ethical standards of the parties concerned. Finally, those who are expected to be the conscience keepers of ethics and morality in public health practice are perhaps the worst offenders in inflicting such a humiliation on the poor peoples of the world.

The line of action for those few who still attach high value to intellectual and moral integrity, and are prepared to pay the sort of price mentioned by Navarro, emerges from the analysis presented in this chapter.

INTELLECTUAL FASCISM

Giving a personal account of studies on class, health, and quality of life during 1965–1997 in the United States, Vicente Navarro notes that "terms such as class, working class (not to mention class struggle), and just plain capitalism were dismissed as ideological. No serious scholar, aware of the penalty it would carry, would dare to use these terms." He has, to my mind very appropriately, used the term "intellectual fascism," whose "destructive powers could be even worse than the fascism I had experienced in Spain," to describe this phenomenon (see Chapter 1).

The intellectual fascism that is being practiced by the rich countries of the world against the poor, dependent countries is of an even more malignant variety. In the field of health, to subserve their commercial and political interests, the ruling classes of the rich and the poor countries have formed an unholy nexus which enables them to impose prefabricated, technocentric, dependence-producing health programs on the poor. These interests are so powerful that even most cogent, well-documented, and well-argued observations calling into question the scientific validity of these programs are simply ignored. When it comes to protecting their interests, the special brand of intellectuals/scholars who are hired by the ruling classes are ruthless, unscrupulous, and nonchalant (2). The Bhopal tragedy of 1984 (3–10), in which the Union Carbide Corporation got away so lightly with the consequences of its criminal neglect—which led to the spraying of the deadly chemical methyl isocyanate on hundreds of thousands of people, leading to the death of thousands and severe health damage to scores of thousands—provides an awe-inspiring case study demonstrating the power of the nexus of the ruling classes.

The ruling classes of the rich countries have also mobilized a number of international agencies and myriad bilateral and "voluntary" agencies or nongovernmental organizations to implement their agenda for action. Suppression of information, doctoring of information, misinformation, and disinformation have been freely used as means to push their agenda. Making use of the market-generated information revolution, they have employed the approach of social marketing (11, 12) to brainwash the helpless masses of the poor so as to sell their programs. The way in which the "experts" employed by the World Bank have twisted and distorted the meaning of health policy formulation almost beyond recognition, by bringing it down to the level of health financing (13), provides a startling instance of this new brand of scholarship from the rich countries.

Lest they "forget" the essence of health policy formulation by hiding themselves in the jungle of the massive, programmed information onslaught, it is worthwhile to "remind" the hired experts about some of its basic concepts. ("Man's struggle against oppression is a struggle between memory and forgetfulness"—Milan Kundera.) Health policy formulation is a highly complex process, requiring optimization of very complex systems. For this purpose, epidemiological, medical and public health, and organizational and management issues are visualized in their social, cultural, and economic contexts so as to crystallize them in the form of policies based on constitutional and other types of political commitments (14). The task becomes even more complicated when it has to be performed in the context of poor, non-Western countries. Western medicine is, after all, Western in origin. Furthermore, it has been grafted onto countries that already had ways of coping with their health problems. The grafting was done usually against the background of colonial conquest, as in the case of India, or in blatant imperialistic settings, as in the case of China. Differences in the ecology of diseases, availability of resources, cultural meanings of health problems and health practices, formulation of appropriate technologies and economic production practices are some other important determining factors. These considerations have received scant attention from the health policy experts hired by rich countries (15).

EARLY EFFORTS TO DEVELOP HEALTH SERVICES IN SOME ASIAN COUNTRIES

Countries of Asia

Asia is a huge continent, with wide variations in geography, population, ethnic composition, and political commitments. For instance, there are Japan and South Korea at one extreme, and Nepal, Bhutan, and Afghanistan at the other. Here I will discuss the role of foreign and international agencies and other organizations in health policy formulation in terms of those Asian countries occupying median positions. A very brief reference will be made to the cases of health service developments on the Indian subcontinent and in China to provide a setting for discussion. Together they account for more than two-fifths of the entire population of the world, and a much higher proportion of the world's poor. Besides, many of the observations made about India and China are also relevant, to varying degrees, to many other Asian countries in "median" positions. It also so happens that information available on development of health service systems in these other Asian countries is very scanty and often of rather unreliable quality.

Health Service Development on the Indian Subcontinent

The long experience of India in developing its health services has escaped the attention of scholars from the rich countries, of both the hired and the "progressive" varieties. Indeed, the former category has actively ostracized the indigenous scholarship, apparently to create "space" for justifying the agenda handed down to them by their paymasters; it has been a most virulent form of intellectual fascism. As pointed out by Navarro (1, 16), and earlier noted by John McKinlay (17) in a slightly different context, these scholars were actively ahistorical, apolitical, and atheoretical. Such an approach subserves the class interests of the rulers. Obviously, this normally would require considerable elaboration (e.g., 18), but in the present context I will present only a bare outline of India's experience.

The British inducted Western medicine in India in the wake of their colonial conquest in the latter half of the 18th century, primarily to strengthen their exploitative machinery—the army, the civil service, the European business class, and a wafer thin, uppermost crust of native collaborators (18). Reciprocally, this further weakened the native working class, which constituted more than 98 percent of the population. They were further pauperized due to colonial exploitation, thus further increasing the disease load, and were made to lose the indigenous coping mechanisms that they had developed over the course of centuries (18).

As a dialectic response, the people of India launched an anti-colonial freedom struggle, which became a mass movement, leading to the overthrow of the colonial rulers in 1947 (19). The reports of the National Health Sub-committee of the National Planning Committee of the Indian National Congress in 1940 (20) and the famous Bhore Committee (21) (which, incidentally, was spearheaded by "foreign" experts such as John Grant and Henry Sigerist) in 1946 provided the basis for the formation of a blueprint for building an egalitarian health service for free India.

After Independence, the ruling class, which had led the freedom struggle, was impelled by those of the working class to fulfill the promises it had made while mobilizing them for the struggle. This was the motive force for ushering in very ambitious health programs to cover the needs of the unserved and the underserved, even though the country faced massive problems—accentuated severalfold in the wake of Partition. A nationwide network of Primary Health Centres (22) for the rural population was established from 1952 to provide integrated health services to entire populations, as part of a still more ambitious Community Development Programme (23). The Primary Health Centres formed the sheet anchor for developing the other important facets of the health service system—for example, people-oriented manpower development (24–27), research (28, 29), regionalization of the health services (30), inclusion of the indigenous systems of medicine (31), and so on. Very well-designed public health research on tuberculosis conducted in India had a far-reaching influence on tuberculosis programs all over the world, including in the rich countries. This research showed that home treatment is as good as sanatorium treatment (32); that the BCG vaccine has little protective value, at least for adults (33, 34); that a substantial proportion of tuberculosis patients in a population were already seeking assistance at Primary Health Centres and other health institutions; and that sputum smear examination is the most reliable diagnostic tool (35–37).

The major political upheaval that followed imposition of the National Emergency in 1975–1977 was instrumental in adoption of the program of entrusting "people's health in people's hands" (38); using community health workers chosen by the people themselves has been another landmark. These movements culminated in enunciation of the National Health Policy in 1982 (39), which proclaimed that:

> The prevailing policy in regard to education and training of medical and health personnel, at various levels, has resulted in the development of a cultural gap between the people and the personnel providing care. The various health programmes have, by and large, failed to involve individuals and families in establishing a self-reliant community . . . the ultimate goal of achieving a satisfactory health status for all our people cannot be secured without involving the community in the identification of their health needs and priorities as well as in the implementation and management of various health and related programmes.

As discussed later, the approach adopted by the special brand of experts hired by the rich countries and their camp followers is diametrically opposed to that envisaged in the National Health Policy. Incidentally, as also pointed out by Navarro, the emphasis on democratization of community health services is also conspicuously missing in the approach adopted by the erstwhile "socialist countries" (including China) and those European countries that have set up national health services (see Chapter 1).

Health Service Development in China

The situation in China is entirely different from that in India. China had the most blatant form of imperialistic exploitation, as symbolized by the Opium Wars; feudal monarchy; the revolution of 1912; the KMT of Chiang Kai-shek and their pathetic, supplicant-level dependence relationship with the United States in almost all spheres; the Japanese war of aggression; the revolutionary movement by the Chinese Communist Party, including the fabled Long March, leading to its ultimate victory and establishment of the People's Republic of China in 1948.

The United Missions Medical College was China's first medical college, started in 1925 (40). In contrast, India had three government-funded medical colleges by 1835 (41). Significantly, the two major ideas in public health that emanated from China—the barefoot doctor and use of the traditional Chinese systems of medicine in the health services (42)—are the outcome of the revolutionary movement, particularly the Long March. Unfortunately, China also adopted the now well-discredited Soviet model, which failed to work. In sheer frustration, Mao had exclaimed, as late as in 1965 (43):

> Tell the Ministry of Public Health that it works only for fifteen percent of the population of the country and this fifteen percent is mainly composed of gentlemen while the broad masses of peasants do not get medical treatment . . . why not change its [Ministry of Public Health's] name into the Ministry of Urban Health, the Ministry of Gentlemen's Health or even the Ministry of Urban Gentlemen's Health?

Deng Xiaoping's move to promote "market socialism" dealt an almost deadly blow to the village commune system, which sustained the barefoot doctors. Even though critical of the Soviet model of health services, Navarro has also observed how the capitalist model adopted by post-Soviet Russia has led to a disastrous collapse of the health service system of that country. Almost grudgingly, he also concedes that "the same process is now underway in China" (see Chapter 1). It is a profound irony that, having brought about the collapse of the earlier socialist system, China is now asking for help from WHO's Division for Intensive Cooperation with Countries and Peoples in Greatest Need "to solve problems in health financing in connection with re-establishment of the country's Rural Cooperative Medical System" (44). China also created a most embarrassing situation for other countries when it accepted the World Bank/WHO-supported tuberculosis program with alacrity, turning a blind eye to the myriad scientific design flaws repeatedly pointed out by scholars from other countries (45–47). That China should now adopt an openly coercive policy of one-child families, while earlier it had described the dangers of population growth as a trait of the capitalist system, is yet another indication of grave flaws in its population policies and planning. Incidentally, no political leader would dare even to think of a similar approach for India, for fear of a backlash from the people.

The "Tiger" and Other Asian Countries

The state of Kerala in India (population 30 million) (48, 49) and Sri Lanka (population 16 million) (50) stand out sharply among all the low-income countries in having remarkably good health and mortality statistics. Other Asian countries such as Pakistan, Bangladesh, Malaysia, Indonesia, Thailand, and the Philippines have also made "progress" in developing their health services.

The four last-named countries were among those specially favored by the world capital for stimulating rapid economic growth during the past two decades. Even at the peak of their growth phase, serious flaws have been observed in their health services in the form of rapid privatization leading to gross overcapacity in private hospitals and almost criminal neglect of the poor because of further decay of the already inadequate health services for the poor (51). In a recent article, Barraclough (51) has described how the conglomerate corporations of Malaysia, which often own plantations, also run the leading private hospitals, using the latest technology. He points out the paradox that the workers on the rubber and palm estates are the poorest in the country. Conforming to laws originating in the colonial period, the services now being provided to them are "woefully inadequate and offer little more than treatment of minor ailments and first-aid." Given such a situation in 1994 in one particularly "successful" "Tiger" country, one can well imagine the health and health service consequences of the severe financial crises that have overtaken these "Tiger" countries since 1997. Although some of these consequences are already visible in the form of a sharp deterioration in health and mortality statistics and an acute scarcity and sharp rise in price of drugs, the full impact of the crises on the health service systems has yet to be systematically assessed.

THE ROAD TO ALMA-ATA AND THE RESPONSE OF THE RICH

The Alma-Ata Declaration: A Watershed in Public Health Practice

This very broad account of the evolution of health service systems in the two Asian giants, and a mere mention of the state of affairs in many other Asian countries, set the stage for understanding and analyzing the practice of intellectual fascism by a syndicate of the world's ruling classes, with those that are rich and powerful setting the agenda for action. The ferment in the development of health services in Asia and elsewhere in the world during the 1960s and 1970s triggered major changes in WHO policies. The Alma-Ata Declaration on Primary Health Care (52) was the culmination of the chain reaction. Health as a fundamental human right, community self-reliance, intersectoral action for health, social control over health services, use of appropriate technology, encouragement of traditional systems of medicine, essential drugs—these are some components of the Declaration. It also contained a detailed definition of Primary Health Care.

The Invention of Selective Primary Health Care

Apparently for tactical reasons, all the rich countries of the world signed the Alma-Ata Declaration even though it shook the very foundations of the conventional thinking on international public health as hitherto practiced by these countries. The Declaration marked a watershed. It was also clear to the rich countries that such a declaration of self-reliance by the poor peoples of the world was against their class interests. They saw its "subversive" character. In Chapter 1, Navarro describes how the use of such radical terminology as "class interests" has long been seen in the United States as "too ideological," with the enjoinment that such things have to be "value free"—forgetting that this is itself a most value-laden term. The retribution for such a daredevil act as the Alma-Ata Declaration was swift and sharp.

As if from "nowhere," the rich nations "invented" the concept of Selective Primary Health Care (53). The justification was that Primary Health Care was good, but was too ambitious; one therefore should be selective in choosing areas that are cost-effective. To legitimize such a fragile stand, they got hold of a very poorly designed, and even more poorly conducted and analyzed, study in Haiti. The principal author was then an "assistant clinical professor of medicine" at Harvard. Such a paper would have been rejected out of hand by even the poorest academic journal in a developing country. That it found ready acceptance for publication in the prestigious *New England Journal of Medicine* speaks volumes about the intensity of intellectual fascism that still prevails in the United States.

More than 80 scholars from schools of tropical medicine and other public health institutions in Europe and from the United States, Africa, and Asia gathered at Antwerp to discuss SPHC. In the Antwerp Declaration (54, 55) they categorically questioned the scientific validity of the concept. *Social Science and Medicine* (56) brought out a special issue with a detailed account of the deliberations at Antwerp. There were articles on the subject in the *Economic and Political Weekly* (Bombay) (57) and the *International Journal of Health Services* (58). *The Journal of the Indian Medical Association* (2) carried a leading article on the subject. All these and many others (e.g., 59–62) failed to make any impression on the exponents of SPHC. The latter went on to organize a high-profile meeting attended by top executives of WHO, UNICEF, the World Bank, and many other agencies, as well as like-minded persons who called themselves public health scholars, at Bellagio, Italy (63), thus getting a resounding endorsement for SPHC. After two years, they organized a similar meeting at Cartagena in Columbia (64) (called Bellagio-II) to get a similar endorsement.

Two main issues stand out from the awesome manifestation of power by the rich countries in imposing their will on the poor. First, although they lay claim to being the inheritors of the European Enlightenment, which involves a deep commitment to the scientific method, they have shown contemptuous disregard for these principles whenever scientific data stood in the way of their commercial and political interests. Second, despite the brave scholars who stood up to the bullies at Antwerp and at other forums, the bulk of public health scholars, who proclaim an allegiance to the scientific method and commitment to social justice, including the Alma-Ata Declaration, found it worthwhile to exercise discretion—the better part of valor. They remained silent on the most blatant desecration of scientific principles and methods, presumably to avoid the anger of the most powerful country and its camp followers. This brand of "intellectuals," who belong to the middle class and attained their positions of importance by putting on a mask of progressivism, can also be said to harbor at least some traits of intellectual fascism, which they try to hide deep within them. They too need to be exposed. Where were they when China started its program of enforcing the norm of a single-child family, or when Indira Gandhi imposed a National Emergency and let loose a reign of terror, and used force to sterilize millions of people against their will (65)? The Vietnam "war hero" and then President of the World Bank, Robert McNamara, visited India at that time and is on record praising India for its achievement in fighting the menace of population explosion (66).

LETTING LOOSE A BARRAGE OF INTERNATIONAL INITIATIVES

UNICEF's Primacy in Imposing International Initiatives

As a follow-up to acceptance of Selective Primary Health Care, the ruling classes exercised their control over international organizations such as UNICEF, WHO, and the World Bank to get them started with formulating some selected programs as "global initiatives" for implementation in the poor countries. The brief accounts of the evolution of health services in India and China and mention of some other Asian countries will provide the context for understanding how different has been the conceptualization, formulation, and implementation aspects of these initiatives undertaken by the triad (WHO, UNICEF, and the World Bank). On the basis of this description it is possible to list some major aspects of their actions.

1. Even the main planks for formulation of these initiatives were profoundly flawed. How can one have a "prefabricated" global initiative when one takes into account the extreme variations among and often within the poor countries? This very obvious determining factor escaped attention, or, more likely, was deliberately overlooked, when the initiatives were formulated. The situation bears an uncanny resemblance to the economic "rescue packages" of the International Monetary Fund (IMF).

2. Selection of health problems for action conformed more to the special interests of the rich countries than to the specific epidemiological situations in the various poor countries.

3. A technocentric approach to problem-solving was adopted, not because it provided the "optimal solution" (67, 68), but because this was "friendly" to the economic interests of the rich countries. The biotechnology, refrigeration, and drug industries, particularly in the private sector, are some examples. There was, besides, the opportunity for the creation of high-salaried employment in rich countries, for hirelings who could then exercise the enormous power bestowed on them to perform the jobs assigned by their paymasters.

4. There is an obvious contradiction in the specific bases of claims that the suggested globe-embracing programs are cost-effective, given the profound variations among and within countries. Presumably because of this, no serious efforts were made to assess cost-effectiveness at the time of program formulation. The claim of cost-effectiveness by once highly respected organizations such as WHO and UNICEF is an example of the blatant spread of almost manifest disinformation. The latest instance of this almost deliberate effort to avoid subjecting their

assumptions to objective evaluation comes from the failure of WHO/WB to set up reliable baseline data on "Annual Rate of Infection" (69) for monitoring the progress of the huge Global Programme for Tuberculosis which they had launched.

5. By their very nature, international initiatives cannot promote community self-reliance.

6. Because countries receive a considerable proportion of the funds from outside, there is the key question of dependence and sustainability—apart from the real danger of vulnerability to political exploitation by the "donors."

7. The "donors" have used their tremendous influence on the pliable ruling classes of the poor countries to get overriding priority assigned to the ill-conceived, ill-designed, and ill-managed global initiatives at the expense of the ongoing work of the health organizations. In India, for example, the primacy given to the programs pushed by the WHO/UNICEF/WB triad, along with an almost frenzied preoccupation with the family planning program, has had a devastating impact on almost every facet of organization, management, and growth of the health services infrastructure. In the case of China, as (under) stated by Navarro in Chapter 1, it was more an overt political decision by the oligarchic ruling class to shift investment away from the people-based health services; privatization was the slogan for socialist market orientation.

8. Above all, these programs are the very antitheses of the Alma-Ata Declaration and, in the case of India, of its National Health Policy (39), which envisaged "involving the community in the identification of its health needs and priorities as well as in the implementation and management of the various health and related programmes."

It is grimly ironic that soon after the leadership given by WHO and UNICEF in writing one of the brightest chapters in public health practice—acceptance of the Alma-Ata Declaration in 1978 by all countries of the world—the ruling classes should have started the international initiatives that opened one of its darkest chapters. The oppressed peoples of the world will have to pay yet another installment to their oppressors before their tormentors are again forced to admit their mistakes and to abandon their ill-conceived misadventures, so that the oppressed can then resume their long, grinding struggle toward access to people-oriented services for their populations (57). Using the hindsight of 1998, it is appalling to find so few who have had the courage of their convictions to call the bluff of the tormentors of the oppressed.

By the early 1980s, the triad of WHO, UNICEF, and the World Bank had started to give a global form to the grossly inadequate but politically and economically important concept of Selective Primary Health Care. UNICEF opened up a barrage of global initiatives on the poor countries of the world. WHO and the World Bank lent the full weight of their considerable prestige and influence in strengthening this menacing trend in public health thinking and action. At first, UNICEF came up with four areas for "special" attention in child health: Growth Monitoring, Oral Rehydration, Breast Feeding Promotion, and Immunization (GOBI) (70, 71). It was soon impelled to add to the list: Fertility Promotion, Feeding Programme, and Female Development, thus making it GOBI-FFF (72). Again, it had to backtrack and focus its attention only on immunization. This project was named the Universal Programme of Immunization (UPI) (73, 74), or simply the strengthening of WHO's pre-existing Extended Programme of Immunization (EPI) (75). It is not difficult to visualize the impact of such a fickle-minded approach on the world's utterly dependent, poorest of the poor countries. At a later stage, there was yet another turnaround, when one of the six diseases—poliomyelitis—was singled out for eradication from the globe (76, 77). Thus, the disturbing signals were already there on the quality of care and on the considerations that had gone into the triad's drawing up policies and plans for acting globally to fulfill the responsibility assigned to the three agencies in their respective constitutions.

In the world of the poor, with virtually no system even to record births and deaths, not to mention a dependable health information and evaluation system, "experts" hired by UNICEF, WHO, and many affluent countries of the world made the pronouncement that six immunizable diseases—tetanus, pertussis, diphtheria, tuberculosis, poliomyelitis, and measles—account for most deaths among infants. It was assumed that a massive program of vaccination against these six diseases would create a strong enough "herd immunity" to eliminate them as public health problems, if not totally eradicating them within five years, presumably as in the case of smallpox (74).

To cope with the mind-boggling task of immunizing hundreds of millions of infants, particularly those living under the most primitive conditions in extremely remote areas of the very large number of the world's poorest countries (where, incidentally, a much higher incidence of the six diseases would be expected), experts from UNICEF/WHO suggested an intensive program of mass communication, using the new technological advances. The globally telecast pop extravaganza organized by the Irish pop star Bob Geldof at London's Wembley Stadium in the form of "Band Aid," and later, a still bigger show at the same place under the label "World Aid" (12), are two outstanding instances of appeals to the "charitable instincts" of the rich to contribute to UNICEF's crusade against the six diseases "to save the lives of the poor." The rank hypocrisy of the over-affluent rich, throwing away hundreds of billions of dollars to sustain their vulgar "entertainment industry," could not have been more blatant. There were, incidentally, few protests from the concerned people of the world at this patently indecent insult to the poor by the rich. These are the modern-day Marie Antoinettes, the only difference being that their number has swollen to the hundreds of millions, brainwashed by the potent weapons provided by the so-called information revolution. UNICEF also hired experts from the marketing field and gave the name "social marketing" to these techniques used to "fight" its crusade against the six diseases. Indeed, in order to sell its ideas, particularly to the burgeoning proportion of the gullible, it claimed that the movement for immunization would lead to "mass mobilization" of the people of poor countries for other health and development work (11, 72).

As I will briefly mention later, the propaganda blitz let loose on the poor countries of the world to promote EPI/UPI has apparently been "forgotten" within a few years, because it has served the purpose for which it was generated. The informatics industry, moving fast on the information highways in the rich countries, has found new pastures for helping to launch new international crusades against other specific diseases (45). The experts also seem to have conveniently "forgotten" about the data that had seriously questioned the very bases of the program (54–62). They, too, seem to have moved on to new pastures, to carry on new crusades. Public health experts at WHO also fully endorsed the UNICEF initiative on EPI/UPI, and WHO undertook to use its far-flung organizational outreach in different countries to push this program (74–76). It has also undertaken the task of running the global program for eradicating poliomyelitis by 2000 (77).

The WHO Global Programme for AIDS (GPA)

The outbreak of the AIDS epidemic in 1982, which later took the form of a pandemic, legitimately thrust on WHO the onerous responsibility for action on a global scale. It developed the Global Programme for AIDS. Despite the bewildering variations in the epidemiological behavior of the disease, including complex social and cultural dimensions that required a very flexible approach to program formulation, the GPA conformed to a set pattern that was principally shaped in the United States (78). As pointed out later, this proved to be its Achilles' heel. At a later stage, implementation of the GPA was entrusted to an inter-agency U.N. organization called UNAIDS.

The WHO/WB Global Programme for Tuberculosis (GPT)

The World Health Organization's declaration of the tuberculosis problem as a "Global Emergency" was a totally surprising move. The database to justify such a sweeping declaration was virtually nonexistent. It has been accepted (e.g., 35–37, 79) worldwide for more than four decades that public health programs against tuberculosis are based on general health services, which are expected to take on the task of diagnosing and treating the bulk of tuberculosis cases in the poor countries. Ironically, allocation of overriding priority to the international initiatives, all down the line, led to the neglect of other services provided at the peripheral or grassroots level. This included tuberculosis work.

What made the very perpetrators of the decline in tuberculosis care work up such an intense concern for the disease as a public health problem is a useful case study for scholars interested in a more detailed study of the political economy of health services. One plausible explanation might be the sudden awakening to the problem in the United States and other rich countries when their AIDS epidemics activated the dormant primary foci in many persons with AIDS, and this led to spread of tuberculosis to others. This triggered alarm bells for the ruling class, which, in the course of its exponential polarization from the poor, has created a sterile/sanitized world for itself. An irrational and therefore very malignant fear of microbes struck terror in the hearts of the rich. One consequence of this mass hysteria against germs, which received support from the once sober and highly respected International Union Against Tuberculosis and Lung Disease (e.g., 45–47, 80), was that these unfounded fears (as will be elaborated later) took the entire world back a century to the days of the long-discarded single-etiology theory of diseases. What is worse, this observation on tuberculosis in the rich countries was extrapolated to the entire world. Already, as the AIDS epidemic seemed to attain a plateau in the rich countries, poor countries were singled out as the "rich" breeding grounds for a devastating spread of the AIDS pandemic. As almost a majority of the adult populations in these countries had acquired primary tubercle foci, a fear complex was actively generated to claim that this would lead to widespread outbreaks of tuberculosis, hence the declaration of the Global Emergency. Incidentally, subsequent experience has shown that both fears proved to be unfounded. Black Africa is very much there, in spite of the rapid phase of spread of AIDS; there is no tuberculosis epidemic even in this region. The incidence/prevalence of AIDS and tuberculosis is a tiny fraction of what was predicted by the WHO/WB experts in North Africa, in Central, West, South, Southeast, and East Asia, and in South America (81, 82). All these facts speak volumes about the technical competence of those who rule over the destiny of the world's health services, particularly in the poor regions.

Sticking tenaciously to the single-etiology theory, despite overwhelming evidence to the contrary, and the (virtual?) "reality" of the Global Emergency, a strategy was developed for the GPT. It consisted of making a massive effort to identify tuberculosis cases in entire populations, then subjecting them to Directly Observed Treatment with Shortcourse chemotherapy (DOTS) (83). Starting with China (45, 46), which did not find anything amiss in the DOTS approach, WHO and the World Bank have come together and managed to successfully "push through" this approach to the poor countries of the world.

WHO's Other Efforts to Launch Global Initiatives

The World Health Organization had also launched two other global programs with considerable fanfare. One was the Diarrheal Disease Control Programme (84), with Oral Rehydration Treatment as its centerpiece. The other program was meant to deal with acute respiratory infections in infants and children (85); it envisaged timely administration of antibacterial drugs to affected children, using paramedical staff in rural and urban areas. Despite the usual promotional efforts of WHO/UNICEF/WB, mercifully, these programs failed right at the take-off stage.

The World Bank had joined WHO to launch yet another international initiative: the Safe Motherhood Initiative (86). Child survival programs were later dovetailed with this initiative. Apart from the question of cost- effectiveness, the success of this initiative, like all the preceding ones, depended on the capacity of the health service systems to undertake the task envisaged in the program.

Global Initiative in Launching "Essential National Health Research"

Some high-profile research administrators, who had earlier headed many key research organizations/committees, both nationally and internationally, in 1987 got together to set up a global Commission on Health Research and Development (87). The report of the Commission, and an account of the subsequent follow-up action and its impact, provide an interesting administrative case study on the intellectual make-up of the key decision-makers who have dominated the field worldwide for the past three or more decades. While the Commission had a self-imposed deadline for its automatic "liquidation" within one year, it could not present the report until 1991. Practice of Essential National Health Research (ENHR) was the centerpiece of the report. The Commission took some more time to hold well-publicized seminars in different parts of the world to promote the report. It received warm endorsement from government leaders and most of academia throughout the world, including the prestigious Nobel Symposium (88). The Swedish Agency for Research Cooperation with Developing Countries (SAREC) (89) and the International Development Research Council of Canada (IDRC) (90) were among the foremost institutions to promote ENHR and the other recommendations. The then Executive Director of UNICEF proclaimed that "in future at least five per cent of UNICEF's budget will be devoted to research." This promise, incidentally, was never kept. SAREC and IDRC also agreed to provide funds for yet another proposal of the Commission to set up a two-year task force, with its office located in Geneva, to encourage developing countries to implement ENHR (88). The materials produced to document progress in the implementation of ENHR (88) leave little doubt that the initiatives could make little impact on the strengthening of health services in the countries of the world. The ENHR movement has not achieved anything more substantial than what was already done by WHO's Advisory Committees on Medical/Health Research at the global and regional levels.

SERIOUS INFIRMITIES IN THE GLOBAL INITIATIVES

It should come as no surprise that virtually every global initiative taken by WHO, UNICEF, and the World Bank since the promotion of Selective Primary Health Care by the rich countries suffered from serious infirmities. Remarkably, even when these infirmities were pointed out to the organizations, they failed even to enter into discussion on the issues raised, not to mention taking any corrective measures. That the infirmities were indeed serious is borne out by the fact that the programs consistently failed to yield the results expected of them. It is not necessary here to present a comprehensive critique of all the programs. Only three of the major ones—the EPI/UPI, GPA, and GPT—will be taken up, and only very briefly.

Even a very broad analysis of the process of policy and program formulation and implementation of EPI/UPI reveals that the apical organizations of international public health have shown scant regard for some of the fundamental principles of public health practice.

1. They have dared to launch a global/universal immunization program without caring to have reasonably reliable, global baseline epidemiological data (91). The specialty of epidemiology should have been the very soul of EPI/UPI. Its absence has made it "soul-less."

2. While using their patently unsubstantiated "estimates," they have tended to "homogenize" the situation even in the 100 or so poor countries, with their widely varying parameters affecting the incidence and prevalence of the six target diseases.

3. With no epidemiological baseline, how is it possible to assess the epidemiological impact of the program? It could well be argued, "from the other side," that the impact, if any, may have been due to the natural histories of the diseases over time.

4. No data have been produced to demonstrate the degree of effectiveness of the vaccines under the ecological/epidemiological conditions prevailing in the different countries.

5. No evidence has been produced to justify why the level of "herd immunity" has been fixed at 85 percent.

6. It is incredible that the program managers claimed that the programs could have been implemented "satisfactorily" in countries such as Chad and Niger, not to speak of Sudan, Somalia, and Sierra Leone, or Colombia, Ecuador or Guatemala. In Asia, Afghanistan, Nepal, Myanmar, Cambodia, and Laos provide the challenging examples. It requires stupendous logistical capabilities to ensure that an epidemiologically adequate proportion of infants receive potent doses of the vaccines in all the countries of the world.

Two academics, specializing in epidemiology, Vance Dietz from the Centers for Disease Control and Prevention and Felicity Cutts from the London School of Hygiene and Tropical Medicine, had an article published in the *International Journal of Health Services* (76) on evaluation of mass immunization campaigns on the basis of a literature review. The fact that not one of the epidemiological issues raised in the foregoing discussion—which, incidentally, have been published in that journal on more than one occasion—received any mention in their review gives a chilling picture of the depth to which the practice of public health principles has fallen during the past three decades. The authors explicitly mentioned that they "did not address the broader issue of comparing different approaches to the delivery of a strategy within the context of primary versus selective health care." Why? They did not even take up the broader epidemiological, sociological, and organizational and management issues raised, even when these issues fell within the severely limited range of the review. In their scheme of things, of course, issues concerning political economy and the less than academically acceptable role of international and other foreign agencies, including their own institutions, were considered "politically improper." Either they have become conditioned to follow the line laid down for them by the dominant intellectual group, or they did not dare deviate from this for fear of inviting retribution from them.

John Bland and John Clements (74) of the WHO/UNICEF/WB establishment have not hesitated to repeat the wild claim, as recently as 1998 in the World Health Forum, that "Today 80 percent of the world's children receive this form of protection against childhood diseases during their first year of life," even though overwhelming data have clearly pointed to the contrary.

It is remarkable, and to a considerable extent frustrating, that neither academics such as Dietz and Cutts nor program managers and experts such as Bland and Clements cared to take cognizance of the well-designed and well-conducted evaluation studies carried out in some of the poor countries by "local" scholars. Dietz and Cutts claimed that these findings did not come within the parameters they had (arbitrarily) set for their literature search. Bland and Clements "blindly" accepted the government data, without caring to question their validity and reliability. Indeed, Dietz and Cutts should have noticed that one of the "local" studies has more than once been discussed in some detail in the references cited by them. These two studies are briefly referred to below.

The EPI/UPI program of India, meant to last five years from 1985, was the largest in the world. WHO and UNICEF joined the Government of India to get the program systematically evaluated in 1989. The results were published in the form of a book, which was widely circulated (92). It showed that the immunization coverage was less than a fifth in the two-thirds of the population that account for most of the poor, as well as for most of the infant mortality in the country; the surveillance system was almost nonexistent. A similar situation existed for potency tests of the vaccines at the time of inoculation. The book described how reports of immunization coverage had been exaggerated by 100 percent or more to please the national and international officers responsible for administering the program. It also reported at least 56 recorded deaths due to the vaccination process itself. There was virtually no outcry, nationally or internationally, against this outrageous consequence of the program. Had even one such death taken place in a rich country, the entire program would have been halted. An in-depth study of the program in the State of West Bengal (93) has reinforced the findings of the national study.

All these startling findings made no impression; there was little follow-up action or correction of the records and reports. Another all-India study, the National Family Health Survey (94), was conducted with the involvement of the U.S. Agency for International Development (U.S. AID) and the East-West Centre at Honolulu in 1992–1993 (that is, well after "completion" of the time limit for the EPI/UPI). This study revealed that at the national level as few as 35.4 percent of eligible children were fully protected, with the coverage hovering around 9 to 22 percent among many of the highly populated states with the poorest records of infant mortality. In this survey, there was no study of the surveillance system, nor was there any check on the potency of the vaccines at the time of inoculation. Apparently, even these admittedly bare data, which called into question the effectiveness of EPI/UPI, did not receive the attention of Bland and Clements (74).

If the situation is so bad in the case of India, which has a fairly extensive network of health services at the grassroots level, the situation in Chad, Niger, and many countries mentioned earlier—as indeed, in all the world's least developed countries (44) and many more—will certainly not be any better. What then was the basis of the claims made by Bland and Clements?

That EPI/UPI was not a temporary aberration becomes clear when one subjects the other global initiatives to academic scrutiny. The "malady" seems to have pervaded the entire academic world of the ruling classes—as, for instance, was encountered by Navarro when he ventured to study class issues in public health policy studies in the 1960s (see Chapter 1). The same trend was followed when WHO, along with a large number of U.N. agencies, set out to design the Global Programme for AIDS, which was principally directed toward the poor countries. Incidentally, the first Union Budget (1992–1993) (13, 95, 96) after India submitted to the IMF conditionalities included a 20 percent slashing of the allocation to health services (including the tuberculosis program), without accounting for inflation. However, the World Bank and WHO "assisted" India in setting up the National AIDS Control Programme (NACP), which accounted for almost a fourth of the total allocation in the same financial year. Following the now familiar line, NACP was formulated under a veil of secrecy and no modification was permitted unless it got clearance from the World Bank Headquarters in Washington, D.C.

Despite the efforts by WHO/WB officials and their Indian camp followers to control information and extensively spread unsubstantiated information, it was possible as early as in 1992 to bring out the monograph *Combating AIDS as a Public Health Problem in India,* which questioned a number of critical assumptions in the formulation of GPA/NACP. Besides addressing matters of interdisciplinary methodology, the monograph raised issues of comparative epidemiology by taking up the history of syphilis. Interestingly, Steve Wing (97) has raised important issues in his article "Whose Epidemiology, Whose Health?" There is an interesting reference to a comparative analysis of the epidemiological behavior of AIDS and syphilis. Among the important issues raised were the profound implications of AIDS changing from a principally homosexual-associated disease in the rich countries to a heterosexual one in the poor countries; the key question of the natural history of the disease, as manifested in the differential incidence in different parts of the world, including among the countries of Sub-Saharan Africa; cultural, social, and economic parameters of the "risk groups" which determine the epidemiology of the disease; and the need for formulation of suitable strategies for different countries, based on these considerations (98–102). From the WHO/WB experts and program managers there was a stony silence on the issues raised in the monograph. Quite predictably, the objectives set before NACP in 1990 remain unfulfilled (103, 104), and very likely AIDS is set on a course broadly similar to that followed by syphilis as a public health problem in India over a period of time. A special category of sickness of mind appears to be afflicting the key decision-makers, who consciously hire an army of properly sanitized and brainwashed personnel to translate their "sick" ideas into action. For the oppressed classes and for all those who are prepared to take up their cause, it appears to be a re-enactment of a form of colonialism, with, as described by Navarro, fascistic overtones.

Justification given by WHO/WB for launching the Global Program for Tuberculosis is even more fantastic and incredibly contradictory. It is simply bizarre. Out of the blue, as it were, in the early 1990s, WHO/WB sounded the maximum-alert bell to proclaim that tuberculosis had become a "Global Emergency" and the GPT was the way to tackle that emergency (105, 106). How did a Global Emergency occur? What was WHO/WB doing when this emergency was building up? Is it reflected in the Epidemiological Intelligence Reports these agencies are constitutionally bound to present? Then why did they cut back the staff of the Tuberculosis Unit at the Headquarters in the 1980s to barely one (45)? Why didn't they raise an alarm when the national tuberculosis programs in the poor countries were being pushed onto the back burner to create "space" for high-priority programs such as EPI/UPI or NACP, with the already crippled health services reeling under the impact of brutal cuts imposed by orders of the IMF? This would be a comical drama had it not been so tragic, costing the lives of hundreds of thousands of the poor, whose voices were stifled by the ruling classes.

A streak of steely determination on the part of WHO/WB in imposing the prefabricated, DOTS-driven agenda of the GPT is reflected in the leading presentation of a *World Health Forum* Round Table, which gives the pre-eminent position to DOTS (83). That even the conversion rates claimed for the new spectrum of drugs used in DOTS are nothing startling is exposed by comments made by the veteran tuberculosis worker of the old school, John Crofton, who was a participant in this Round Table Discussion (79, 83). He stated "We demonstrated in Edinburgh in the 1950s that 100 percent cure of pulmonary tuberculosis, with no relapse, could be a reasonable aim (even with the drugs then available: streptomycin, isoniazid and para-amino salicylic acid)."

The GPT was particularly painful for tuberculosis workers in India, who have been instrumental in making such a mark in tuberculosis research and action worldwide over the past four decades. A meeting of key tuberculosis workers called by the Tuberculosis Association of India and the Government of India in 1992 to discuss the poor state of the country's National Tuberculosis Programme came out with well-argued and eminently implementable lines of action (107). Once again, a comprehensive document was prepared pointing out major epidemiological, sociological, economic, and administrative flaws in the GPT (108). To initiate dialogues, this too was extensively circulated to various agencies by the Voluntary Health Association of India, specifically including the chief executives of WHO, UNICEF, and the World Bank and aid missions of some of the major "donors." However, as in the previous cases, they remained unmoved; they refused to enter into discussion on scientific aspects of the program. A detailed account of the efforts made to bring them round to scientific discussions is also included in this document (108).

The cloak of secrecy shrouding the "selling" of the program to India has been a particularly unpleasant feature (108). The WHO/WB experts actively avoided entering into discussion with their counterparts at the National Tuberculosis Institute, Bangalore, and others actively involved in the conceptualization, formulation, and implementation of India's National Tuberculosis Programme. Instead, they interacted extensively with the then director-general of the Indian Council of Medical Research, who had been a tuberculosis microbiologist, and the then director-general of health services of the Government of India, who was a specialist in orthopedics. Both these functionaries were later offered positions in the South-East Asian Regional Office of WHO.

CONCLUSIONS: A FRIGHTENING SPECTACLE OF DISTORTION OF THE PRINCIPLES AND PRACTICE OF INTERNATIONAL PUBLIC HEALTH BY WHO, UNICEF, AND THE WORLD BANK

A very large area has been covered in this chapter to demonstrate how imposition of an enormous, high-priority, prefabricated health service agenda by the rich countries on the poor ones has virtually decimated the somewhat promising growth of people-oriented health services in a country such as India. Poor people will have to struggle for their right to access to services that are specifically designed to conform to their epidemiological, sociological, cultural, and economic requirements. For this purpose, they will not only have to fight the misconceived and mismotivated interventions in the form of international initiatives; their struggle will also include restructuring of the entire health/health service system to be in tune with their requirements. This will be a long, grinding struggle.

It may also be mentioned in passing that the overriding priority assigned to a Malthusian family planning program for over four decades by the ruling classes, both national and international (109–116), has also had a devastating impact on the growth and development of health services in India (114). In his book *Birth Control and Foreign Policy* (117), Nicholas Demerath, Sr., has given a well-documented account of the various ways in which India's family planning program has been influenced by the U.S. Government (U.S. AID) and other U.S. agencies, such as the Population Council, the Ford Foundation, the Population Crisis Committee, the Council of Foreign Relations, and programs sponsored by numerous universities, church organizations, the International Planned Parenthood Federation, and other voluntary associations. So powerful has been the population lobby in the United States that it forced the publishers, Harper and Row, to hastily withdraw Demerath's book from bookstore shelves all over the world. It has now become a collector's item.

From the standpoint of sociology of knowledge, it is interesting to note that no other scientific specialty, not even the cousins of public health such as clinical medicine/surgery, microbiology, and health statistics, has undergone such a far-reaching distortion. What a macabre situation, reflecting the nature of international and national power plays of our time. This is indeed the darkest chapter in the history of public health. In conclusion, five major areas of such distortion are summarized.

1. The "public health" practiced by exponents of the international initiatives is starkly ahistorical (16, 17). They seem to consider themselves the inventors of the wheel. So carried away were they with the "new" thinking injected into their heads by the ruling class that they seemed to have no use for the pioneering work in public health done in earlier years by many profound and dedicated scholars. C. E. A. Winslow's classic definition of public health way back in 1920 (118); Henry Sigerist's emphasis on the history of medicine (119–121) to develop a perspective for building health services, as in the report of India's Bhore Committee (21); John Grant's efforts to promote regionalization of health services and take public health research and practice to rural field stations (40, 122); the pioneering works of Rene Sand (123), John Ryle (124), and Iago Galdston (125) in giving content to the important specialty of social medicine; John Gordon's pathbreaking field research at Khanna in India on the epidemiology of child mortality and morbidity (126); Hugh Leavell's insightful ideas on the development of strategies for intervention in the epidemiological behavior of a health problem based on analysis of its natural history of disease in an individual (127–129); Edward McGavran's exposé on an epidemiological approach to solving a public health problem (130); Milton Roemer's contributions to health manpower development (131); George Foster's pioneering work on medical anthropology (132); P. V. Benjamin and Halfdan Mahler's dedicated efforts to establish the National Tuberculosis Programme in India (35) and the latter's role in getting the Alma-Ata Declaration on Primary Health Care all over the

world—these are but a few of the works of just some of the pioneers. The public health experts hired by WHO/WB/UNICEF have been selectively bred and properly programmed to be unaware, or at least to pretend to their paymasters that they are unaware, of the work of such pioneers.

2. The scientific term "epidemiology," which forms the foundation of public health practice, has been grossly misused by the new breed of experts. On the basis of the unrepresentative nature of the data used and their highly questionable reliability and validity, and the very limited data on causative relationship, validity and reliability of impact measurement, and the time trends, we can reject out of hand the scientific bases of almost all the international initiatives taken by the triad. Epidemiology, besides, includes the crucial areas of natural histories of diseases over time (133–139) and in the individual, as emphasized by Leavell (128). The experts have chosen simply to ignore other important areas, such as the social meaning of epidemiological data, the politics and political economy of health, and concepts of health administration elaborately developed in poor countries like India for over six decades (18, 129). In their zeal to sell their wares, they have also grossly distorted the concept of health economics, by confusing it with health financing (13). This amounts to practice of public health quackery. A similar fate was meted out to a well-established research tool—operational research (67, 68, 140–146). Developed in the course of World War II, it has very specific connotations and has enormous application to public health practice, as it seeks to optimize complex systems. These specifications too were simply ignored, and operational research has been grossly vulgarized (e.g., 69).

3. Suppression of information, use of doctored information, spread of misinformation and disinformation, and lack of effective evaluation/surveillance are expected outcomes when programs are meant to serve power managers, required by their paymasters to satiate the ever increasing hunger of the marketplace.

4. Directors-general of two top public health institutions in India extended their support to the GPT, even though serious flaws in the program were repeatedly brought to their notice. After they endorsed the WHO/WB program, they found highly lucrative positions in WHO. It is not necessary to speculate here about other instances. This marks the rock-bottom of the moral and ethical standards of the practices of the parties concerned.

5. Those who are expected to be the conscience keepers of ethics and morality in public health practice—teachers in public health schools/institutes, key public health administrators in national and international institutions, nongovernmental organizations, and political leaders/activists responsible for safeguarding and promoting the health of the people—are perhaps the worst offenders in inflicting such humiliation on the peoples of the world. Apparently attracted by the financial rewards, many of these professionals actively associated themselves with the not so ethical and moral ventures. Many others looked the other way, fearing retribution for exclaiming that the emperor had no clothes. And there must have

been a very substantial number of this "intelligentsia" who could not move themselves to find out what was happening. The situation certainly did not compare in depth with that in Hitler's Germany or even Franco's Spain, but the resemblance is uncanny. It shows how cheaply the leaders of the profession can be bought, to lend their support for patently unscientific, unethical, and immoral programs which have cost literally hundreds of thousands of lives of the world's poor.

The line of action for those few who still attach a high value to intellectual and moral integrity, and are prepared to pay the sort of price mentioned by Navarro (1), emerges from the analysis made in this report. The Indian subcontinent and China must take the responsibility for rediscovering their lost heritage, to set the tone for alternative, people-oriented health services for the long-exploited, deprived peoples of the world.

REFERENCES

1. Navarro, V. A historical review (1965–1997) of studies on class, health, and quality of life: A personal account. *Int. J. Health Serv.* 28(3): 389–406, 1998.
2. Banerji, D. Hidden menace in the Universal Child Immunization Programme. *J. Indian Med. Assoc.* 84(8): 229–232, 1986.
3. Indian Council of Medical Research. *Projectisation of ICMR Supported Research at Gandhi Medical College, Bhopal and at Other Collaborating Institutes.* New Delhi, 1985.
4. Medico Friend Circle. *The Bhopal Disaster Aftermath: An Epidemiological and Socio-medical Survey.* New Delhi, 1985.
5. Morehouse, W., and Subramanian, M. *The Bhopal Tragedy.* CGPA, New York, 1987.
6. Sadgopal, A. *Comments on ICMR's Epidemiological Report of the Gas-Exposed Localities of Bhopal.* Submitted to the Supreme Court Committee, New Delhi, June 28, 1986.
7. Indian Council of Medical Research. Scientific studies on Bhopal gas victims: Part-A. *Indian J. Med. Res.* 86(Suppl), 1987.
8. Narayana, T. *The Health Impact of the Bhopal Disaster: An Epidemiological Perspective.* LSHIM, London, 1987.
9. Banerji, D. Bhopal tragedy and Sarkari scientists. *Econ. Polit. Wkly.* 20(32): 1330, 1985.
10. Banerji, D. An epidemiological and sociological study of the Bhopal tragedy: A preliminary communication. *Medico Friend Circle Bull.* 114, June 1985.
11. Manhoff, R. K. Social marketing and nutrition education: A pilot project in Indonesia. *Assignment Children* 65/68: 95–113, 1984.
12. Grant, J. P. Marketing child survival. *Assignment Children* 65/68: 3–9, 1984.
13. World Bank. *Health Sector Financing: Coping with Adjustment Opportunities for Reforms.* Population and Human Resources Division, Washington, D.C., 1992.
14. Banerji, D. *A Socio-cultural, Political and Administrative Analysis of Health Policies and Programmes in India in the Eighties: A Critical Appraisal,* p. 9. Lok Paksh, New Delhi, 1990.

15. Banerji, D. Social and cultural foundations of health service systems of India. *Inquiry* 12(2, Suppl.): 70–85, 1975.
16. Navarro, V. Comment: Whose globalisation? *Am. J. Public Health* 88(5): 742–743, 1998.
17. McKinlay, J. B. *Issues in the Political Economy of Health Care.* Tavistock, London, 1984.
18. Banerji, D. *Landmarks in the Development of Health Services in the Countries of South Asia,* pp. 29–53. Nucleus for Health Policies and Programmes, New Delhi, 1997.
19. Kulke, H., and Ruthermond, D. *A History of India*, pp. 236–316. Routledge, London, 1990.
20. National Planning Committee, Sub-committee on National Health (Sokhey Committee). *Report*, edited by K. T. Shah. Vora, Bombay, 1948.
21. Government of India, Health Survey and Development (Bhore) Committee. *Report* (Bhore Committee), Vol. IV. Manager of Publications, Delhi, 1946.
22. Dutt, P. R. *Rural Health Services in India: Primary Health Centres,* Ed. 2. Central Health Education Bureau, New Delhi, 1965.
23. Bhattacharya, S. N. *Community Development: An Analysis of the Programme in India.* Academic Publishers, Calcutta, 1970.
24. Taylor, C. E., et al. *Doctors for the Villages: Study of Rural Internship in Seven Medical Colleges.* Asia Publishing House, Bombay, 1978.
25. Banerji, D. Social orientation of medical education in India. *Econ. Polit. Wkly.* 8: 485–488, 1973.
26. Government of India, Group on Medical Education and Support Manpower. *Health Services and Medical Education: A Programme for Immediate Action.* Ministry of Health and Family Planning, New Delhi, 1975.
27. Government of India, Central Health Council and Central Family Welfare Council. *National Medical and Health Education Policy.* Agenda Item No. 3. Ministry of Health and Family Welfare, New Delhi, 1981.
28. Pandit, C. G. *Fifty Years of Progress: Indian Research Fund Association and ICMR.* Indian Council of Medical Research, New Delhi, 1961.
29. Pandit, C. G. *My World of Preventive Medicine.* Indian Council of Medical Research, New Delhi, 1981.
30. Government of India, Health Survey and Planning (Mudaliar) Committee. *Report.* Ministry of Health, New Delhi, 1962.
31. Government of India, Central Council of Health. *Indian System of Medicine and Homeopathy.* Agenda Item No. 6. Ministry of Health and Family Planning, New Delhi, 1974.
32. Tuberculosis Centre, Madras. A concurrent comparison of home and sanatorium treatment of pulmonary tuberculosis in India. *Bull. World Health Organ.* 29: 5, 1959.
33. Baily, G. V. J. Trial of BCG vaccines in South India for tuberculosis prevention. *Indian J. Med. Res.* 72 (Suppl.), July 1980.
34. World Health Organization. *BCG Vaccination Policies: Report of a WHO Study Group.* WHO Technical Report Series Number 652. Geneva, 1980.
35. Banerji, D. A social science approach to strengthening India's National Tuberculosis Programme. *Indian J. Tuberculosis* 40: 61–82, 1993.

36. Nagpaul, D. R. District Tuberculosis Programme in concept and outline. *Indian J. Tuberculosis* 14(4): 186–198, 1967.
37. Banerji, D. Tuberculosis as a problem of social planning in India. *NIHAE Bull.* 4(4): 9–25, 1971.
38. Government of India. *Annual Report 1977–78.* Ministry of Health and Family Welfare, New Delhi, 1978.
39. Government of India. *Statement of National Health Policy.* Ministry of Health and Family Welfare, New Delhi, 1982.
40. Siepp, C. (ed.). *Health Care for the Community: Selected papers of Dr. John B. Grant.* Johns Hopkins University Press, Baltimore, Md., 1963.
41. Ramasubban, R. *Public Health and Medical Research in India: Their Impact During the British Colonial Policy.* SAREC Report No. 4. SAREC, Stockholm, 1982.
42. Sidel, V. W., and Sidel, R. The health care delivery system in the People's Republic of China. In *Health by the People,* edited by K. N. Newell, pp. 1–13. WHO, Geneva, 1975.
43. Lampton, D. N. *The Politics of Medicine in China: The Policy Process, 1949–1977.* Dowson, Folkstone, England, 1977.
44. Jancloes, M. The poorest first: WHO's activities to help the people in greatest need. *World Health Forum* 19(2): 182–187, 1998.
45. World Health Organization Tuberculosis Unit. *First Programme Report (1989–90) and Future Plan (1991–1995).* Geneva, 1991.
46. World Health Organization. *Tuberculosis Programme: Report of the Second Meeting of the Coordination, Advisory and Review Group.* WHO/TVS/CARG/91.4. Geneva, 1991.
47. World Health Organization. *WHO Report on Tuberculosis Epidemics, 1995.* WHO TB/95/183. Geneva, 1995.
48. Mari Bhat, P. N., and Irudayarajan, S. Demographic transition in Kerala. *Econ. Polit. Wkly.* 28(23), 1992.
49. Jagadeesan, C. K. Exploring an enduring myth: The 'Kerala Phenomenon.' *Health for the Millions* 23(2): 13–15, 1997.
50. World Health Organization. *Intersectoral Linkage and Health Development,* edited by G. Gunatillake. WHO Offset Publication No. 83. Geneva, 1984.
51. Barraclough, S. Growth of corporate private hospitals in Malaysia: Policy contradictions in health system pluralism. *Int. J. Health Serv.* 27(4): 643–660, 1997.
52. World Health Organization. *Primary Health Care: Report on the International Conference on Primary Health Care, Alma-Ata, USSR, September 6–12, 1978.* Geneva, 1978.
53. Walsh, J. A., and Warren, K. S. Selective primary health care: An interim strategy for disease control for developing countries. *N. Engl. J. Med.* 301: 967–974, 1979.
54. Institute of Tropical Medicine, Antwerp. *Proceedings of the Meeting on Selective Primary Health Care, November 29–30, 1985.* Antwerp, 1985.
55. Institute of Tropical Medicine. *Manifesto.* Antwerp, 1985.
56. Editorial. The debate on selective or comprehensive primary health care. *Soc. Sci. Med.* 26(9): 877–878, 1988.
57. Banerji, D. Technocentric approach to health: Western response to Alma Ata. *Econ. Polit. Wkly.* 21(28): 1233–1234, 1986.

58. Banerji, D. Crash of the Immunization Programme: Consequences of a totalitarian approach. *Int. J. Health Serv.* 20(3): 501–510, 1990.
59. Grodos, D., and de Bethune, X. Les interventions sanitairs sélectives: Un piège pour les politiques des santé du tiersmonde. *Soc. Sci. Med.* 20: 879, 1988.
60. Newell, K. N. Selective primary health care: The counterrevolution. *Soc. Sci. Med.* 26(9): 903–906, 1988.
61. Wisner, B. GOBI versus PHC? Some dangers of selective primary health care. *Soc. Sci. Med.* 26(9): 693–699, 1988.
62. Banerji, D. Primary health care: Selective or comprehensive. *World Health Forum* 5: 312–315, 1984.
63. Rockefeller Foundation. *Protecting the World's Children: Vaccines and Immunization Within Primary Health Care, Conference Proceedings, Bulletin I.* New York, 1984.
64. Rockefeller Foundation. *The Task Force for Child Survival: Protecting World's Children, Bellagio II.* New York, 1986.
65. Banerji, D. Will forcible sterilisation be effective? *Econ. Polit. Wkly.* 11(18): 665–668, 1976.
66. Government of India. *Centre Calling* XII: 4–5, April-May 1977.
67. Churchman, C. W., et al. *Introduction to Operation Research.* John Wiley, New York, 1957.
68. Andersen, S. Operations research in public health. *Public Health Rep.* 79(4), 1964.
69. Government of India, Tuberculosis Division, Directorate General of Health Services. *National Tuberculosis Control Programme: Current and Revised Strategy: A Brief.* Ministry of Health and Family Welfare, New Delhi, 1995.
70. Grant, J. P. Child survival and development revolution. *Assignment Children* 61/62(1): 21–31, 1983.
71. Mandl, P. E. Achieving nation-wide programme coverage: Innovative strategies and methods. *Assignment Children* 65/68, 1984.
72. Vittachi, V. T. CSDR: Dialectics of development. *Assignment Children.* 69/72: 19–31, 1985.
73. Grant, J. P. Universal child immunization by 1990. *Assignment Children* 69/72: 3–11, 1985.
74. Bland, J., and Clements, J. Protecting the world's children: The story of WHO's immunization programme. *World Health Forum* 19(2): 162–173, 1998.
75. World Health Organization. 41st World Health Assembly. *World Health Forum* 3: 470–480, 1980.
76. Dietz, V., and Cutts, F. Use of mass campaigns in the Extended Programme of Immunization: A review of reported advantages and disadvantages. *Int. J. Health Serv.* 27(4): 767–790, 1997.
77. Mann, J. Global AIDS: Epidemiology, impact, projections, global strategy. In *AIDS: Prevention and Control: World Summit of Ministers of Health on Programmes for AIDS Prevention,* Jointly Organized by WHO and the United Kingdom, 26–28 January, 1988, pp. 3–13. WHO, Geneva, 1988.
78. Crofton, J. Don't let us wait another 40 years: Discussion on the Round Table on 'Tuberculosis control: Is DOTS the breakthrough of the 1990s?' *World Health Forum* 18(3–4): 233–234, 1997.

79. World Health Organization. *Expert Committee on Tuberculosis: Eighth Report.* Geneva, 1964.
80. Fox, W. Tuberculosis in India: Past, present and future. *Indian J. Tuberculosis* 37: 175–213, 1990.
81. Banavalikar, J. N., et al. HIV seropositivity in hospitalized pulmonary tuberculosis patients in Delhi. *Indian J. Tuberculosis* 44(1): 17–20, 1997.
82. Banerji, D. *Combating AIDS as a Public Health Problem in India.* Voluntary Health Association of India and Nucleus for Health Policies and Programmes, New Delhi, 1992.
83. Kochi, A. Round Table: Tuberculosis control—is DOTS the breakthrough of the 1990s? *World Health Forum* 18(3–4): 225–232, 1997.
84. World Health Organization and UNICEF. *The Management of Diarrhoea and Use of Oral Rehydration Therapy*, Ed. 2, pp. 1–15. A Joint WHO/UNICEF Statement. Geneva, 1985.
85. World Health Organization. *Programme for Control of Acute Respiratory Infections.* Programme Report WHO/RI 89(3). Geneva, 1989.
86. World Health Organization. *Maternal Care for Reduction of Perinatal and Neonatal Mortality.* A Joint WHO/UNICEF Statement. Geneva, 1986.
87. Commission on Health Research and Development. *Health Research: Essential Link to Equity and Development.* Oxford University Press, New York, 1990.
88. Council for Health Research for Development. COHERD/ENHR Evaluation in Progress. *Newsletter COHERD* 6: 2, July–September 1996.
89. Swedish Agency for Research Cooperation with Developing Countries. *Annual Report 1988–89.* Stockholm, 1989.
90. International Development Research Centre, Canada. *Twenty Years of Development Through Research.* Ottawa, 1990.
91. Government of India. *Universal Immunization Programme by 1990: Report of a Task Force.* Ministry of Health and Family Welfare, New Delhi, 1984.
92. Gupta, J. P., and Murali, I. *National Review of the Immunization Programme in India.* National Institute of Health and Family Welfare, New Delhi, 1989.
93. Banerji, D. *National Review of Immunization: The Case of West Bengal.* Centre of Social Medicine and Community Health, Jawaharlal Nehru University, New Delhi, 1989.
94. International Institute of Population Studies. *National Family Health Survey in India: An Introductory Report.* Bombay, 1994.
95. Tuasidhar, V. B. Expenditure compression and health sector analysis. *Econ. Polit. Wkly.* 27(45), 1993.
96. Duggal, R. Public health budgets: Recent trends. *Radical Health* 1(3): 177–182, 1995.
97. Wing, S. Whose epidemiology, whose health? *Int. J. Health Serv.* 28(2): 241–252, 1998.
98. Mann, J. [Quoted in] Women and AIDS: The unprotected sex. *Women's Health J.*, April–June 1990.
99. Mann, J. Global AIDS: Critical issues in the prevention in the 1990s. *Int. J. Health Serv.* 21(3): 553–559, 1991.
100. Moss, A. R., and Baccheti. Natural history of HIV infection. *AIDS* 3: 55–61, 1989.
101. Peterman, T. A., et al. Epidemiology of AIDS *Epidemiol. Rev.* 7: 1–21, 1985.

102. World Health Organization. *Global Programme on AIDS: Current and Future Dimensions of the HIV/AIDS Pandemic. A Capsule Summary.* WHP/GPA/RES/SFI/92.1. Geneva, 1992.
103. Editorial. *Health for the Millions* 22(6): 1, 1996.
104. Banerji, D. AIDS threat to India: A response. *Health for the Millions* 22(6): 23–27, 1996.
105. Anil, P. TB: A global emergency? In *A National Consultation on Tuberculosis,* pp. 22–23. Voluntary Health Association of India, New Delhi, 1994.
106. Jhunjhunwala, B. C. Efficacy of the Revised National Tuberculosis Programme. In *National Consultation on Tuberculosis,* pp. 12–21. Voluntary Health Association of India, New Delhi, 1994.
107. Nagpaul, D. R. Editorial: Surajkund deliberations. *Indian J. Tuberculosis* 39: 1–2, 1992.
108. Banerji, D. *Serious Implications of the Proposed Revised National Tuberculosis Programme for India.* Voluntary Health Association of India and Nucleus for Health Policies and Programmes, New Delhi, 1997.
109. Banerji, D. Population planning in India: National and foreign priorities. *Int. J. Health Serv.* 3(4), 1973.
110. Banerji, D. Will forcible sterilization be effective? *Econ. Polit. Wkly.* 11(18): 665–668, 1976.
111. Community response to the intensified family planning programme. *Econ. Polit. Wkly.* 12(6–8): 261–266, 1977.
112. Banerji, D. Family planning in the nineties. *Econ. Polit. Wkly.* 27: 883–887, 1992.
113. Minkler, M. Thinking the unthinkable: The prospects of compulsory sterilization in India. *Int. J. Health Serv.* 7(2): 237–248, 1977.
114. Banerji, D. Health services and population policies. *Econ. Polit. Wkly.* 11(31–33): 1247–1252, 1976.
115. Banerji, D. India's forgotten people and the sickness of the public health service system: A prescription for the malady—A summary in three parts. *Health For The Millions* 23(3–5), 1998.
116. Bergstrom, S. Welfare as a need in Indian population policy. *Tropical Doctor.* Pt. 1: 182–184, October 1982.
117. Demerath, N. J. *Birth Control and Foreign Policy.* Harper and Row, New York, 1976.
118. Winslow, C. E. A. The untilled fields of public health. *Science* 51(8): 23–33, 1920.
119. Marti-Ibanez, F. *Henry Sigerist on the History of Medicine.* MD Publications, New York, 1960.
120. Sigerist, H. E. *Civilization and Disease.* Cornell University Press, Ithaca, N.Y., 1943.
121. Sigerist, H. E. *History of Medicine.* Oxford University Press, New York, 1961.
122. Grand, J. B. International planning of organizations of medical care. In *Health Care for the Community: Selected Papers of Dr. John B. Grant,* edited by C. Siepp. Johns Hopkins University Press, Baltimore, Md., 1963.
123. Sand, R. *The Advance of Social Medicine.* Staples Press, New York, 1980.
124. Ryle, J. A. *Changing Disciplines.* Oxford University Press, London, 1948.
125. Galdston, I. *The Meaning of Social Medicine.* Harvard University Press, Cambridge Mass., 1954.
126. Wyon, J. B., and Gordon, J. *The Khanna Study: Population Problem in Rural Punjab.* Harvard University Press, Cambridge, Mass., 1971.

127. Leavell, H. R. Levels of application of prevention medicine. In *Preventive Medicine for the Doctor in his Community: An Epidemiological Approach,* edited by H. R. Leavell and E. G. Clerk, pp. 14–38. McGraw-Hill, New York, 1965.
128. Leavell, H. R. Basic unity of private practice and public health. *Am. J. Public Health* 43: 1501–1506, 1953.
129. Leavell, H. R. Health administrator in the making. *NIHAE Bull.* 1: 15–19, 1968.
130. McGavran, E. G. What is public health? *Can. J. Public Health* 441–451, 1953.
131. Fulop, T., and Roemer M. I. *International Development of Health Manpower Policy.* WHO, Geneva, 1982.
132. Foster, G. M. *Medical Anthropology.* John Wiley, New York, 1978.
133. Dubos, R., and Dubos, J. *The White Plague.* Little Brown, Boston, 1952.
134. Dubos, R. *Mirage of Health, Utopias, Progress and Biological Change.* Anchor Books, New York, 1959.
135. McDermott, W. Demography, culture and economics and the evolutionary stages of medicine. In *Human Ecology and Public Health,* Ed. 4, edited by E. D. Kilborne and W. G. Smille, pp. 7–28. Macmillan, London, 1969.
136. McKeown, T. *Role Medicine: Dream, Mirage or Nemesis?* Nuffield Provincial Hospitals Trust, London, 1976.
137. Grzybowski, S. Epidemiology of tuberculosis with particular reference to India. *Indian J. Tuberculosis* 42: 195–200, 1995.
138. Chakraborty, A. K. Tuberculosis situation in India: Measuring it through time. *Indian J. Tuberculosis* 40: 215–226, 1993.
139. Grigg, E. R. N. Arcana of pulmonary tuberculosis. *Am. Rev. Tuberculosis Pulmonary Dis.* 78: 151–172; 426–453; 583–603, 1958.
140. Mishra, B. D. *Organization for Change: A Systems Analysis of Family Planning in Rural India.* Radient Publishers, New Delhi, 1982.
141. World Health Organization, South-East Asian Regional Office. *The Concept of Health Services Research.* New Delhi, 1983.
142. World Health Organization, South-East Asian Regional Office. *The Concept of Health Services Research.* New Delhi, 1985.
143. Luck, G. M., et al. *Patients, Hospitals and Operational Research.* Tavistock, London, 1971.
144. Banerji, D. Administration of family planning programme: A plea for an operational research approach. *Management in Government* 1(2): 46, 1969.
145. Banerji, D. Operational research in the field of public health. *Opsearch* 9: 13–16, 1972.
146. Banerji, D. *Research in Delivery of Health Care in Countries of SEARO.* WHO/SEARO, New Delhi, 1976.

PART IV
Neoliberalism and Social and Health Policy

CHAPTER 11

THE MEXICAN SOCIAL SECURITY COUNTERREFORM: PENSIONS FOR PROFIT

Asa Cristina Laurell

A wave of social policy counterreforms has swept Latin American countries and other parts of the world during the last decade (1). In the subcontinent these reforms are part and parcel of structural adjustment. Although structural adjustment programs (SAPs) are generally presented as economic policy, in reality they correspond to a global reorganization of society based on neoclassical economic theory and neoliberal ideology (2). This global project comprises a conception of how to satisfy needs (3) that is translated into specific social policy. There is thus much more to "social reform" than a simple pragmatic or technical adaptation of social programs to increase efficiency and diminish costs in order to reduce the public budget deficit. The main thrust of this reform is to "commodify" social services and benefits, to increase the role of the family, and to reduce the responsibilities of the state in the production of welfare (4). "Reform" in the context of social policy tends to be associated with an increase in citizens' social entitlements. Since the neoliberal reform implies the opposite—a reduction of social services and benefits granted by the state and a strong individualistic and market orientation—it could be described as a counterreform.

From the economic perspective, what is at stake in this reform is the moving of social services and benefits into the direct sphere of private capital accumulation (5). This explains why public social security is a primary target for reform: in most Latin American countries it is responsible for the major health service institutions and pension funds. The direct relationship between SAPs and "social reform" is reflected in the fact that most reform programs are directly or indirectly conducted and frequently financed by the World Bank (6). Thus the basic ideas that inspire the Latin American social security reform are to be found in the World Bank's *Investing in Health* (7) and *Averting the Old Age Crisis* (8). Although the application of the reform varies with the previous configuration of nations' social security institutions, the fundamental pattern is the same (9).

The Mexican case is paradigmatic of the neoliberal social security reform because it involves pensions, workers' compensation, health services, and child care. This chapter analyzes the process that provided the justification for reform, its general characteristics, and the new pension scheme that highlights the new conception of social policy. The health service component of this reform, which necessarily has to be interpreted in the general context of the broader health system reform (10), will be the subject of a separate study.

BASIC CHARACTERISTICS OF SOCIAL SECURITY IN MEXICO

The Mexican Constitution mandates (11) that all wage and salary earners have a right to social security provided by public institutions and guided by the principles of integrality, solidarity, and redistribution.[1] To this end there are two large social security institutes, the Mexican Social Security Institute (IMSS) for private sector workers and the Institute of Social Security and Services for State Workers (ISSSTE) for public employees. It is important to note that the reform has so far involved only the IMSS, the most important social security institute covering about 85 percent of the insured population. However, official documents such as the *National Development Plan, 1995–2000* indicate that a similar reform of the ISSSTE is on the agenda (12). There are presumably two reasons to postpone this. First, the ISSSTE does not directly involve private business, which has been pressing for reform (13). Second, public employees constitute a well-organized segment of the labor force and are likely to take political action if confronted with retrenchment of their rights, particularly since their pension scheme is more generous and linked to years of service rather than to age (14). Their entitlement losses would thus be more important.

Until 1997, when the new IMSS legislation came into force (15), the IMSS and ISSSTE were decentralized state institutions in charge of financing and delivery of services. They provided all services and administered all benefits using salaried staff and their own infrastructure. Subcontracting with the private sector was therefore very uncommon. The social security institutes have by far the most important network of health care facilities in Mexico, distributed throughout the country (approximately 40,000 hospital beds, 1,300 operating rooms, 50,000 physicians, and a total of 300,000 employees) (16). This network was established by investing the pension funds in health centers, clinics, and hospitals with the idea that common social funds should be applied to socially useful ends.

The principle of integrality is understood as a system of payments and entitlements that should provide protection against adversity and contribute positively

[1] Although the new legislation abandons these basic principles, the Constitution was not changed and the government claims that the reform does not affect its spirit.

to social and physical well-being. The ordinary social security scheme consequently includes old-age and disability pensions for insured workers; pensions for widows and dependent children; workers' compensation; medical care for insured workers and their families; child care for insured female workers; cultural, sports, and recreation centers; and housing programs financed by special low-interest funds. The difference between the IMSS and the ISSSTE is that public employees have more generous entitlements than private sector workers, particularly in pensions, housing, and low-interest loans (14).

The principle of solidarity is understood as solidarity between active and inactive workers (the retired and disabled) via the pension scheme, between sick and healthy workers, and between all workers and women with preschool children. This is closely related to the principle of redistribution since health insurance and child care are financed by a tripartite payroll tax that represents a fixed percentage of wages or salaries. This means that workers contribute according to their income, but they and their dependents have equal rights to receive health care according to needs. Given the wage structure, 80 percent of insured workers receive, on average, more health services than they paid for. This tax has an income ceiling at 25 times the minimum wage, which makes it regressive above this income level because the contribution is a fixed sum and not a percentage of salaries. However, just 1 percent of the insured benefit from this rule (17).

The main restriction of Mexican social security is that it covers only 55 percent of the population (18) as a result of the nation's labor market structure. Since it is only mandatory for dependent workers, self-employed and informal sector workers are in practice excluded. This clearly represents a serious inequity, particularly because those left out are generally among the poorest. However, insured workers cannot be seen as a "privileged group" given that 70 percent earn only three times the minimum wage (about U.S. $300) or less (17), which corresponds to a condition of absolute poverty (19). Another source of segmentation is that public employees have more generous entitlements than private sector workers.

It should be stressed that although social insurance is contingent on a formal labor relation and is segmented according to type of employment (public or private), it is not a variable fringe benefit. This is because it does not depend on collective or individual bargaining agreements or bargaining power, and within each social security institute all workers have the same rights. One could even argue that historically, the Mexican strategy to build a universal welfare state was founded on the social security system since its coverage increased very rapidly: in the 1960s the growth in the number of insured workers was 13 percent annually, in the 1970s, 11 percent; and in the 1980s, 5 percent (see Table 2). Furthermore, starting in the 1970s the IMSS, using its administrative capacities, developed a separate state-subsidized health care system for the poor uninsured population. These services, known as IMSS-Solidaridad, were much more efficient and comprehensive than those run by the Ministry of Health and covered an estimated 10.5 million Mexicans in rural areas (18).

THE SOCIAL SECURITY CRISIS: PUBLIC INCOMPETENCE OR NEOLIBERAL FAILURE?

In the mid-1980s the fairly well-functioning social security institutes started to deteriorate, and a decade later the idea of crisis became common in government speeches. Pensions, eroded by inflation, had become totally insufficient to grant even a modest living, and the formerly high-quality health services were declining.

There is general agreement that the key problem is insufficient funding, particularly of health services. This has repercussions for pension funds because the deficit in health insurance has been covered with these funds, which do not receive any revenues on their investments in clinics and hospitals (20). However, the explanations given for those financial difficulties differ. Government officials argue that they are due to a demographic and epidemiological transition and suggest that these problems have been amplified by inefficient use of resources (17). Employer organizations are more explicit on this point, stating that public institutions are inefficient by nature, which, together with unrealistically generous entitlements, has not just caused a crisis but has also burdened employers with high labor costs, making them uncompetitive in the global marketplace (13). This last argument has no objective base given that the average industrial wage in Mexico is around $300 a month and indirect labor costs amount to 24.7 percent of total labor costs, compared with, for instance, 35 percent in Japan, 45 percent in the United States, 65 percent in Germany, and 74 percent in Sweden (10). The arguments of government and employer organizations were thus built up to justify a social security reform that aims at downsizing entitlements, shifting costs away from employers, and privatization.

A closer look at the funding problem reveals a quite different picture and indicates a close relationship between the decay of social security and the neoliberal economic policies adopted in 1983. The two foremost causes of declining social security funds are the continual wage reduction and the prolonged stagnation of formal job creation, both inherent to SAP policies (21). With declining salaries and growing underemployment, no social security or insurance scheme, be it public, private, or mixed, can be sustained, much less extended, since all the schemes are funded by salaries of employed workers through either general or payroll taxes or premiums.

The minimum wage has declined steadily since 1982, and by 1995 the reduction was about 60 percent (Table 1). The industrial wage shows a similar but less dramatic pattern, and by 1995 it had decreased to less than half of its 1982 level (22). This has had a direct impact on social security funding because premiums are a fixed percentage of workers' wages. Calculated with official data, the income loss suffered by the IMSS due to wage reduction from 1983 to 1994 was about 215 billion pesos, 5.4 times its total revenue for 1994 (10). Simultaneously,

Table 1

Trends in wages and employment in Mexico, 1982–1995[a]

	1982	1984	1986	1988	1990	1992	1994	1995
Wages (1982 = 100)								
Minimum wage	100	77	70	57	49	45	44	39
Industrial wage	100	70	80	61	57	56	55	43
Employment, percent[b]								
Formal	89.9	84.6	79.1	75.0	72.2	69.3	64.4	57.7
Informal	1.1	6.5	9.2	13.2	19.4	21.4	26.0	30.8
Open unemployment	8.0	8.9	11.7	11.8	8.3	9.3	9.6	11.5
Insured workers, IMSS and ISSSTE, percent[b]	36.5	37.2	36.6	37.6	40.5	38.3	37.8	34.7

[a]Source: Calculated with data from references 22–24.
[b]Percentage of economically active population.

government subsidies were gradually diminished and supposedly transferred to selective poverty programs.[2]

The stagnation of the formal labor market and the rapid growth in informal jobs (Table 1) have had a double impact on social security funding. They provoked a slow down of the growth rate of coverage, which for the IMSS declined from a yearly average of 9.7 percent in the 1970s to 5.1 percent in the 1980s to –0.8 percent in the first half of the 1990s (Table 2) (23, 24). The corresponding figures for all insurance are 11.1, 4.8, and –0.4 percent. Thus the strategy of expanding the base of contributors to extend coverage and to finance social security was reversed. This in turn created an imbalance between active insured workers and pensioned workers (23), putting the pay-as-you-go pension scheme under severe strain.

Contrary to what is usually argued, this situation has little to do with the demographic transition because the total Mexican dependency ratio—that is, the ratio of the population below 15 and over 65 years to the population between 15 and 64 years—has actually declined steadily during the last three decades, from 1.050 in 1970 to 0.661 in 1994, as a result of falling birth rates. The broad dependency ratio—the ratio of the over-64 population to the age group from 15 to 64—has changed very slowly, from 0.068 in 1980 to 0.069 in 1994 as calculated with census data (10). This means that Mexico as a country would be in a favorable demographic phase if the potentially active population were employed

[2] Although the government argued that subsidies to social security were diminished in order to finance social programs targeted to the poor, there is no empirical evidence to support this claim (10).

Table 2

Social security coverage, IMSS and ISSSTE, Mexico, 1961–1995[a]

Year	IMSS insured workers			ISSSTE insured workers			Total		
	Number, thousands	Yearly variation, %	Average yearly variation per decade, %	Number, thousands	Yearly variation, %	Average yearly variation per decade, %	Number, thousands	Yearly variation, %	Average yearly variation per decade, %
1961	1,419			133			1,552		
1970	3,121		12.0	431		22.4	3,552		12.9
1971	3,233	3.6		469	8.9		2,702	4.2	
1972	3,581	10.8		532	13.5		4,113	11.1	
1973	3,901	8.9		617	16.1		4,518	9.9	
1974	4,020	3.1		856	38.7		4,876	7.9	
1975	4,306	7.1		1,013	18.3		5,319	9.1	
1976	4,338	0.7		1,087	7.3		5,425	2.0	
1977	4,554	5.0		1,213	11.6		5,767	6.3	
1978	5,157	13.2		1,438	18.6		6,595	14.4	
1979	5,500	6.7		1,408	−2.1		6,908	4.7	
1980	6,369	15.8	9.7	1,435	2.0	20.6	7,804	13.0	11.1

1981	7,112	11.7		1,532	6.7		8,644	10.8	
1982	7,037	–1.1		1,584	3.4		8,621	–0.3	
1983	7,059	0.3		1,651	4.2		8,710	1.0	
1984	7,630	8.1		1,828	10.8		9,458	8.6	
1985	8,132	6.6		1,857	1.6		9,989	5.6	
1986	7,986	–1.8		2,004	7.9		9,990	0.0	
1987	8,757	9.7		2,097	4.7		10,854	8.7	
1988	8,917	1.8		2,098	0.1		11,015	1.5	
1989	9,926	11.3		2,097	–0.1		12,023	9.1	
1990	10,764	8.4	5.1	2,012	–4.1	3.1	12,776	6.3	4.8
1991	11,333	5.3		2,019	0.3		13,352	4.5	
1992	11,369	0.3		2,046	1.4		13,415	0.5	
1993	11,317	–0.5		2,107	3.0		13,424	0.1	
1994	11,561	2.2		2,150	2.0		13,711	2.1	
1995	10,892	–5.8	–0.8	2,162	0.6	1.4	13,054	–4.8	–0.4

[a]Source: Calculated with data from references 23 and 24.

and contributed to social security. The inability of the economic model to create even a modest increase in formal employment during periods of growth is what generates an imbalance between active workers and the retired, a relation that went from 38 active workers per retiree in 1980, to 20 per retiree in 1994 (23).

There is no consistent empirical evidence to demonstrate the alleged negative impact of the epidemiological transition on health care costs. Thus no significant change has occurred in the frequency of registered morbidity among patients attended by the IMSS, and cancer and cardiovascular diseases represent only 8 percent of all hospitalizations (16).

The financial difficulties of the IMSS were initially compensated for by dramatic cuts in the salaries of its personnel. For instance, physicians lost 80 percent of their income in ten years and other categories about 70 percent (25). This, together with the gradual wear and tear of equipment and installations and a lack of day-to-day supplies, led to a devaluation of institutional work. Simultaneously, the demand for service increased because of the general impoverishment of the insured, which in turn created barriers to immediate access. Despite these adverse conditions, the IMSS and ISSSTE continue to be by far the most important providers of health services in Mexico and are actively used by at least 40 percent of the population, including workers and their dependents (16), who belong to the low or low-middle income brackets. Estimations from official data (16) also show an optimal use of existing resources that contrasts with the low utilization in private establishments (10, p. 44).

After a long period of monetary stability, Mexico's inflation increased an average of 30 percent a year from 1977 to 1982 and became exorbitant from 1983 to 1989 with a yearly average increase of 83 percent (23), which severely eroded pensions that were not inflation-indexed. A vigorous movement of retirees managed to negotiate an annuity level of not less than the minimum wage, but this amount is insufficient to grant even a modest living (19). Measures do need to be taken to modify the undeniable deterioration of social security institutions. The case in point, however, is that social security institutions face a crisis that has its structural roots in the economic model adopted more than a decade ago and has little to do with public inefficiency or demographic variables. The government has not clearly stated in the debate over reform that one of the social costs of its economic policy is its incompatibility with the maintenance of social protection for workers, let alone its extension to a larger population. On the contrary, it is claimed that the reform will resolve financial problems, increase entitlements, and create the conditions necessary for including a larger part of the population.

FROM PUBLIC SOLIDARITY TO PRIVATE INDIVIDUALISM

The New Social Security Act (15), which was passed by Congress in 1995 and came into force in July 1997, discloses a radical conceptual shift away from the historical principles of Mexican social security and is clearly inspired by neoliberal thought. The basic scheme moves from public financing and provision to private administration; from an integral scheme to separate insurance for specific contingencies; from solidarity to individualism; from redistribution and equal rights to equivalence between premium and entitlements.

This shift is clear-cut in the pension reform—modeled on the Chilean scheme—which eliminates the pay-as-you-go scheme based on publicly administered common funds with guaranteed annuities. The old scheme is replaced by a mandatory one of individual retirement accounts managed by private financial intermediaries, the so-called *Administradoras de Fondos de Retiro (Afores).* These accounts must be used at retirement to purchase old-age and survivor annuities from private insurance companies, and the amount of each pension depends on the individual savings and is therefore uncertain. Although the funds dedicated to covering disability pensions and workers' compensation continue to be collective, the annuity must be purchased from an insurance company and in doing so the individual retirement account is expropriated.

The tendency to privatize and individualize health insurance is less sweeping since it is conceived as a selective process designed for high- and middle-income employees. The two most relevant changes in legislation are a new premium formula and the possibility of choosing between public and private health insurance and services within the compulsory system. The new financing scheme establishes "equal pay for equal services"—that is, the same premium for all instead of a fixed percentage of individual income, which is highly regressive and abolishes solidarity between high- and low-income groups. The private option in compulsory health insurance is implemented by means of the so-called "agreements of premium reversal" that oblige the public social security institute to return the compulsory quota to those who have private health insurance.

The new legislation similarly broadens the possibilities of privatizing child care, presumably in order to cut costs. The cultural, sporting, and other recreational activities implemented as part of the integral social security scheme will be paid for with the child care insurance funds. These activities were previously financed by pension funds, which becomes impossible with the establishment of individual retirement accounts. In practice this means that these facets will decline because child care has traditionally been underfunded. Although social security funds for housing are administered by an independent institute, the National Workers' Housing Fund (INFONAVIT), shortly after passage of the new Social Security Act legislation was changed in order to add workers' housing quotas to their retirement accounts (26). This probably augurs a future "reform" that would abolish workers' constitutional right to proper housing, transferring the present 5 percent payroll tax to the retirement account in order to supplement insufficient resources.

A PENSION SCHEME FOR THE BENEFIT OF FINANCIAL GROUPS

The new pension scheme reveals the neoliberal conception of social policy. Economic objectives prevail over social goals: the emphasis is on privatization, domestic saving, and expansion of the financial market. Furthermore it establishes a strict equivalence between the amount saved and the annuity, which is therefore uncertain. It also tightens the eligibility rules: 1,250 weekly contributions must be accumulated to qualify for a pension, compared with 500 in the previous scheme (15). This reform follows the broad guidelines of the World Bank (8), adopting its implicit assumptions, both unproven and controversial, about the inefficiency of public institutions and the key role of mandatory individual saving for economic growth (27, 28).

The reform entirely restructures the previous pensions scheme and establishes three separate kinds of insurance: old-age retirement insurance, life and disability insurance, and workers' compensation insurance (15). In the new scheme the first of these is the most important. As mentioned earlier, the pay-as-you-go scheme is being replaced by a fully funded scheme of individual retirement accounts that eliminates intergenerational transfers and risk-sharing among workers. However, the law guarantees a minimum annuity for eligible retirees equal to the legal minimum wage, which means that the state will eventually complement the individual assets with public tax funds. The tripartite premium for this insurance is 6.5 percent of the worker's wage with a state subsidy corresponding to 5.5 percent of the legal minimum wage. The mandatory quota for housing, 5 percent of the wage, is also deposited in the individual retirement account but is not subject to variable interest rates. Workers may also deposit voluntary savings in their accounts.

Workers are not allowed to continue in the old scheme and are obliged to make a contract with an *Afore* (see below). Unlike the case of Chile, pension quotas paid previous to the enforcement of the new law are not recognized in Mexico, presumably because this would increase the "transition cost" substantially. Government officials argue that this virtual expropriation of workers' funds has a compensating device since those eligible workers who contributed to the old scheme may on retirement choose between annuities calculated by the old or the new rules. If the worker opts for the old rules, the government will provide additional funds if those accumulated in the worker's individual account are not sufficient to supply the corresponding annuity. Meanwhile, however, private pension funds will receive premiums and charge commissions for years.

The Winners: Private Pension Funds and Insurance Companies

The Social Security Act creates three special financial bodies that will manage the whole pension scheme: the *Administradora de Fondos de Retiro (Afore),* the *Sociedad de Inversión de Fondos de Retiro (Siefore),* and special insurance companies dedicated to handling annuities. The *Afore* manages the retirement accounts and invests the savings in financial markets through one or various associated *Siefores* (trust funds). The role of the specialized insurance companies is to sell old-age, survivor and/or disability pensions to insured workers. In this way the new financial bodies will replace the IMSS in all functions related to pensions, with the exception of the administration of funds collected from life and disability insurance and workers' compensation. The IMSS will additionally channel general tax revenues to complete the sum needed to purchase a guaranteed minimum annuity for eligible persons.

The new pension scheme is designed to achieve the largest transfer of public funds to private financial groups ever experienced in Mexico, because the scheme hands over the control of mandatory pension funds to *Afores, Siefores,* and insurance companies. In order to grasp the magnitude of the transaction, consider the following data. The IMSS estimates that these pension funds will accumulate an amount equal to 25 percent of the GNP in ten years, 45 percent in 20 years, and 60 percent in 30 years (29). Control over these large quantities of capital confers on these financial agents unprecedented economic and, consequently, political power that can only be partially moderated by legislation (30).

Although legally any "physical or moral" person could constitute an *Afore-Siefore* or pension insurance company, in practice all of them belong to the dominant Mexican financial groups that as a rule have international partners such as Aetna, Cigna, Geo New York Life, ING America, GE Capital, Citibank, Dresdner Pension Fund Holdings, and Santander Investments, among others. The foreign partners frequently hold 49 percent of the stocks, which is the legal ceiling (10, p. 66). Although the Congress of the Union, including prominent legislators of the official party, tried for economic and political reasons to prevent the new pension scheme from being dominated by international financial capital,[3] this is actually happening. The only restriction so far is that funds cannot be invested abroad.

The pension business is very attractive quite apart from controlling large amounts of capital, since the *Afores* charge insured workers a commission. According to the regulations (31) established after approval of the Social Security Act, this fee could be a percentage of the premium, a percentage of the accumulated assets of the retirement account, and/or a percentage of the revenues of the invested funds. All but two of the *Afores* charge a percentage of the premium ranging from 0.9 to 1.99 percent of the workers' wage, which corresponds to between 14 and 30 percent of the pension quota. In addition, most of them

[3] With a last minute maneuver, the agreed upon legal text was changed by the Ministry of Finance to allow foreign investment in *Afores-Siefores,* using the argument that restrictions would violate international trade agreements.

charge a percentage of the accumulated assets that ranges from 0.65 to 3.5 percent, and one charges 20 percent of the revenue. These data notoriously contradict the claim that private management of pension funds is more efficient, since the IMSS spent 0.63 percent of workers' wages on administration (17). The reason for this inefficiency is that an *Afore* has high commercialization and promotion expenses (27) and is intended to make a profit. Although it is argued that the commission might decrease over time, the evidence from Chile shows that this has not been the case: competition tends to increase that kind of expense (32). Thus one of the main objections made by experts to individual retirement accounts is that they are the most expensive pension alternative (30, 33–35).

Charging a percentage of the premium gives the *Afore* a secure income that does not depend on its investment expertise or the performance of financial markets. The financial risks are thus passed on to the insured who, given the mandatory character of the scheme, have no choice but to sign a contract that explicitly states that his or her funds may decrease or increase due to market fluctuations (10, p. 70). Thus the "liberty of choice" is a fallacy since all *Afores* have the same rule in their contracts.

It has been argued that competition among the different *Afores* will work against the inefficient ones since the insured workers can choose a different trust fund. This presupposes that workers have the expertise to make informed long-term financial decisions, which is quite unrealistic (28). Furthermore, the Mexican legislation does not include regulations such as the Chilean law that cancels the authorization of trust funds that fail to make correct investment decisions (30).

The second type of charge—a percentage of the accumulated assets in the account—has an element of risk-sharing between the insured and the *Afore* but also grants a relatively stable income to the latter. Actually, the *Afore* runs a financial risk similar to that of the insured workers only when the fee constitutes a percentage of profits. Significantly enough, just one *Afore* has chosen this option alone but charges 33 percent of revenue.

The second phase of the pension scheme, the management of annuities, is entirely transferred to specialized insurance companies. The dominant trend in the integration of the new system is that the main financial groups incorporate an *Afore-Siefore* and an insurance company. They will thus control the whole pension cycle, and predictably most workers will purchase their annuity at retirement from the insurance company of the same financial group as their *Afore*.

These insurance companies are even more favored than *Afores* by the new Social Security Act because not just the old-age pension but also the survivors, disability, and workers' compensation insurance must be purchased from them. When the contract is signed, the funds of the individual retirement account are transferred to the insurance company, which will manage them for an average of 16 years. This new legislation will therefore have a radical impact on the Mexican insurance market. The mandatory pension premiums will initially be roughly equal to the premiums paid for all other private insurance (10, p. 72).

The design of the Social Security Act is a splendid example of direct state intervention to create entirely new markets and to favor special interest groups, in this case financial trusts. What used to be a social concern and a public responsibility has now become the terrain of private business. This is not accidental, as can be illustrated by the World Bank opinion that the great achievements of the Chilean pension reform are the enlargement of capital markets, growth of the trust fund industry, and renewal of the insurance industry (36).

The Grand Underwriter: The State

State intervention is not limited to legislation but also implies a long-lasting commitment to subsidizing the privatization of the pension scheme with tax money. Thus the so-called "transition cost" of the new scheme is estimated by the Ministry of Finance to be between approximately 1 and 1.5 percent of GNP[4] for half a century (37) and has to be paid by the federal government—that is, by insured and uninsured tax payers.

The transition cost is an absolute condition and an inevitable result of the shift from a pay-as-you-go scheme to a fully funded scheme of private retirement accounts. This is because the former scheme is built on a match between income and outlay: part of the contributions of active workers is used to pay the pensions. Under this logic it is not necessary to accumulate financial assets equal to the future pensions (fully funded pensions) but only to have sufficient actuarial reserves to grant the annuities in case of fluctuations in incomes over and above immediate pension commitments.

The new scheme based on private retirement accounts establishes a completely different logic: the premiums of active workers cannot be used to pay current annuities for two related reasons. First, a basic requirement of this scheme is to capitalize these accounts in order to accumulate sufficient assets to grant the future annuity. Second, the premiums are managed by private trust funds and invested in financial markets with the criterion of maximizing profit. This obliges someone to pay the current pensions and complement the amount necessary to purchase an annuity for those who paid part of their quotas to the pay-as-you-go scheme. The payment of these two expenses constitutes the transition cost, and nobody but the state could or would be willing to commit funds to this end. In practice, of course, this means the tax payers are charged the bill.

[4] The large number of uncertain events (wage and employment levels, GNP growth, interest rates, etc.) involved in the estimation of the transition cost makes a more precise forecast unfeasible.

The Mexican retirement scheme has some additional state subsidies that were adopted to legitimize the new legislation, which faced strong public resistance (13). It thus includes a "social quota" of 5.5 percent of one minimum wage, a guaranteed minimum annuity, and the right of workers that belonged to the previous scheme to choose the most favorable annuity calculated by the old or the new rules at retirement. All subsidies will be financed by the state.

It must be stressed that the establishment of private retirement accounts is not feasible unless the state underwrites the costs of transition and additional benefits. This is why the contention is that the state subsidizes private financial groups and not workers, who would actually be better off with the pay-as-you-go scheme as will be discussed below. In this context two additional facts must be contemplated. The estimated transition cost of 1 to 1.5 percent of GNP should be compared with the total government social expenditure—less than 10 percent of GNP, including education, health, social security, poverty programs, and housing (38). Since the Mexican government considers a balanced budget an essential priority, some other social programs will have to be cut in order to finance pensions. On the other hand, the expenditure for a universal minimum pension for all senior citizens—0.8 percent of GNP—would currently be less than the transition cost of the selective scheme of private retirement accounts (10, p. 110).

The Losers: Working People

As a means for granting income security to senior citizens, the pension reform has some very serious inconveniences since it grants neither higher annuities nor the opportunity to extend pension coverage to a larger part of the population, but rather the reverse. By definition the quantity of an annuity based on a private retirement account is uncertain, depending as it does on the individual savings accumulated. These, in turn, depend on the amount and the number of weekly premiums deposited, the commission charged for management, and the interest rate on the account. None of these components can be safely predicted over a period that corresponds to a working life, and therefore nobody can make more than an informed guess about the future annuity (27, 28, 30, 34, 36, 39, 40). This is why there is such a broad range of estimations of the annuities that will result from the new Mexican pension scheme, some of them quite biased for commercial or political motives. However, a minimum of scientific (actuarial) veracity obliges one to include at least the three elements mentioned above, which also comprise the possible "wage career"—that is, wage increases experienced during a working life. In general, the main uncertainty concerns the average interest rate that financial markets will deliver over the coming decades, particularly with the reality of the impact on the global financial market of regional or national financial crises, such as those experienced in 1995 in Mexico and presently in Asia. Although the initially high returns on Chilean private pension funds have been much publicized by politicians and financial trusts, even optimistic experts, supportive of the scheme, estimate real annual rates of 4 to 5 percent, while more moderate experts predict rates of 2 to 3 percent based on historical empirical evidence (27, 28, 30, 41, 42). The yearly interest rate without commission charges reported in Mexico was 6.08 percent. This means that, on average, workers' retirement account savings were 15 to 20 percent less than their contributions (43).

In the case of Mexico, a second important source of uncertainty is that related to the formal labor market since its slow growth and the frequent lay-offs make it very difficult to estimate the average period of unemployment a worker will experience during her or his working life. Given that the unemployed discontinue their contributions to the retirement account, while *Afores* continue to charge a commission, a job loss diminishes savings. Existing data show that on average workers used to contribute to social security for about nine weeks out of ten, but this refers to a period of sustained economic growth with a rapidly expanding labor market. The former "density of contributions" is therefore likely to decline. It is revealing that official data have reported that 28 percent of retirement accounts were inactive eight months after the new scheme began (44). This has also been the trend in Chile: in 1995, more than a decade after reform and despite a favorable economic situation, 43 percent of workers with retirement accounts were not active contributors (30).

The most technically adequate estimation of future annuities of the new Mexican pension scheme, considering all the necessary elements, has been presented by the National Association of Actuaries. This study is based on the assumption of 35 years of continuous contributions at 6.5 percent of the wage and the "social quota," a charge of 25 percent of the total premium, and an average interest rate of 3.5 percent. Depending on the "wage career" the annuity would range from 3.3 to 22.7 percent of the pre-retirement income. Even more important, nobody would obtain the guaranteed minimum annuity equal to a minimum wage, which means that the state would have to subsidize all annuities with important implications for the transition cost. As a comparison, with the previous pay-as-you-go scheme someone who had contributed over 35 years would have an annuity corresponding to, at worst, 98.75 percent of pre-retirement income and, at best, 99.7 percent (45).

A second estimate (39), based on three times the minimum wage, 40 years of continuous contribution including the quota for housing, a charge of 25 percent of the premium, and a wage increase of 2.2 percent, is more favorable. Thus the annuity would be 29.3 percent of the pre-retirement income with an average interest rate of 2.5 percent, 59.6 percent with an interest rate of 5 percent, and 127.2 percent with an interest rate of 7.5 percent. However, assuming that the housing quota is not capitalized, which is currently the case, the corresponding annuities would be 24.3, 42.6, and 82.2 percent of the pre-retirement income.

These data reveal two important points. On the one hand, they confirm the prediction that future annuities will fall short of an acceptable standard of income security for senior citizens, given that a minimum-wage income (U.S. $100) is below the absolute poverty line. On the other hand, these data show that the retirement quota, strictly speaking (6.5 percent of income and the "social quota"), is clearly insufficient and needs to be complemented with the 5 percent contribution for housing in order to give certain sustainability to the new scheme. If the social insurance payroll tax is to be maintained at its present level, which is a government commitment to employers, it will be necessary to abolish the right to adequate housing and incorporate the corresponding 5 percent into the retirement account. Even so, a reasonable annuity could only be achieved with an average interest rate of at least 5 percent, which by no means is guaranteed.

Although the new legislation lays down that annuities are to be inflation-adjusted once a year, how this will actually be implemented by the private insurance companies is unclear. Pension experts are skeptical about whether this is feasible with a private and individualized scheme (27, 28). Ultimately the state would have to intervene to uphold this promise in the case of rising inflation, directly by subsidizing insurance companies or indirectly by issuing government bonds with a guaranteed interest rate above inflation (27).

Something the new legislation does not do is set clear-cut rules to compute the purchasing cost and amount of the annuity that should regulate the pension contracts. This might lead to discriminatory practices against entire population groups, particularly women. Since women live longer on average, their annuity would be less than that of men given the same retirement savings unless insurance companies are forbidden to differentiate by sex and other individual characteristics (27, 30).

This question highlights another objection to the new social insurance legislation: insufficient regulation that leaves a substantial margin for discretionary decisions. Among other legal anomalies, the government department in charge of regulation, *Comisión Nacional de Sistemas de Ahorro para el Retiro* (CONSAR), is given the power to decree "general rules" (31), which are understood as laws in Mexican legal practice. This is a clear intrusion of the executive power into a field that corresponds to Congress (46). Apart from the notorious lack of public and private accountability arising from this, it also puts those insured in a precarious legal situation from which there is no escape given the compulsory character of the system.

Contrary to government claims, the new scheme is also likely to bring about a retrenchment of coverage because it changes the eligibility rules. In the previous scheme, a worker who had contributed 500 weekly pension quotas had the right to receive a life-long pension at the age of 65 and free medical care. With the new legislation 1,250 weekly contributions must be accumulated to qualify for a pension, and 750 weekly contributions to preserve the right to free medical care (11). As pointed out above, the characteristics of the Mexican labor market reduce the possibilities of making continuous contributions, and this will restrict the number of eligible workers. Presently the average number of weekly contributions by retirees is 1,196 (17).

Under these circumstances, the percentage of senior citizens entitled to receive an annuity is likely to decline. So the new Social Security Act cancels the slow trend toward a universal pension scheme in Mexico. This will have dramatic social consequences for an impoverished population in a society where traditional forms of care for the elderly are breaking down with urbanization and the disintegration of the extended family.

Domestic Saving, Economic Growth, and Employment

The final argument of those who believe in pension reform is that none of these objections are valid since the large increase in domestic saving will lead to rapid economic growth and more jobs. This is a point of polemic among economists, however, with no consistent empirical evidence to prove a causal relationship between the rates of saving, investment, and GNP growth (39, 40).

An initial problem to be elucidated is whether compulsory pension saving leads to an increase in global national saving or just brings about a change in the proportions between the private and public share. In the case of Mexico, the reform will probably lead to a drop in public saving given its high transition cost. Unless the state reduces other expenditure it will have to finance the privatization of pensions with loans, which has already happened in 1997 with a World Bank credit of $900 million. Depending on what option is chosen, there will then be a direct public "un-saving" or a reorientation of public spending. This might, in turn, lead to a decrease in public investment with negative effects on growth or to a reduction in social spending.

The assumption that savings are immediately invested in production can also be challenged. Generally speaking a mere supply of financial assets does not automatically generate a credit demand for production: companies take credit decisions based on the expected demand for their products in the market. Given the prolonged retrenchment of the Mexican domestic market caused by a sustained wage reduction, few elements would lead one to believe that an increase in domestic saving will invigorate the economy (35). Recent studies on the dynamics of the Mexican economy (47, 48) show that large profits, obtained primarily through wage depression, have increased neither the rates of productive investment nor job creation. Rather, the scarcity of domestic profitable investment opportunities has provoked capital flight and a boom in luxury consumption, generally of imported goods, concentrated in the tiny minority favored by the neoliberal model. The expected "trickle-down" has not occurred.

This concrete evidence challenges the assumption that mandatory pension saving, channeled through new financial intermediaries, will create a "virtuous circle" of "saving-investment-employment." Even worse, the Mexican financial market may not have the capacity to absorb the new credit supply and this would force a change in legislation to allow the trust funds to invest abroad, as happened in Chile (30). The only other alternative would be for the government to provide bonds and pay a high enough interest rate to grant the expected return on the retirement accounts (27).

This logic reveals an insoluble contradiction in the pension reform that makes the simultaneous accomplishment of two of its stated goals unachievable. It is not possible at one and the same time to attain both acceptable annuities from individual retirement accounts and investment of pension funds in productive activities. The reason is simple: to grant a fair annuity presupposes very high interest rates attainable only through financial speculation, while productive investment requires "cheap" credit, that is, low interest rates. A choice is inevitable: either the pensions of two or three generations are sacrificed, or productive investment and jobs are sacrificed for quite some time. This paradox emanates from the specific form of the new pension scheme and the logic of neoliberal economics. In contrast, different forms of pay-as-you-go schemes would allow payment of fair annuities and contribution to growth and job creation by investing the actuarial reserves in strategic productive projects or social infrastructure (20).

These are the reasons why the social security reform is actually a counterreform viewed from a social perspective and mirrored in the new pension scheme. It does not solve any of the problems that supposedly inspired it. There is no empirical evidence that it will increase pension coverage or grant old-age income security to insured workers. The alleged positive impact on economic growth and job creation is equally uncertain. The values of solidarity and income redistribution through public action are replaced by the values of the marketplace, individual capacity, and private profits. This trajectory is only possible using the power of the state to promote private goals at the expense of common interests. Even worse, this counterreform is a concession to a tiny minority that exercises its economic power to socialize risks and losses and privatize profits, a behavior alien to classical liberal thought and even more to the ethical and social values of the 20th century. It is a counterreform that is stepping into the 21st century with the imposition of the 19th century's failed ideas, looking ahead with a return to the past.

REFERENCES

1. Navarro, V. *Neoliberalismo y Estado de Bienestar.* Ariel, Barcelona, 1997.
2. Sader, E., and Gentili, P. *Pósneoliberalismo: Las politicas Sociais e o Estado Democrático.* Paz e Terra, São Paulo, 1995.
3. George, V., and Wilding, P. *Welfare and Ideology.* Harvester Wheatsheaf, London, 1994.
4. Esping-Anderson, G. After the golden age? Welfare states dilemmas in a global economy. In *Welfare States in Transition,* edited by G. Esping-Andersen, pp. 1–31. Sage, London, 1996.

5. Laurell, A. C. Crisis, neoliberal health policy, and political processes in Mexico. *Int. J. Health Serv.* 21: 457–470, 1991.
6. Paul, S., and Paul, J. The World Bank, pensions, and income (in)security in the global South. *Int. J. Health Serv.* 25: 697–726, 1995.
7. World Bank. *Investing in Health.* Washington, D.C., 1993.
8. World Bank. *Averting the Old Age Crisis.* Oxford University Press, New York, 1994.
9. Laurell, A. C. La politica de salud en el contexto de las politicas sociales. Paper presented at the IV Congreso Latinoamericano de Ciencias Sociales y Medicina, Cuernavaca, Mexico, 1997.
10. Laurell, A. C. *La Reforma contra la Salud y la Seguridad social.* Ed. ERA, México DF, 1997.
11. Instituto Nacional Electoral. *La Constitución Politica de los Estados Unidos Mexicanos.* Article 123. México DF, 1997.
12. Poder Ejecutivo Federal. *Plan Nacional de Desarrollo, 1995–2000.* México DF, 1995.
13. Laurell, A. C. *La Reforma de los Sistemas de Salud y Seguridad Social: Concepciones y propuestas de los distintos actores sociales.* Fundación F. Ebert, México DF, 1995.
14. *Ley del Instituto de Seguridad y Servicios Sociales de los Trabajadores del Estado.* Porrúa, México DF, 1990.
15. Ley del Seguro Social. *Diario Oficial de la Federación.* December 21, 1995.
16. Sistema Nacional de Salud. *Boletín de Información Estadística,* 14. Instituto Nacional de Estadística, Geografía e Informática and Secretaría de Salud, México DF, 1994.
17. Instituto Mexicano del Seguro Social. *Diagnóstico.* México DF, 1995.
18. Laurell, A. C., and Ruiz, L. *¿Podemos Garantizar el Derecho a la Salud?* Fundación F. Ebert, México DF, 196.
19. Boltvinik, J. *Pobreza y Estratificación Social en México.* Colegio de México-INEGI-IIS-UNAM, México DF, 1995.
20. Garcia Saínz, R. La reforma de la reforma. In *Alternativa de Reforma de la Seguridad Social,* edited by M. L. Mussot, pp. 211–244. Universidad Autónoma Metropolitana–Fundación F. Ebert, México DF, 1996.
21. Valenzuela, J. C. *¿Qué es un Patrón de Acumulación?* Facultad de Economía UNAM, México DF, 1990.
22. Martínez, I. *Economía y Democracia.* Grijalvo, México DF, 1995.
23. Salinas, C. *Informe de Gobierno. Anexo Estadístico.* Poder Ejecutivo Federal, México DF, 1994.
24. Zedillo, E. *Informe de Gobierno. Anexo Estadístico.* Poder Ejecutivo Federal, México DF, 1995.
25. Herrera, M. Austeridad y lucha sindical en el IMSS. *Chemizal* 3: 57–66, 1990.
26. López Angel, C. Afore-Infonavit, el despojo. *La Jornada Laboral* 75: 2.
27. Beattie, R., and McGillivry, W. A risky strategy: Reflections on the World Bank Report *Averting the Old Age Crisis.* In *Proceedings of the Conference on Financial Security in Retirement.* International Labour Organization and International Social Security Association, Geneva, 1995.
28. Du Boff, R. The welfare state, pensions, privatization: the case of social security in the United States. *Int. J. Health Serv.* 27: 1–23, 1997.
29. Instituto Mexicano del Seguro Social. *Aportaciones para el debate.* México DF, 1996.

30. Ruíz-Tagle, J. El nuevo sistema de pensiones en Chile: una evaluación preliminar. *Comercio Exterior* 46: 703–709, 1996.
31. Ley de los Sistemas de Ahorro para el Retiro. *Diario Oficial de la Federación,* May 23, 1996.
32. BANAMEX. Administradoras de fondos de retiro: reforma en México y los ejemplos chileno y argentino. *Examen de la Situación Económica de México* 884: 102–114, 1996.
33. Hazas Sánchez, A. Futuro del sistema pensionario de los trabajadores sujetos a la nueva ley del IMSS. In *Alternativas de Reforma de la Seguridad Social,* edited by M. L. Mussot, pp. 153–198. Universidad Autónoma Metropolitana–Fundación F. Ebert, México DF, 1996.
34. Bonilla, A. 1995: Reformas de los sistemas de pensiones. In *Memorias de la Reunión Internacional de Expertos en Seguridad Social.* Centro de Desarrollo Estratégico para la Seguridad Social, México DF, 1995.
35. López, A. C. El ahorro interno en los planes de ajuste estructural. In *Memorias de la Reunión Internacional de Expertos en Seguridad Social.* Centro de Desarrollo Estratégico para la Seguridad Social, México DF, 1995.
36. Lacey, R. La reforma de la jubilación en América Latina: los retos y el papel del Banco Mundial. *Comercio Exterior* 46: 683–691, 1996.
37. Secretaría de Hacienda y Crédito Público. *Informe sobre la Situación Económica, las Finanzas Públicas y la Deuda Pública.* México DF, 1996.
38. Zedillo, E. *Informe de Gobierno. Anexo Estadístico.* Poder Ejecutivo Federal, México DF, 1997.
39. Kurczyn, S. Reforma del sistema de pensiones mexicano: principales aspectos macroeconómicos. *Comercio Exterior* 46: 741–754, 1996.
40. Lo Vuolo, R. Reformas previsionales en América Latina: el caso argentino. *Comercio Exterior* 46: 692–702, 1996.
41. Gillion, C., and Bonilla, A. Analysis of a national private pension scheme: The case of Chile. *Int. Labour Rev.* 131: 2, 1992.
42. Bustos Castillo, R. Analysis of a national private pension scheme: The case of Chile. *Int. Labour Rev.* 133: 3, 1993.
43. *El Financiero,* July 15, 1998.
44. *Excelsior,* March 3, 1998.
45. Instituto Mexicano del Seguro Social. *Ley del Seguro Social.* Article 167. México DF, 1993.
46. de Buen, N. Principios de la seguridad social mexicana. In *Alternativas de Reforma de la Seguridad Social,* edited by M. L. Mussot, pp. 17–40. Universidad Autónoma Metropolitana–Fundación F. Ebert, México DF, 1996.
47. Valenzuela, J. C. Estancamiento económico neoliberal. In *México ¿Fin de un Régimen?,* edited by J. C. Valenzuela, pp. 15–36. Universidad Autónoma Metropolitana, México DF, 1995.
48. Huerta, A. *La Economía Mexicana más allá del Milagro.* Diana-UNAM, México DF, 1991.

CHAPTER 12

REMAKING MEDICARE: THE VOUCHER MYTH

Jonathan Oberlander

An increasingly prominent option for Medicare reform is to transform the federal health insurance program for the aged and disabled into a voucher system. Under such a scheme, Medicare beneficiaries would receive a fixed-dollar contribution from the government to purchase health insurance. Proponents anticipate the introduction of vouchers would trigger a large-scale movement of program beneficiaries from the present Medicare system into private health insurance plans. Vouchers would thus represent a privatization of federal health insurance and a radical change in the philosophy and operation of Medicare.

Once promoted by only a small coterie of conservative health economists, during the 1980s Medicare vouchers were thought to be an "impossible dream" by even their own advocates (1). Now, however, vouchers have been endorsed by a growing number of health policy makers and analysts, as well as by the American Medical Association and *The New York Times* (2, 3). The political ascendance of Medicare voucher plans is largely due to the election of a Republican Congressional majority in 1994. The Republican leadership's anti–welfare state, pro-market ideology has created a receptive climate for long-time voucher advocates. Meanwhile, Washington-based policy analysts have followed the political winds in putting forward their own voucher proposals, a bandwagon recently joined by the Congressional Budget Office (4).

Interest in vouchers is also driven by well-publicized alarm over financial problems in Medicare. In the short term, Medicare faces a trust fund "crisis" and pressures from deficit reduction. Medicare's hospitalization insurance trust fund is projected to be insufficient to pay out all benefit costs (commonly, but incorrectly, referred to as "bankruptcy") by as soon as 2001. Moreover, Medicare is one of the fastest growing components of the federal budget. Most balanced budget plans consequently call for substantial reductions in the rate of growth in program expenditures. In the long run, Medicare's financial problems are expected to worsen with the retirement of the baby-boom generation beginning in the second decade of the 21st century and the accompanying decline in the number of active workers per retiree. At the program's current rate of growth, the fear is that the working population will not be able to support the growing numbers of Medicare beneficiaries. These demographic pressures, some observers allege, make Medicare "unsustainable in its current form" (5).

There is reason to believe, however, that both Medicare's current financing problems and the longer-term demographic "crisis" are exaggerated. The present shortfall in the Medicare trust fund can be redressed through modest adjustments in program policies (6). The retirement of the baby-boomers will exert substantial financial pressures on the program. Yet other countries have successfully dealt with similar demographic pressures without the dire consequences now being predicted for the United States. Furthermore, as international experience suggests, vouchers hardly represent the only (or best) alternative for a health insurance system to manage the medical care costs of an aging population. In fact, not one of the industrialized nations with older populations and lower health expenditures than the United States uses vouchers to control health care costs.

In large part, the warnings of impending "bankruptcy" and "crisis" represent emotionally loaded images intended by program critics to raise public anxiety in order to permit radical restructuring of Medicare (7). Indeed, voucher advocates have taken advantage of, and intentionally fueled, the current climate of crisis surrounding Medicare to sell vouchers as a solution to the program's financial problems. Vouchers, though, are touted by their supporters for more than fiscal prowess. Advocates also claim vouchers would benefit Medicare enrollees by increasing the range of choices available to program beneficiaries and by decentralizing power over health coverage decisions from federal bureaucracies to individual consumers (8). In addition, vouchers are believed to promote fair market competition by rewarding cost-conscious behavior from medical providers, health plans, and beneficiaries (9). Vouchers, then, combine the assurance of fiscal control with the symbolism of individual empowerment and market efficiency.

Given the powerful appeal of these claims, the recent enthusiasm for transforming Medicare into a voucher system is not surprising. I argue here, however, that such enthusiasm is misplaced and that many of the claims made for vouchers are false. Vouchers would not work as advertised by their advocates. And their adoption would pose substantial risks for beneficiaries as well as the Medicare program. In particular, I show why the elderly and disabled Medicare population is ill-suited for a voucher system and how vouchers would exacerbate patterns of inequality in access to medical care. I also emphasize the serious problems that would arise in a voucher system due to the absence of working risk-adjustment technology.

The first section summarizes the claims made for vouchers and reviews how they might operate in Medicare. The second section examines potential problems with a Medicare voucher system and explains why these problems are sufficiently serious to warrant rejection of vouchers as program policy. I conclude by examining the implications of this analysis for other public policy issues and outlining an alternative for Medicare reform.

A MEDICARE VOUCHER SYSTEM

How Vouchers Would Work

A Medicare voucher system would embody the principles of "managed competition" developed by Alain Enthoven and would resemble the health insurance system currently used by federal employees (the Federal Employees Health Benefits Plan, FEHBP) (10). Rather than providing federal insurance for a defined package of medical services, as Medicare currently does, the federal government would give program beneficiaries a voucher ("defined-contribution") to purchase health insurance. The government, through the Department of Health and Human Services or the Health Care Financing Administration, would then contract with private insurance companies that wished to compete for Medicare enrollees. Participating health plans might encompass health maintenance organizations (HMOs), preferred provider organizations, point of service plans, and indemnity insurers. Health plans could be required to offer a standard minimum benefit package while being permitted to vary coverage above the minimum, as well as their cost-sharing arrangements and organization of medical services. The current Medicare program would compete with private plans for enrollees.

Health plan marketing would be centralized through an annual enrollment process, or "open season," supervised by the federal government. During open season, beneficiaries would select the health plan they wanted from those participating in the Medicare insurance system. Medicare enrollees would receive comparative information on health plans from the government sponsor, or private intermediaries and consumer groups, to assist them in making informed choices. This information might include comparisons of premium costs, covered benefits, and cost-sharing arrangements in different plans, as well as quality indicators such as member satisfaction and disenrollment rates. Participating plans would have to accept any beneficiary during open season, and beneficiaries would have to remain in health plans for the entire year. In addition to organizing annual enrollment and operating a public Medicare plan, the federal government would monitor the behavior of private insurers to assure they did not violate prohibitions on selective marketing or enrollment of healthier beneficiaries ("cherry-picking"). Finally, the government would pay health plans the voucher amount once they had been selected for the upcoming year by a Medicare beneficiary. These payments could be adjusted for enrollee characteristics such as age and disability status ("risk adjustment") to pay health plans elevated rates for beneficiaries expected to incur higher than average medical expenses.

Beneficiaries would receive the same fixed-dollar voucher regardless of the plan in which they enrolled. They would therefore bear the financial consequences of their health insurance choices. If the premium of the plan they selected cost less than the value of the voucher, they could receive a cash rebate or premium give-back. If, however, they chose a plan charging premiums in excess of the dollar amount of the voucher, they—not Medicare—would pay the difference, creating strong incentives for beneficiaries to select low-cost health plans.

The Case for Vouchers

Consumer Choice. Vouchers are claimed by their proponents to have four major advantages over traditional Medicare. First, vouchers would enhance consumer choice in health care. Ninety percent of Medicare beneficiaries are currently enrolled in the federally operated indemnity insurance plan. While Medicare permits beneficiaries to join HMOs, the program has been slow to contract with other types of managed care plans. Nor can Medicare beneficiaries use their coverage to enroll in private indemnity insurance. Voucher advocates contend that Medicare, as presently organized, constitutes a public monopoly on health insurance for program beneficiaries (1, pp. 25–26).

A Medicare voucher system would seek to end that monopoly. The range of health insurance choices available to beneficiaries would be expanded and the program opened up to private insurers. Medicare enrollees could choose plans that matched their preferences for premium cost, benefit coverage, and cost-sharing. Beneficiaries who were comfortable with managed care organizations could join them, while those who preferred indemnity insurance would be free to choose that type of plan. Proponents argue that a voucher system would decentralize authority over Medicare coverage; individuals, rather than the government, would make decisions about what type of health coverage was best for them (1, p. 33).

In addition to increasing the range of consumer choice, vouchers would also, according to their advocates, improve the quality of choice. Medicare beneficiaries currently have little access to data on the hospitals and physicians they use. A voucher system would provide beneficiaries with detailed information on health plan characteristics and performance. This information would enable beneficiaries to compare health insurance products on a variety of dimensions in order to select an appropriate plan.

Fiscal Control. A second advantage claimed for vouchers is that they would introduce firm fiscal controls on federal Medicare expenditures. Medicare spending is currently open-ended; program expenditures in any given year depend on the quantity and cost of services provided to Medicare beneficiaries. In large part, this is because Medicare is an entitlement (11). By virtue of their eligibility for the program, beneficiaries are entitled to (and Medicare is obligated to pay for) any medical services delivered by licensed medical practitioners. Although there are regulatory controls on federal payments in some parts of the program (the Prospective Payment System for hospitals and the Medicare Fee Schedule for physicians), there is no prospective budget imposing a hard limit on total Medicare spending (12).

A voucher system would dramatically alter Medicare's budgetary and entitlement status. In contrast to the present open-ended system, vouchers would establish a prospective cap on federal Medicare spending that would simply be the product of the number of Medicare beneficiaries and the value of the federal voucher. Proponents argue that federal Medicare expenditures would consequently be made predictable and controllable. The rate of growth in Medicare expenditures would be controlled by restraining the dollar amount of the voucher. Federal spending on any individual beneficiary would be limited to that amount. As noted earlier, the fiscal control offered by vouchers is thought to make the specter of the retirement of the baby-boom generation less threatening. In fact, some analysts claim that vouchers represent the only feasible option for restructuring Medicare to absorb the baby-boomers (5).

Competition. Third, vouchers are believed to produce the supposed benefits of market competition: reduced costs, enhanced quality, and greater efficiency. A voucher system would introduce incentives to engage in cost-conscious behavior for health plans, medical providers, and beneficiaries. Health plans would compete against each other to gain shares of the Medicare market. Competition for beneficiaries could take place in quality, cost, and satisfaction, with plans lowering premiums, expanding benefit coverage, and improving services to attract enrollees. In such a competitive environment, health plans are assumed to have incentives to innovate in the organization and delivery of medical care services. Inefficient plans that failed to maximize benefits per cost or had poor quality would be driven out of business (9, pp. 70–75, 89–92). These competitive pressures would shift down to physicians, who would come under pressure from health plans to deliver cost-effective and high-quality care to their patients or risk losing contracts.

Since they would receive fixed-sum vouchers, beneficiaries would also have incentives for cost-conscious behavior. A central tenet of voucher plans is that consumers "should bear the financial costs of their [health insurance] choices" (5, p. 22). Beneficiaries who chose low-cost health plans could receive cash rebates, while those who enrolled in plans costing more than the Medicare voucher would pay the balance. A beneficiary who wanted the right, for instance, to self-refer to see a specialist, and consequently wanted to enroll in an indemnity insurance plan, could do so but would have to pay for this "extra" option. Medicare beneficiaries in a voucher system would thus face trade-offs in cost, convenience, and benefits when choosing insurance plans. Voucher proponents believe this system rightly rewards those who enroll in cost-effective health plans while penalizing those who select less efficient medical providers.

Regulatory Relief. A fourth argument made for vouchers hinges on their presumed ability to reduce the regulatory burden on the federal government and to avoid the political pathologies associated with regulation. Vouchers are claimed to assign government a simpler, less intrusive role than it allegedly plays in the current Medicare system. No longer would the primary role of the federal government be to offer a defined-benefit package or to regulate payments to hospitals and physicians. Instead, its main task in a voucher system would be to monitor the competition by private insurance plans; government would move from regulator to referee. Federal policy makers, rather than micro-managing Medicare policy, would let private plans decide on their own how to pay providers, what benefits to cover, and how to organize medical care delivery (8).

According to voucher proponents, by redirecting federal payments from a price schedule to a flat per beneficiary voucher, the incidence of "gaming"—where affected actors attempt to get around government regulations—would be lessened (9, pp. 93–95). Hospitals currently operate sophisticated computer programs to determine which diagnostic categories earn them the most money, so patients can be assigned profitable diagnoses ("upcoding"). And physicians often unnecessarily break a single office visit into multiple visits and services ("unbundling") in order to protect their incomes. Medical providers also react to price controls by increasing the volume and complexity of the services they deliver ("behavioral offset"), weakening the effectiveness of regulation. Since a voucher system would not contain any government price regulation other than the basic voucher amount, it is assumed providers would have little opportunity or incentive to engage in regulatory gaming.

Proponents also contend that vouchers would avoid the bias in regulatory politics toward an imbalanced political market dominated by the concentrated interests of regulated industries. Industries greatly affected by regulatory policies exert considerable efforts to "capture" government agencies and shape regulation to their benefit (9, pp. 110–114). They may be aided in this enterprise by their ability to offer policy makers financial resources and political support, as well as their willingness—in contrast to the general public or consumers—to pay the information costs necessary to monitor regulatory developments. Advocates argue that a voucher system would temper these dynamics by focusing attention on a single decision—the setting of the voucher amount—thereby lowering information costs and offsetting some of the medical industry's political advantage. Because regulation in a voucher system would not involve price controls and would modify the behavior of health plans only at the margin, it is also believed that regulated entities would make attempts to engage in pressure politics, since they would "derive little financial benefit from changing or evading the rules" (9, p. 94).

REASSESSING VOUCHERS

At first glance, vouchers appear to offer an attractive option for Medicare reform. As presented by their supporters, vouchers promise to control Medicare costs, enhance beneficiaries' choice of medical care, substitute market efficiency for ineffective government regulation, and make the program "safe" for the retirement of the baby-boomers. As the ensuing discussion demonstrates, however, the actual performance of a Medicare voucher system is likely to fall considerably short of this promise. Rather than being a panacea for Medicare's problems, a voucher system would undermine many of the program's existing strengths.

The Illusion of Choice

While vouchers are commonly promoted as expansions of consumer choice, in reality they would significantly reduce the medical care choices available to Medicare beneficiaries. In fact, voucher systems are explicitly designed to force individuals to leave indemnity insurance for managed care plans such as HMOs, though this goal is frequently shrouded in the rhetoric of a "choice-based system" (13). Under current arrangements, Medicare beneficiaries are free to choose any physician they want. A voucher system would take that freedom away. Beneficiaries who wished to enroll in insurance plans that guaranteed free choice of physicians would have to pay financial penalties if the premiums of those plans cost more than the voucher. In private health insurance markets, indemnity plans—those allowing free choice of providers paid on a fee-for-service basis—tend to be more expensive than managed care organizations that limit selection of medical providers. It is virtually certain this pattern also would hold in a Medicare voucher system. Beneficiaries who wished to remain in the present Medicare program would thus be forced to pay a supplemental premium and consequently, the "choice" offered by vouchers would be loaded against indemnity insurance. This choice would be particularly illusory for poorer beneficiaries who lacked the money to select more expensive plans. And if voucher payments did not keep pace with the costs of medical care, or if competition did not produce the savings anticipated by its advocates, a growing proportion of Medicare enrollees would be forced over time either into low-cost (and potentially low-quality) health plans or to pay a greater share of their income toward health insurance. In this sense, vouchers represent not an expansion of choice but an attempt to shift the costs of medical care onto the elderly and the disabled.

Moreover, if the premium differentials between indemnity insurance and lower-cost managed care plans became extreme, beneficiaries might not have any choice at all as indemnity plans were priced out of reach for all but the wealthiest Medicare enrollees. This is precisely what has happened in some private and public sector insurance plans that have adopted voucher frameworks. Indemnity plans are at particular risk in voucher systems because sicker individuals are less likely than healthier enrollees to leave these plans for managed care organizations. This adverse selection can induce a "death spiral" in which indemnity plans are left with sicker, and consequently more expensive, insurance pools and therefore must charge higher and higher premiums to cover their costs. Eventually, these selection dynamics may boost premiums so high as to drive the plans out of business, as happened with Aetna's high-option FEHBP plan in 1989 (14). The introduction of vouchers, then, may cause Medicare beneficiaries to lose their ability to choose the one type of health plan that guarantees them free choice of medical provider.

Finally, many Medicare beneficiaries would not enjoy the almost unlimited choice of health insurance that voucher advocates envision because much of the United States does not have the population density or health care infrastructure to support a local Medicare market of competing health plans. And even in those areas with sufficient populations and resources to support competing plans, choice of private options could turn out to be less diverse than expected if the current trend of health insurance mergers continues and creates monopolies or oligopolies in Medicare markets (13).

Managed Care and the Chronically Ill

It is, of course, no accident that the financial incentives introduced by a voucher system encourage consumers to exit indemnity insurance. Voucher proponents regard such insurance as inefficient, rewarding of wasteful care, costly, and inimical to competition in health care markets (9, pp. 21–23). Moving Medicare enrollees into managed care, especially prepaid insurance plans such as HMOs, is therefore a primary goal of voucher proposals. It is argued that HMOs, often depicted as the epitome of cost-effective medical care, could reduce federal Medicare expenditures, offer health coverage broader than traditional Medicare, and improve the quality of medical care services (15).

HMOs do have features—such as coordination of health services—that may benefit some Medicare enrollees. And for many services, HMOs can provide medical care that costs less than that delivered in fee-for-service settings without harming quality. However, there is significant evidence documenting HMOs as not appropriate for all segments of Medicare beneficiaries, particularly those with chronic conditions (16). A recent report from the Medical Outcomes Study concluded that over a four-year period, chronically ill elders in HMOs were twice as likely to experience a decline in their health status as were chronically ill elders in fee-for-service Medicare, and that low-income elderly fared particularly poorly in prepaid settings (17). These findings corroborate other studies that have found worse outcomes in HMOs for home health care and for patients with persistent joint pain (18). In part, the worse outcomes are due to the reliance of HMOs on primary care gatekeepers, which may adversely affect the care of elders who have multiple conditions that can be better diagnosed and treated by specialists. Utilization of capitated payment arrangements by HMOs may also endanger the health of their Medicare enrollees. Capitation creates incentives for medical providers to undertreat sick, expensive patients and to dump such patients on other health plans and providers.

In extolling the virtues of HMOs, voucher advocates fail to note these problems. Managed care does not work equally well for all patients and would therefore pose risks to the health of some Medicare beneficiaries. Vouchers, then, would effectively create financial pressures for some segments of the Medicare population to join insurance plans that would provide them with inadequate health care. Moreover, the burden of such pressures would fall disproportionately on the most vulnerable of Medicare beneficiaries, the chronically ill and the poor, making these incentives particularly troubling.

The Limits of Consumerism

Voucher advocates envision that in a competitive health system, Medicare beneficiaries would become effective consumers of medical care. When confronted with financial incentives, beneficiaries would supposedly respond by shopping for the "best-buy" in health insurance: carefully calculate their preferences for cost, quality, and convenience; weigh the differences between health plans on these dimensions; and seek out information to make more informed choices. This consumer role, which requires patients to be cost-conscious, well-informed, and aggressive, would represent a substantial transformation from the traditionally passive role of medical care patients (19).

The problem is, the Medicare population is ill-suited to assume the consumer role that a voucher system would assign to it. Studies have found the elderly less likely to be effective consumers of medical care than the general population (19, pp. 1025–1031). Program beneficiaries have consistently demonstrated widespread confusion about Medicare coverage and cost-sharing arrangements. And the one area where Medicare beneficiaries presently select private insurance—the Medigap market—provides little optimism for turning the elderly into rational consumers. Medicare beneficiaries, confused about their existing coverage and the benefits of Medigap, and sometimes duped by the marketing practices of insurance companies, have purchased overlapping policies they did not need or did not cover what they expected (13). Similar patterns of "irrational" consumer behavior by the elderly have been found in the health plan choices of retirees in the FEHBP; many federal retirees select high premium plans even though those plans offer them little extra benefit for the additional cost (14, p. 5).

If elders cannot navigate the Medigap market, there is little reason to believe they would fare better in a voucher system that increased the range, complexity, and consequences of their medical care choices. For elderly who were long retired and accustomed only to indemnity insurance, the panoply of new insurance options would seem bewildering. Beneficiaries who were seriously ill and those who were lower-income and less educated would similarly be in a poor position to judge alternative health plans or to engage in consumer behavior. The wide choice of health plans offered by a voucher system would be meaningless for much of the Medicare population.

The Risk-Adjustment Dilemma

A properly functioning voucher system depends on effective risk adjustment: that is, the ability to predict individuals' expected medical costs and adjust payments to health plans accordingly. In theory, risk adjustment would help ensure access to medical care for sicker enrollees that insurers might otherwise shun by paying elevated rates on their behalf. It would also be critical to promoting fair market competition between health plans. Without risk adjustment, plans could gain a competitive advantage by attracting healthier risks, rather than innovating or providing cost-effective care. In a risk-adjusted world, healthier enrollees would bring lower payments, taking away the financial benefits of "cherry-picking." Risk adjustment is consequently a fundamental requirement of an efficient and fair voucher-based health insurance system (9, pp. 119–121).

The problem is that a working risk-adjustment system does not currently exist. It is extremely difficult to define actuarial categories that accurately predict individual medical expenses. Medicare's troubled experience with risk adjustment is indicative of the general problem. The present Medicare risk-adjustment system has managed to explain less than 1 percent of the variance between beneficiaries' medical expenses (20). As a result, Medicare substantially overpays HMOs contracting with the program for treating beneficiaries who are healthier than the program average, causing the federal government to lose money on Medicare HMO patients (15). While alternative risk-adjustment models have been proposed, none has yet worked in practice or accurately predicted the huge variation in individual medical expenses. Even when researchers refined the Medicare risk-adjustment formula by incorporating additional variables to reflect beneficiary health status and prior utilization of medical services, a paltry maximum of only 10 percent of the variance in individual expenditures could be explained (21). Some of the health insurance systems cited as exemplars by voucher proponents—including the FEHBP—do not even attempt risk adjustment. Given the enormity of the task and the technological limitations inherent in actuarial science, there is little chance an ideal individual-level risk-adjustment system will emerge anytime soon, if ever.

The dilemma of risk adjustment, then, is that voucher systems depend crucially on a nonexistent technology. As a result, a Medicare voucher system would likely be implemented *without* effective risk adjustment. Voucher advocates downplay this omission by claiming it can be dealt with in implementation and does not pose a serious problem for their model (5). There is strong reason to doubt these claims: the limitations of risk adjustment will not somehow magically disappear during implementation and would pose a significant threat to the successful operation of a voucher system.

Four problems may emerge in a voucher system without effective risk adjustment. First, efficient and socially desirable health insurance plans could go out of business because of adverse selection. In the idealized world of voucher advocates, the market works with Darwinian efficiency: plans that deliver poor quality, are unable to maximize productivity or control costs, or do not offer products demanded by consumers will fail economically. Health plans that "lose" in a voucher system, in other words, deserve to lose because they are inefficient. However, without workable risk adjustment, plans may lose simply because of their risk pool. If a health plan attracts disproportionately sick enrollees and is not properly compensated through risk adjustment, its premiums will rise and it may suffer the "death spiral" described previously. Similarly, plans may succeed by attracting healthier risks that enable them to offer low premiums, thus forgoing the pursuit of organizational innovation and cost-effective medical care that voucher advocates expect. Under these conditions of risk-based competition, the market will not fairly reward efficiency and punish inefficiency as it is supposed to in a voucher system. Instead, it will reward those insurers who are the most clever at enrolling good risks while punishing those who provide coverage to sicker individuals—hardly desirable social policy (22).

A second, closely related problem is that without working risk adjustment, a voucher system may produce considerable instability as health insurers subject to adverse selection go out of business. Health plans caught in "death spirals" of increasingly sick insurance pools and rising premiums can go bankrupt within relatively short periods of time. Moreover, these "death spirals" may be mobile. If, for example, an indemnity plan fails because of adverse selection, those selection effects may simply be transferred to the next plan likely to attract sicker enrollees, such as a preferred provider organization. Consumers in a voucher system could therefore find themselves forced to change plans and doctors as their previous choice disappears, while administrators would have to devise efforts to stabilize the system.

A third problem is that in the absence of effective risk adjustment, one of the central rationales for vouchers—making people pay more for choosing expensive health plans—unravels. Voucher proponents believe it is fair to charge enrollees higher amounts for more expensive plans because these plans are less efficient than lower-cost medical care organizations. Why should the government, voucher advocates ask, subsidize Medicare beneficiaries for inefficient and "cost-unconscious" behavior? This efficiency argument is central to the justification for transforming Medicare from a defined-benefit into a defined-contribution program. Yet without good risk adjustment, there is no way to know whether the high premium amounts paid by enrollees who choose more expensive plans are due to differences between plans in their efficiency or in the health status of their insurance pools. Nor is this only a theoretical possibility. In the FEHBP, health plans that differ only 5 percent in their covered benefits differ 100 percent in premiums; the wide disparity is predominantly due to differential risk selection (23). Under a voucher system, Medicare beneficiaries would consequently pay the price not for selecting inefficient health plans, but simply for being in the wrong risk pool. In the absence of effective risk adjustment, then, there seems to be no compelling normative justification for imposing financial penalties on enrollees in more expensive plans.

A fourth and final problem is that access for sicker Medicare beneficiaries could suffer if risk-adjusted payments proved insufficient to cover their actual costs. In this circumstance, plans would have a strong incentive to shun sicker enrollees because they would be revenue losers and would potentially threaten the competitive position of their insurers. A voucher system would formally prohibit selective marketing and other techniques used by health plans to discourage beneficiaries from selecting that plan or renewing their coverage. However, in the past, plans have used a variety of tactics to induce disenrollment of costly beneficiaries, including creating barriers to care for particular services, and it is by no means clear that regulators could consistently deter plans from this behavior.

In sum, the absence of working risk-adjustment technology is not merely another implementation matter. Rather, it is a crucial flaw undermining both the stable operation and normative justification of voucher systems.

The Challenge of Regulating Vouchers

Despite claims by their proponents, vouchers are highly unlikely to produce significant reductions in the regulatory burden on the federal government. The primary argument for vouchers as a source of regulatory relief is that the government would get out of the business of setting price schedules and controlling the volume of services delivered by medical providers. Instead, federal regulators would settle into a simpler role of paying health plans their voucher amounts, as well as monitoring the enrollment process. However, most voucher plans assume the government would continue to operate a public Medicare program, meaning that the type of federal regulation currently in use would continue, with the added responsibilities (and considerable administrative costs) of regulating the voucher system.

Those responsibilities, contrary to the image of the federal government as a mere "referee" that must only intermittently intervene in the "game," would be formidable. Two of the regulatory challenges in a voucher system have already been mentioned: operating an effective risk-adjustment system and preventing plans from selectively enrolling healthier beneficiaries and disenrolling the seriously ill. Neither of these tasks would be easily accomplished, and both would require considerable resources to monitor individuals' experiences with health plans, risk selection among plans, marketing behavior, and the internal operations of medical care organizations. It is by no means clear that the costs of this type of regulation would be less than those in Medicare's current regulatory regimen. In fact, the costs of regulating a market-based voucher system may well be greater than those of a regulatory health system (24).

Voucher advocates commonly argue that government regulation of medical care prices and volume is doomed to fail because it works against the natural economic incentives (i.e., higher income or maximizing profits) of health providers (5, pp. 110–114). Yet prohibitions on "cherry-picking" raise exactly the same issue, with no greater likelihood of success. The costs of medical care in the Medicare population are highly concentrated, with 10 percent of beneficiaries accounting for 70 percent of program spending in 1995, at a per person average expenditure of $28,120, compared with an average of $4,020 for the overall Medicare beneficiary (25). The payoff for health plans to avoid this group is extremely high; regulations requiring health plans to accept all-comers thus run directly counter to the economic interests of insurers. Vouchers would clearly not eliminate the tensions between financial incentives and regulation.

Similarly, vouchers are unlikely to reduce significantly the incidence of "gaming" in Medicare. Voucher advocates rightly note that hospitals and physicians sometimes respond to federal payment regulations by delivering more services, unbundling one service into multiple visits, and altering diagnoses to correspond with higher payment categories. However, a voucher system would generate its own set of regulatory games. For example, health plans could be expected to devote considerable effort to identifying categories of beneficiaries whose risk-adjusted voucher payments, due to actuarial imperfections, exceeded their actual medical care costs (22). Computer programs that now detect profitable diagnosis categories would simply be reprogrammed to detect profitable risk-adjustment categories.

Nor will a voucher system take the politics out of regulation. Voucher advocates assert that the political activities of the regulated would be reduced because there would be only one major regulatory decision—the setting of the basic voucher amount—to influence, and rules in a voucher system would affect the behavior of medical plans only at the margin. This story seems highly improbable. As already noted, medical plans would have a strong financial stake in the formulation and implementation of rules governing enrollment, marketing, benefit coverage, and risk adjustment. Their financial performance would also be substantially determined by the amount of the federal voucher, and they could be expected to lobby aggressively to shape its outcome. Private insurance companies would become the prime stakeholders in Medicare policy and could be expected to exert their considerable political influence on federal policy makers in pursuit of more profits and less regulation (26). Finally, the introduction of risk adjustment would engender its own politics, with various groups of patients and medical lobbies vying to get their illness a higher risk-adjustment category so as to make patients more attractive to health insurers (24, pp. 215–216).

In sum, a voucher system would move the focus of regulation from hospitals and physicians to health insurers and medical plans. Regulatory gaming would change from upcoding and unbundling to locating profitable risk-adjustment categories. And regulatory policies would center on marketing regulations and the voucher amount rather than on price schedules. Vouchers, then, would not reduce regulation in Medicare, only change its character.

Political Fragmentation

Medicare is a universal social insurance program. All workers who pay into the system through mandatory payroll taxes are eligible, regardless of income, for program benefits. And virtually all beneficiaries are enrolled in a single insurance program. As a result, Medicare has a cross-class program constituency, with program beneficiaries encompassing the middle class and the wealthy, as well as lower-income persons. The universal model of social program contrasts with means-tested welfare programs, such as AFDC, serving only the poor. That contrast is by design; Medicare's programmatic architects believed universal social insurance was politically stronger than welfare programs (27). Programs targeted exclusively to the poor often turned out to be poor programs, both in terms of administration and inadequate benefits, because the poor lacked political clout. Social insurance sought to protect the poor by putting them in the same program with middle-class and wealthier beneficiaries, thereby giving these politically more powerful classes a stake in maintaining the program. During Medicare's three decades of operation, the universal scope of its constituency has made it difficult for policy makers to cut back program benefits or to impose substantial new costs on beneficiaries.

A voucher system would unravel the universal fabric of Medicare politics. Instead of all beneficiaries joining the same program, enrollment would fragment as many enrollees left public Medicare to join private health insurance plans. This fragmentation could prove especially hazardous for the traditional Medicare program if it disproportionately lost wealthier beneficiaries to private insurance. Without these beneficiaries, the constituency for maintaining and improving program benefits would weaken considerably (1, pp. 42–44). Moreover, if current enrollment trends in managed care were to hold in the future, the public Medicare program would be left with a sicker insurance pool. A public program of the poor and sick not only would be politically weak, it would also more than likely incur high costs because of the health care needs of its clientele, triggering political pressures as the program appeared (unfairly) to be less efficient than its private sector counterparts.

Vouchers would also exacerbate inequality in the health care experiences of Medicare beneficiaries. There is, of course, inequality in the present Medicare system, largely due to the limited scope of benefits and differential access to Medigap and supplemental insurance policies. A voucher system, though, would significantly worsen this pattern. Wealthier beneficiaries would have a wider choice of insurance plans than they now have, while poorer beneficiaries could be forced to join only those plans whose premiums were covered by the government voucher. Discrepancies in benefit coverage would widen; some voucher proposals would permit insurance plans to offer less than the current Medicare benefit package. In this case, Medicare could quickly deteriorate into a tiered system of medical insurance with excellent coverage for those who could afford to supplement the voucher and mediocre coverage for those who could not. This tiering could weaken the constituency for increasing the annual voucher amount. Affluent beneficiaries might have little reason to support voucher increases designed to enable lower-income enrollees to purchase bottom-end insurance with improved benefit packages.

Finally, a voucher system might make it easier to impose benefit cuts and cost increases on Medicare enrollees. Voucher advocates believe it would be politically easier to hold down cost increases in a defined-contribution than to curtail defined benefits or raise premiums. If they are right, the ability of beneficiaries to resist benefit cuts would be weakened and the quality of Medicare coverage would erode over time. For proponents, the great virtue of a voucher system is that rationing of medical services would be carried out by health insurers such as HMOs in the political obscurity of the private sector, making politicians less accountable to program-based pressures. For beneficiaries, this "virtue" is a substantial danger, since it may be harder to influence the health care decisions of private insurers than public officials. In sum, the politics of vouchers might place beneficiaries in a disadvantaged position in fighting to protect the value of Medicare insurance.

CONCLUSION

This chapter raises serious doubts about the desirability of transforming Medicare into a voucher system. The Medicare population, because of the high number of elderly and disabled persons who are seriously or chronically ill and their limited consumer sophistication, is ill-suited to succeed in a competitive insurance environment. The attraction of broader choice offered by vouchers would therefore prove illusory for many Medicare beneficiaries. Furthermore, the highly concentrated distribution of medical care costs among the Medicare population, and the absence of effective risk adjustment to control for the effects of this concentration on health plan premiums, pose formidable, perhaps insurmountable, barriers to implementing a workable voucher system in the program. Under these circumstances, introducing vouchers into Medicare would unfairly penalize beneficiaries who enrolled in more expensive health plans; threaten the availability of indemnity insurance (and the existence of public Medicare) that guarantees free choice of provider; and create an unstable system of risk-based competition in which health plans were rewarded for attracting healthier enrollees, rather than pursuing efficiency or innovation. Finally, a voucher system would have adverse distributional consequences, exacerbating existing inequalities in access to medical care and undermining the universal and cross-class political coalition that has supported Medicare. In sum, vouchers for Medicare are neither feasible nor desirable (22).

These arguments have implications beyond the Medicare case. Some European countries, in efforts to strengthen cost containment and enhance efficiency and accountability, are interested in applying the principles of Alain Enthoven's "managed competition" scheme to their own health systems. The analysis in this chapter suggests that such interest should be accompanied by a healthy dose of skepticism about the benefits of such a framework. In the United States, the current Medicare reform debate is part of a broader political argument over the adoption of vouchers in a variety of public policies, including education and housing. Many of the arguments developed here might also apply to these other policy areas. For example, the illusion of choice in a voucher-based health insurance system probably has parallels in "school choice" systems. And the harmful effects of transforming public Medicare into private health insurance are analogous to the perils inherent in current proposals to privatize Social Security. In both cases, proposed market-based reforms would subject retirees to substantial risk, while exacerbating inequality and fragmenting the universal political coalition of social insurance that protects lower-income elderly.

That vouchers are undesirable for Medicare should not be taken to mean that fiscal control of Medicare expenditures is an undesirable goal. On the contrary, reducing the rate of growth in Medicare is important to maintaining the program, absorbing the coming demographic bulge in beneficiaries, and pursuing other social priorities and government programs. Restraining the growth of Medicare expenditures is particularly vital in order to prevent burdensome increases for beneficiaries in program premiums and cost-sharing payments. In one crucial respect, I believe voucher advocates are correct: long-term control of Medicare expenditures is unlikely without the introduction of budgetary limits on program spending. However, vouchers are not, as their advocates often suggest, the only option for budgeting Medicare. One alternative would be to impose a global budget on Medicare expenditures in much the same manner that the single-payer and all-payer health systems in Canada and European countries control their health spending (28). This approach would rely on regulating payments to medical providers, rather than shifting costs to elderly and disabled patients as voucher advocates propose, as the means of stabilizing Medicare expenditures. By adopting a single-payer style budget, Medicare could achieve fiscal control while avoiding the risks to beneficiaries inherent in a voucher system.

Acknowledgments — I gratefully acknowledge the help of Mark Schlesinger in thinking about this project. I have also benefited from numerous conversations on this subject with Theodore Marmor. My thanks also to John Ellwood, Carroll Estes, Meredith Minkler, Timothy Prinz, Michael Schoenbaum, and Harold Wilensky for their helpful comments. This chapter was prepared with the support of the Robert Wood Johnson Foundation, Princeton, New Jersey.

REFERENCES

1. Bovbjerg, R. R. Vouchers for Medicare: The impossible dream. In *Lessons from the First Twenty Years of Medicare*, edited by M. V. Pauly and W. L. Kissick, pp. 25–48. University of Pennsylvania Press, Philadelphia, 1988.
2. Rich, S. AMA's Medicare plan borrows from GOP. *Washington Post*, December 5, 1996, p. A11.
3. Rich, S. The new consensus. *New York Times*, December 11, 1996, p. A26.
4. Congressional Budget Office. *Reducing the Deficit: Spending and Revenue Options*. U.S. Government Printing Office, Washington, D.C., 1996.
5. Aaron, H. J., and Reischauer, R. D. The Medicare reform debate: What is the next step? *Health Aff. (Milwood)* 14: 8–30, 1995.
6. Moon, M., and Mulvey, J. *Entitlements and the Elderly*. Urban Institute Press, Washington, D.C., 1996.
7. Estes, C. L. Social security: The social construction of a crisis. *Milbank Q*. 61: 445–461, 1983.
8. Elhauge, E. Vouchers: Medicare's only hope. *The New Republic*, November 13, 1995, pp. 24-27.
9. Enthoven, A. C. *Health Plan: The Only Practical Solution to the Soaring Cost of Medical Care*. Addison-Wesley, Reading, Mass., 1980.
10. Butler, S. M., and Moffit, R. E. The FEHBP as a model for a new Medicare program. *Health Aff. (Milwood)* 14: 47–61, 1995.
11. Wildavsky, A. *The New Politics of the Budgetary Process*, Ed. 2. Harper Collins, New York, 1992.
12. Moon, M. *Medicare: Now and in the Future*. Urban Institute Press, Washington, D.C., 1993.
13. Light, D. W. Homo economicus: Escaping the traps of managed competition. *Eur. J. Public Health* 5: 145–151, 1995.
14. Evans, A. *The Federal Health Benefits Program, Managed Competition and Considerations for Medicare*. National Academy on Aging, Washington, D.C., 1995.
15. Brown, R. S., et al. Do health maintenance organizations work for medicare? *Health Care Financ. Rev*. 15: 7–23, 1993.
16. Schlesinger, M. On the limits of expanding health care reform: Chronic care in prepaid settings. *Milbank Q*. 64: 189–215, 1986.
17. Ware, J. E., et al. Differences in 4-year health outcomes for elderly and poor, chronically ill patients treated in HMO and fee-for-services systems. *JAMA* 276: 1039–1047, 1995.
18. Shaughnessy, P., Schlenker, R., and Hittle, D. Home health outcomes under capitated and fee-for-service payment. *Health Care Financ. Rev*. 16: 187–221, 1994.

19. Hibbard, J. H., and Weeks, E. C. Consumerism in health care. *Med. Care* 25: 1019–1032, 1987.
20. Newhouse, J. P. Rate adjusters for Medicare under capitation. *Health Care Financ. Rev.*, Annual Suppl. 1986, pp. 45-55.
21. Newhouse, J. P. Reimbursing health plans and health providers: Efficiency in production versus selection. *J. Econ. Lit.* 34: 1236–1263, 1996.
22. Luft, H. S. On the use of vouchers for Medicare. *Milbank Q.* 62: 240–242, 1984.
23. Jones, S., Cohodes, D. M., and Scheil, B. The risks of ignoring insurance risk management. *Health Aff. (Milwood)* 13: 108–122, 1994.
24. Morone, J. A. The ironic flaw in health competition. In *Competitive Approaches to Health Care Reform*, edited by R. J. Arnould, R. Rich, and W. D. White, pp. 207–222. Urban Institute Press, Washington, D.C., 1993.
25. Kaiser Family Foundation. *Medicare Chart Book*. Menlo Park, Calif., 1995.
26. Navarro, V. *Dangerous to Your Health: Capitalism and Health Care*. Monthly Review Press, New York, 1993.
27. Marmor, T. *The Politics of Medicare*. Aldine, Chicago, 1973.
28. Marmor, T., and Oberlander, J. Rethinking Medicare Reform. Paper presented at the Health Consumer Summit on Medicare and Universal Coverage, Washington, D.C., April 25–26, 1997.

CHAPTER 13

A SLIPPERY SLOPE: ECONOMISTS AND SOCIAL INSURANCE IN THE UNITED STATES

Richard B. Du Boff

On a range of issues, mainstream economics in the United States carries with it a narrow policy perspective which relies on the free market rather than social choice to address economic problems, promotes saving and profitable accumulation rather than expansion of wages, and stresses undifferentiated productivity growth rather than the utilization and distribution of productivity gains. It is treacherously easy to slip into this dominant mode of public policy analysis, which is pervasive when it comes to virtually anything having to do with "government interference" in the economy, as it is called in some economic textbooks authored by liberals (1, pp. 66, 69; 2, p. 89). (Here the term "liberal" is used in the American sense, meaning somewhat left-of-center politically.) The public sector is seen as an agency outside "the market," and distinct from "consumers" or "households" or "firms." It is as though the government in question has never been involved in, or any way responsible for, the degree of economic development that has taken place—and as though it is not composed of elected officials collecting taxes and administering programs mediated through a democratic process.

This may explain why, on so many occasions, economists who consider themselves liberal or left of center reach out to their conservative colleagues to forge a "consensus," even when one does not exist, and why they minimize differences between themselves and their adversaries in public forums (3). Only through concerted effort can they avoid assimilating positions formulated by conservative economists and mass-merchandized by aggressive, well-financed organizations devoted to the promotion of right-wing social and economic policy.

SOCIAL SECURITY IN PLAY: A TALE OF TWO LIBERALS

Social Security "reform" may be the best example in the late 1990s. For years Social Security was sacrosanct, the "third rail" of American politics (touch it and you're dead). That began to change in 1981–1983, when conservatives believed that the Reagan presidency would create a climate favorable for cutting back Social Security or eliminating it altogether. In the 1990s, the attacks were renewed, and intensified, with dire predictions of a disaster in the making: the retirement of the baby boom generation starting in 2012 will bankrupt the system and leave an empty trust fund for later generations, whose current payroll taxes will get them nothing in return when they retire.

Paul Krugman, an economist at Massachusetts Institute of Technology and a declared liberal, is known as a critic of standard free trade theory and a defender of John Maynard Keynes against monetarists and other practitioners of laissez-faire economics. He is also a keen student of the income inequalities that have widened so dramatically in the United States since the late 1970s, and has written on this subject in left-of-center publications (4, 5). But when attacks on the integrity of Social Security escalated in 1993 and 1994, led by The Concord Coalition, The Cato Institute, Third Millennium, and other conservative organizations with heavy media exposure, Krugman simply absorbed their position. He passed it on in his own work (6, pp. 72–73), as well as in his review (7) of a book by Peter Peterson, former Nixon Secretary of Commerce, investment banker, and self-styled "Republican fat cat." Peterson is the chief spokesman of the Concord Coalition and for years has been criticizing Social Security as an "entitlement dole . . . welfare for the well-off elderly" (8, pp. 31, 63). It may be that Krugman, and other liberals, accept such propositions as compatible with a liberal concern over income disparities, in this case "well-off elderly" taking resources away from people who do need them. If so, it would be, for an economist of Krugman's stature, an extraordinarily superficial analysis of the sources of economic inequality and deprivation in the United States. But in its skeptical view of a government program, it is not inconsistent with positions Krugman himself has taken, namely, that grafting nonmarket allocation mechanisms onto basically efficient free markets ultimately fails, and that in the end this might succeed only in making matters worse (9, 10).

Krugman's fellow MIT economist Lester Thurow is in the same mold, although his positions may be more consistently liberal. He often raises hackles among mainstream economists by writing books with broad, socially relevant themes that expose the narrowness of their research. In *The Future of Capitalism: How Today's Economic Forces Shape Tomorrow's World* (11, pp. 6–10), Thurow contends that "the world's economic topography" has been altered by a shifting of "five economic tectonic plates"—the end of communism, the global economy, the new "brainpower" technologies, "a multipolar world" with no dominant power, and the demography of "growing, moving, and getting older."

These themes seem unexceptional, until one encounters the last, especially its "getting older" segment and its treatment of Social Security. At once what happened is evident: Thurow added a fifth "tectonic plate" because he must have realized that he had to address the controversies swirling about the "welfare state" in capitalist nations since the 1970s. Hastily, and opportunistically, he reached out for the most common currency—the right-wing argument that the welfare state has caused government spending to spiral out of control and that a major culprit in the United States is Social Security. In Chapter 5 of *The Future of Capitalism*, this argument is rehashed. Portions of it were reprinted in a *New York Times Magazine* article, "The Birth of a Revolutionary Class" (12), which could prove more damaging to progressive economic policies than any other popular article published so far in the 1990s. Diatribes against Social Security are commonplace, but this one comes from a prominent liberal, an editorial contributor to *Dollars & Sense* and *The American Prospect* and a founding scholar of The Economic Policy Institute in Washington. We can now expect to see Thurow's *New York Times* article cited regularly in campaigns to do away with Social Security. Thurow has bestowed upon the neoconservative right a priceless gift—support, from a man associated with the U.S. left, for their campaign to destroy the greatest single accomplishment of social legislation in the United States.

THUROW ON SOCIAL SECURITY: THE SOUND AND THE FURY

Thurow paints a lurid picture of "a large group of affluent, economically inactive, elderly voters" who are "bringing down the social welfare state, destroying government finances, altering the distribution of purchasing power and threatening the investments that all societies need to make to have a successful future" (12, p. 46). In blaming the elderly for this catalogue of economic troubles, Thurow builds his case on inflammatory rhetoric and misuse of statistics, as this sentence further demonstrates: "Adjusting for things like household size, taxes and noncash benefits like health insurance and school lunches, the elderly have a median per capita income of a whopping 67 percent above that of the population as a whole" (12, p. 47).

In his book, Thurow (11, p. 98) supports this claim by citing U.S. Bureau of the Census data—which include, as income, "imputed return on equity in owned homes" and "medical programs" (13, Table 10-D15). While noncash benefits like these are included in a definition of "income" which is useful for some purposes, they vastly overstate the economic well-being of senior citizens. For nonwealthy elderly who occupy homes worth more than they paid for them, there is no easy way to convert these paper gains into higher current incomes. Nor do Medicare and Medicaid increase spendable income, but do for the elderly what should be done for everyone in any decent and rational society. Removing "imputed return" and "medical programs" from Thurow's figures cuts his 67 percent difference by more than half.

But Thurow's figures, no matter how adjusted, are irrelevant. They cover all households having any members 65 years of age or older, with many of these households also containing younger people who have higher incomes than most independently housed elderly. In the Census Bureau publication Thurow cites (13), Table 1 shows that for households headed by a householder (in whose name the home is owned or rented) under 65 years of age, median money income in 1993 was $35,957, while for households actually headed by someone 65 or older, it was $17,751, including Social Security benefits. ("Median" income is the midpoint of the whole distribution: half of all income receivers get more, half get less. It is a better measure of economic status because, unlike a "mean" or an average, it is not affected by extreme values.) By these figures, per capita money incomes of the elderly appear to be about 7 percent higher than for the rest of the population—which includes 15- to 23-year-old householders with median incomes half those of householders 24 to 64 years of age. Take out Social Security, and the incomes of two-thirds of the elderly would drop 40 percent or more; a third of the elderly would lose 65 percent of their incomes or more (14, p. 28).

When Thurow deals with wealth (or assets), he is equally unreliable: "Those 65 to 74 have an average net worth of $222,000 versus $66,000 for those 35 to 44" (12, p. 47). His source is an article by economist Edward Wolff, an authority on the distribution of wealth (15). Thurow fails to inform his readers that Wolff's data are for 1983, that Wolff never makes the age-group comparison or presents the figures that Thurow does (and leaves unexplained), and that in 1983 average net worth peaked for the 65 to 69 age group (at $339,000 per household, including homes) and dropped by 40 percent for those aged 70 to 74, putting that group well below net worth for the entire 45 to 64 age group. In *Top Heavy*, his latest study of the distribution of wealth in the United States, Wolff reports that for 1962 to 1989, the only households that increased their share of total assets were those with heads of household in the 45 to 69 age group. Although they were wealthier than those below 45 years of age, the 70 and over group lost the most ground of all (16, pp. 16–17).

Well, Thurow might reply, even if the elderly are not so "affluent" after all, they are "one-issue voters who exercise a disproportionate impact on the political process." The result is that "today, spending on entitlements plus interest payments on the national debt (most of it accumulated in recent years to make payments to the elderly) take 60 percent of total tax revenue" (12, p. 47).

To begin with, comparing "spending on entitlements" alone with "total tax revenue" is an arithmetic trick that inflates the share of entitlements in the federal budget, because tax receipts are continually running lower than spending. For example, if total revenues are 100, total spending 125, and entitlements 20, the latter are 20 percent of revenues. But they are 16 percent of outlays, with which they should be compared in the company of other major budget outlays. In addition, Thurow's statement lumps all entitlements together as one huge problem, never distinguishing among them. Thurow is in fine company here: Peter Peterson and his Concord Coalition partners are making careers out of this kind of Social Security bashing.

Table 1

Total federal government outlays in the United States:
Annual averages, 1975–76 through 1995–96[a]

	1975–76	1985–86	1995–96
Total federal outlays, billions	$352.1	$968.4	$1,545.8
Percent of outlays in major program groups			
Social Security	19.4%	19.8%	22.0%
Medicare and Medicaid	6.1	9.3	16.7
Means-tested (except Medicaid)	5.8	4.2	6.1
Military and international	27.4	29.0	18.8
Physical resources[b]	10.6	6.0	2.6
Net interest	7.1	13.7	15.3
All other	23.6	18.0	18.5

[a]Source: reference 17, Tables 3.1, 8.1, 8.5.
[b]Includes energy, environment, transportation, community and regional development.

Figures in Table 1 provide the information that serious students of these issues need. The largest entitlements are Social Security, Medicare (which covers the elderly and the disabled), and Medicaid (the state-federal health program for the poor). Together they now account for nearly 39 percent of federal outlays, and about 70 percent of all entitlements. The next largest entitlements are Civil Service and military retirement and disability, and unemployment compensation (totalling 12 percent of entitlements and included in "All other" in Table 1), followed by means-tested programs, largely food stamps, family support assistance (AFDC), supplemental security income (SSI), and earned income tax credits. While Social Security, which includes disability benefits, has been increasing faster than total federal outlays over the past two decades, the only entitlements growing very much faster are Medicare and Medicaid. On that subject, few words suffice: Thurow seems to believe that a health care system which is the costliest of any high-income nation (14 percent of gross domestic product) yet excludes nearly 20 percent of of its people can be cured by cutting benefits for the elderly, rather than replacing the entire system.

The figures in Table 1 also belie Thurow's comment that the national debt has been forced up "to make payments to the elderly." In one swoop Thurow rewrites fiscal history to shift blame for the deficits of the past 15 years from Reaganomics to the elderly. Those deficits are mainly the result of the 1981–1983 tax cuts, only partially reversed by the tax increases of 1990 and 1993. On the expenditure side of the ledger, only the rising cost of health care and larger interest payments are contributing to the ongoing budget deficits. The more than doubling of the interest share of outlays since 1975 (Table 1) came not only from the deficit-driven increase in the national debt, but also from the historically high interest rates imposed by the Federal Reserve to "fight inflation." Higher interest rates also bring slower economic growth and higher unemployment, and in turn lower tax revenues, widening budget deficits, and a bigger interest bill yet. That Thurow can overlook this vicious circle is a tribute to the slipshod character of his article and the book from which it is drawn: elsewhere in *The Future of Capitalism,* Thurow assails the "war on inflation" waged by Federal Reserve Chair Alan Greenspan and his fellow central bankers and the "real human havoc" it has wrought (11, Chapt. 9).

THE FUTURE OF SOCIAL SECURITY: NO EXIT?

If Social Security spending is growing any faster than total outlays, the increases in the taxes that support it more than make up for rising benefits being paid to retirees. In 1995, Social Security payroll tax receipts were $399 billion, while Social Security benefits amounted to $339 billion, meaning that the system ran a surplus of $60 billion. Without it, the 1995 federal deficit would have been $224 billion instead of $164 billion (18, pp. 3, 7).

Here Thurow makes a bad case worse (12, p. 47):

> advocates for the elderly argue that Social Security is running a surplus and, hence, needs no restructuring. But that is an illusion. If the Government is running an overall deficit, it is irrelevant if one sector has a "surplus" because it is credited with collecting more taxes than it needs. What matters is what is driving the expenditure side of the budget.

This is an amateurish evasion: if Social Security is in surplus, there is no way it could add to the deficit except to allow *non–Social Security expenditures* to be larger than otherwise. It is also a bizarre application of public finance. Apparently Thurow would cut Social Security benefits while leaving intact the structure of payroll taxes, which are specifically and legally dedicated to Social Security.

To this, Thurow delivers the standard response: Social Security's surplus will disappear once the "baby boomers" start retiring in 2012, so that "the current 15 percent Social Security tax rate would have to be boosted to 40 percent by 2029 to provide the benefits that have been promised" (11, p. 47). His source (12, pp. 99, 345) is purely second-hand—an article in *Fortune* (19). Its author predicts the demise of Social Security by referring to economist Laurence Kotlikoff's "generational accounting," which purports to measure the costs of government borne by each generation of people over their entire lifetimes (20). Each generation's "net tax rate" equals total taxes paid minus total government benefits received, compared with lifetime earned income. Social Security enters into both taxes and benefits, along with a host of other government programs. The net tax rate is supposed to be small for older people today, crushing for generations born after 1980. But the estimates required for these calculations are more than heroic. They involve, among other things, how much income an age cohort will earn over their entire working lives, what gets included in their benefits, what taxes and debts are passed on to future generations, and how all these future sums are to be discounted to determine what they are worth today. By one reckoning, reasonable changes in just three assumptions (interest rates, spending on education, health care costs) can reduce lifetime net tax rates from 84 percent to 20 percent (21). By another, longstanding fiscal practices that are likely to be repeated in some way (modest adjustments in taxes and benefits, continued rolling over of the federal debt) make Kotlikoff's assumptions look even more arbitrary (22, Chapt. 6).

Thurow completely overlooks the more widely accepted way of estimating the future costs of Social Security. The *1996 Annual Report* of the Social Security Trustees forecasts that by its "best estimate of the future course of the population and the economy," the Social Security deficit (benefits exceeding tax collections) will be 2.2 percent of taxable payroll over the next 75 years, equivalent to a payroll tax increase today of 1.1 percentage points for workers and employers, over the 6.2 percent they each now pay (18, pp. 4, 113). (The total rate at present is 12.4 percent. Thurow's "current 15 percent" rate is wrong: it includes payroll taxes for Medicare.) In fact, the Trustees' "best estimate" is based on the assumption that over the next 35 to 70 years the economy, and its taxpaying capacity, will grow at a rate of 1.8 percent per year—more slowly than in any other 30 to 40 year period in U.S. history and well below the historical trend of 3 percent per year (23, pp. 5–10). If the economy grows at the lower rate experienced during the past two decades, 2.5 percent per year, actuarial balance could be achieved by 2070 with an immediate tax increase of only 0.5 percent of taxable payroll (18, pp. 54–55, 113).

An alternative would be to raise payroll taxes in steps, which would require somewhat larger increases (for example, 1 percent every 10 to 15 years). Even these increases hardly seem onerous in a rich country which has the smallest share of gross domestic product going to taxes of any high-income nation—less than 32 percent (24, p. A32). Nor would it be necessary, or desirable, to raise the tax rate for all workers. Actuarial balance might be achieved by removing the income ceiling on the payroll tax ($65,400 in 1997) and levying it on all incomes without upper limit. This solution certainly seems desirable in the light of recent history and projected trends. One reason why Social Security shows a long-term deficit is that the proportion of total compensation subject to the FICA tax is predicted to drop, from 82 percent at present to 77 percent in 2030 as incomes grow faster at the upper end of the income distribution (25, p. 83). Already the Social Security Trustees have noted that since 1984 the ratio of taxable earnings to all earnings in Social Security–covered employment has dropped, "due to the higher proportion of total covered wages earned by very high wage earners"

(18, p. 152). As Thurow himself observes, "No country not experiencing a revolution or a military defeat with a subsequent occupation has probably ever had as rapid or as widespread an increase in [income] inequality as has occurred in the United States in the past two decades" (11, p. 42).

To borrow a term from Thurow, the "disconnect" between his eloquent writing on economic inequalities and his mindless assault on Social Security and the elderly who rely on it is gaping. Another example: "No public interest is served by making parents rich at the cost of making children poor" (12, p. 47). Thurow thus joins the rank of those who blame Social Security for child poverty. In other words, the highest child poverty rate of all high-income nations by far (more than a fifth of all children living in poverty) is caused by Social Security benefits which are more modest than those of other high-income nations.

The disconnect is no less impressive for military spending. Unlike "expenditures on the elderly," Thurow states, military spending is not "squeezing government investments in infrastructure, education and research and development," because it is "down to less than 4 percent of gross domestic product, and even if America were willing to take defense spending down to zero, the day of reckoning would be postponed by only a few years" (12, p. 47). There will be no "day of reckoning" for Social Security unless politicians, helped by articles like Thurow's, act to dismantle it instead of taking the modest steps needed to preserve it. Furthermore, while the military's share of the federal budget has declined since the 1980s, a Cato Institute analyst points out that its current level of $265 billion per year is at least three times as much as Russia spends, and twice the amount spent by Britain, France, Germany, and Japan combined (26). That sum would appear to "squeeze" a wide range of desperately needed social outlays—especially since (to quote Thurow again) "there is no credible military threat to the United States that even the American military can imagine when justifying their budgets" (11, p. 64).

SOCIAL INSURANCE: THE DARK SIDE OF THE MOON

For all of Thurow's contributions to left-of-center publications, his moorings have never been firm. In the United States, the corporate business counterattack against "big government" is more than two decades old, but for Thurow the only problem raised by U.S. corporations is how to make them "world class" competitors in the global economy. In the struggle over the federal government budget, the only political force Thurow recognizes is the elderly, and the only class war being waged is the war of the old against the young.

Thus, while the ferocity of Thurow's attack on Social Security may be unexpected, his instinctive reaction toward it should not be. It is another example of an ad hoc, one-at-a-time treatment of "problems" placed on the public agenda by private capital, the major media, and the political establishment. Economists like Thurow question the prevailing state of affairs within the framework of capitalist institutions and have never thought about comprehensive nonmarket solutions to a whole array of social and economic problems. Nonmarket mechanisms invoke the logic of collective action, the antithesis of the individual choice theoretics in which the vast majority of economists are trained and through which they must communicate if they wish to be considered "professional" by their colleagues. Social insurance is a leading example of such a nonmarket mechanism. It is hardly surprising that many economists do not grasp the concept, or cannot accept it as their primary frame of reference for dealing with economic insecurity.

Social insurance is universal insurance, covering several independent risks for all citizens without exception and financed by contributions (taxes) that are not directly related to benefits. It cannot be compared with a private insurance contract covering only one contingency at a time as a single market (life or disability or home protection or anything else). Social Security in the United States, like its counterparts elsewhere, is portable from job to job and covers more than retirement: it provides disability insurance and benefits to survivors of those who die before retirement. Its benefit formula keeps millions of elderly out of poverty, since it is weighted in favor of workers with lower lifetime earnings and guarantees that they will not outlive their savings. This adds up to more lifetime insurance than all types of life insurance combined, especially when one considers that unemployment insurance is also part of the Social Security system.

For most of us, life is a lottery; we cannot know what will become of us before we die. Pooling resources so that everyone shares the major risks of life, and free market failures, is the essence of social insurance. This is why comparing "rates of return" on FICA contributions for one generation of beneficiaries against another, or calculating "unfunded liabilities" that present generations are alleged to be passing on to their followers, is irrelevant (unless it is assumed that succeeding generations will live in an economy significantly less productive, and poorer, than today's—an unlikely prospect) (27, p. 37):

> This sort of group-by-group analysis of who gets what, on average, misses the basic point of social insurance. At birth, none of us knows for sure where we will end up socially or economically. We may be low- or high-wage earners. We may marry or not. Our spouses may work or not. Our working spouses may be low- or high-wage earners. We may incur misfortune. The current [Social Security] scheme ensures us that however things turn out in life, our retirement benefit will not be too awful, and our dependents will be provided for if we expire before retirement.

Social Security is part of the public sector, which, in a capitalist society, is the only means for sustaining us as a collection of diverse human beings with different fates, but with common basic needs. The idea was well put by a noted liberal economist—characteristically, however, on one selective occasion. It came in 1981, at the opening of the Reagan offensive against the welfare state (28):

> Societies do not work unless there is a feeling of mutual obligation and willingness to sacrifice for the common good. . . . Regardless of how privately wealthy we are, a good life cannot be had in the midst of social disintegration. What Reaganomics forgets is that government plays an important role in creating feelings of mutual obligation and respect. Those feelings don't just exist on their own. They have to be carefully cultivated. They can easily be exterminated by what seem to be relatively trivial problems.

Fifteen years later, on another occasion far-removed, the author—Lester Thurow—addressed the relatively modest problem of Social Security in terms repudiating the essence and spirit of his critique of Reaganomics. The ideas he expressed in 1981 were in total eclipse. It is an object lesson in what can happen when one reacts to problems in a piecemeal fashion, without a clear vision of a society freed from the grip of capitalist priorities.

Note — This chapter is an expanded version of an article published in *Monthly Review,* Vol. 48, No. 5, 1996, pp. 1–9.

REFERENCES

1. Samuelson, P. A., and Nordhaus, W. *Economics*, Ed. 15. McGraw-Hill, New York, 1995.
2. Baumol, W., and Blinder, A. *Economics*, Ed. 7. Dryden Press, Fort Worth, Tex., 1997.
3. Gordon, D. M. Twixt the cup and the lip: Mainstream economics and the formation of economic policy. *Soc. Res.* 61(1): 1–33, 1994.
4. Krugman, P. The rich, the right, and the facts. *The American Prospect* 11: 19–31, 1992.
5. Krugman, P. The spiral of inequality. *Mother Jones* 21: 44–49, November/December 1996.
6. Krugman, P. *Peddling Prosperity: Economic Sense and Nonsense in the Age of Diminished Expectations*. W. W. Norton, New York, 1994.
7. Krugman, P. Demographics and destiny. *New York Times Book Review*, October 20, 1996, p. 12.
8. Peterson, P. *Facing Up: How to Rescue the Economy from Crushing Debt and Restore the American Dream.* Simon & Schuster, New York, 1993.
9. Burkett, P. The bankruptcy of mainstream economics. *Monthly Rev.* 44(5): 18–26, 1992.
10. Kuttner, R. Peddling Krugman. *The American Prospect* 28: 78–85, 1996.
11. Thurow, L. C. *The Future of Capitalism: How Today's Economic Forces Shape Tomorrow's World.* William Morrow, New York, 1996.
12. Thurow, L. C. The birth of a revolutionary class. *New York Times Magazine*, May 19, 1996, pp. 46-47.
13. U.S. Bureau of the Census. *Income, Poverty, and Valuation of Noncash Benefits: 1993*. Current Population Reports, Series P60-188. Government Printing Office, Washington, D.C., 1995.

14. Pattison, D. The distribution of OASDI taxes and benefits by income decile. *Soc. Sec. Bull.* 58: 21–33, 1995.
15. Wolff, E. Changing inequality of wealth. *Am. Econ. Rev.* 82(2): 552–558, 1992.
16. Wolff, E. *Top Heavy: A Study of the Increasing Inequality of Wealth in America.* Twentieth Century Fund Press, New York, 1995.
17. *Historical Tables, Budget of the United States Government. Fiscal Year 1997.* Government Printing Office, Washington, D. C., 1996.
18. Social Security Administration. *1996 Annual Report of the Board of Trustees of the Federal Old-Age and Survivors Insurance and Disability Insurance Trust Funds.* Washington, D.C., 1996.
19. Dowd, A. Needed: A new war on the deficit. *Fortune* 130: 191–200, November 14, 1994.
20. Kotlikoff, L. *Generational Accounting: Knowing Who Pays, and When, for What We Spend.* Free Press, New York, 1993.
21. Baker, D. *Robbing the Cradle? A Critical Assessment of Generational Accounting.* Economic Policy Institute, Washington, D.C., 1995.
22. Eisner, R. *The Misunderstood Economy: What Counts and How to Count It.* Harvard Business School Press, Boston, 1994.
23. Du Boff, R. The welfare state, pensions, privatization: The case of Social Security in the United States. *Int. J. Health Serv.* 27: 1–23, 1997.
24. *OECD Economic Outlook* 60, 1996.
25. Bipartisan Commission on Entitlement and Tax Reform. *Final Report to the President.* Government Printing Office, Washington, D.C., 1995.
26. Bandow, D. Dole's military card. *New York Times*, July 6, 1996, p. 19.
27. Mashaw, J., and Marmor, T. The great Social Security scare. *The American Prospect*, 29: 30–37, 1996.
28. Thurow, L. C. Holes in Reaganomics. *New York Times*, November 8, 1981, Sec. 4, p. 21.

PART V
Debate on Pathways of Social Inequalities and Health

CHAPTER 14

INCOME INEQUALITY, SOCIAL COHESION, AND CLASS RELATIONS: A CRITIQUE OF WILKINSON'S NEO-DURKHEIMIAN RESEARCH PROGRAM

Carles Muntaner and John Lynch

Research on social inequalities is going through a period of resurgence in public health and epidemiology. Using the MEDLINE database of biomedical publications, Lynch and Kaplan have recently noted a steep increase during the last ten years in the number of articles per month that list social class, socioeconomic factors, income, or poverty as descriptors. Although the relevance of class analysis (e.g., pragmatic, functionalist, neo-Weberian, or neo-Marxist) is still debated in epidemiology (2–4) (along with other forms of research on social inequalities such as those due to gender, race/ethnicity, age, migration, or sexual orientation), the growing evidence of an increasing polarization of the U.S. social structure in terms of gradational measures of class (i.e., income, wealth) (5, 6) has become difficult to ignore. There are several possible explanations for the "class denial" that affected the biomedical and public health literatures between the mid-1970s and the mid-1980s. Political changes in the control of government funding can have a major impact on the content of scientific production. During the 1980s, the Reagan administration launched a backlash against social science in the government (7). For example, the National Institutes of Health section headed by Elliot Liebow that had funded research on social inequalities (studies on economic cycles, unemployment, and health) (8) was shut down. In spite of notable exceptions (9), few government epidemiologists and demographers conducted studies on social inequalities in health in the 1980s. Indeed, some of the most influential articles in the early 1990s by U.S. researchers came from other disciplines (10, 11). The British Black report (12, 13) could be considered the milestone that helped spur this new interest in class inequalities in health. Ten years later, in the early 1990s, several studies based on data collected at the National Center of Health Statistics provided evidence that class inequalities in health were substantial in the United States as well (10, 11). It is within this period of resurgence that Wilkinson and other investigators in Europe and the United States have built an original research program on social inequalities in health (14).

The main thrust of the program's empirical studies involves correlations between national mortality and morbidity rates and national measures of income inequality (e.g., Gini coefficient, percent share of total household income received by the least well-off 50 percent of the population), which are typically strong (correlations range between .6 and .8) (14, 15). A second aspect of this research program is the attribution of the effects of income inequality on population health to the breakdown of social cohesion (e.g., cooperation, reciprocity, trust, civic participation), in the Durkheimian[1] tradition of social integration and suicide. Although the relationship between income inequality and health is backed up by many empirical studies, the role of social cohesion as mediator of this relationship is mostly an untested hypothesis, to which Wilkinson arrives after reviewing a large body of research on social relations and health spanning several disciplines (including epidemiology, sociology, political science, anthropology, and behavioral neuroscience). However, recent work by Kawachi and colleagues (20, 21) provides some empirical support for the idea that social cohesion (i.e., organization membership) mediates the effects of income inequality on health.

In the following sections we begin by reviewing several contributions of Wilkinson's model on income inequality and social cohesion to the field of social inequalities in health. We then propose several amendments to the model, drawing mostly from research on class relations and class formation.

CONTRIBUTIONS OF WILKINSON'S MODEL OF INCOME INEQUALITY AND SOCIAL COHESION

An important contribution of Wilkinson's model is that it provides a sociological alternative to other explanations for social inequalities in health that have emphasized health behaviors such as smoking, overweight, drinking alcohol, using drugs, and being sedentary (e.g., 22, 23), in particular among the poor (24), or that advance subjective interpretations for social inequalities based on perceived status or prestige (e.g., 25). Income inequality is an emergent property of populations, a social fact that cannot be attributed to any single person, as income

[1] Wilkinson's program can be characterized as "neo-Durkheimian" (e.g., 14, pp. 15, 170–172) because of its emphasis on solidarity and morality (i.e., social cohesion) and health and its use of social facts (i.e., national mortality rates) (see 16). This characterization is a stereotype, such as "neo-Weberian" or "neo-Marxian," but helps in tracing some relevant antecedents of Wilkinson's research. Wilkinson's model appeals to social facts such as the national distribution of income and the density of a social network rather than to individual characteristics (a person's income, a person's sociability score). Ecological studies are also part of the history of social epidemiology in the United States (17, 18). For example, social epidemiologists have studied aggregated social indicators (e.g., unemployment rate) in relation to morbidity and mortality rates (19).

inequality only emerges from relations among individuals. Income inequality can only be defined in relational terms—it is literally the income or share of income of an individual or group relative to another individual or group (26). However, most research on income and health in the United States has looked exclusively at the health effects of low absolute levels of income (i.e., poverty) while reducing the health effects of poverty to personal attributes (such as culture of poverty, genetic or racial inferiority, low self-esteem, lack of "values," inability to delay gratification) (27, 28).

Wilkinson's analyses of developed capitalist countries that have gone through the epidemiologic transition (e.g., Europe, Japan, the United States, Canada, Australia) show that population health is strongly associated with the distribution of income, even after taking into account average disposable personal income, absolute levels of poverty, smoking, racial differences, and provision of health services. In these countries, relative income is more closely associated with mortality within countries than are absolute income differences between them (14). (An exception is research by Judge and colleagues (29) which finds little support for an association between income inequality and mortality in rich nations.) Income inequality has also been associated with mortality in some poor countries. For example, in a combined analysis of rich and poor countries, Waldmann (30) found that comparing countries where the income of the poor is equal, those where the rich are wealthier are more likely to have higher infant mortality rates. Studies on income inequality also confirm that behavioral risk factors (e.g., smoking) are minor determinants of the social gradient in mortality (14, Chapt. 5).

When looking for explanations for the effects of income inequality on individuals, Wilkinson follows his own data-driven approach by examining findings from a variety of disciplines (research on social change, social capital, social isolation, child development, and stress, among other topics). He rejects some of the assumptions about human behavior associated with rational choice (e.g., that people behave only in pursuit of self-interest) (14, pp. 25, 145, 211).[2] Wilkinson's stance is important as rational choice has dominated theory on social inequalities during recent decades (31–33). Wilkinson's own empiricist inclination leads him toward social psychology when searching for the consequences of income inequality among individuals (e.g., social isolation) and rejecting a model of human behavior with weak empirical support (34–37) that has often been used to justify social inequalities.

Another major contribution of Wilkinson's work is that he has established a realist alternative to the use of socioeconomic status in contemporary social epidemiology. Research on social inequalities in health can now concentrate on

[2] The assumptions of rational choice vary among social scientists. They can encompass complex attributes such as cognitive proficiency, utility maximization, and autonomy (e.g., 31), or restrict assumptions to a minimum such as in "persons have at any point in time a set of ranked options for action and they choose the one that ranks first" (Roemer, personal communication).

income inequality or other objective indicators of social inequalities (38, 39), rather than perceptions of status, control, or prestige. Concepts of status and prestige refer to subjectively perceived social ranking (40) rather than to objective inequalities as measured by income or credentials (e.g., 11 years of schooling signals lack of a high school diploma) that are independent of respondents' perceptions.[3] In spite of high correlations between socioeconomic status, income, and occupational prestige[4] and the availability of composite measures of status that incorporate income (41), using income inequality is important as status conveys the notion that social inequalities are not real, or blurs the distinction between objective and subjective inequalities (38).

Although Wilkinson concludes that what matters most for determining the health of populations is the quality of social relations (i.e., social cohesion) (14, p. 211), a public health implication of his research is that income should be redistributed more equitably to reduce mortality and morbidity rates. This epidemiologic evidence that supports an egalitarian distribution of national incomes is a welcome addition to health policy recommendations that target poverty (42–44). Thus, research on social facts leads to different social policies than research on health behaviors (14, pp. 184–185). Drawing on Rose's work on the failure of the high-risk approach to prevention (e.g., the number of people at high risk for dementia in a population is a function of the average cognitive ability in the whole population) (14, p. 19), Wilkinson presents a compelling case against the risk behavior approach to prevention (e.g., 45) while advocating the reduction of income inequalities.

A CRITICAL APPRAISAL OF THE INCOME INEQUALITY AND SOCIAL COHESION MODEL

Income Inequality

International Relations, Income Inequalities, and Health. By restricting its analysis of income inequalities to Europe and the United States, Wilkinson's model does not explain how the large international (between-country) variation of income affects the health of nations. More "developed" countries constitute only

[3] When researchers do not provide a rationale for what determines differences in education or income, they probably should use terms such as "social stratification" that do not convey the subjective nature of status. The functionalist school in American sociology has used measures of socioeconomic status based on the regression of income and education on occupational prestige scores. One could understand this practice in an academic environment that had trouble admitting the reality of social inequalities in health. Contemporary research on social inequalities in health already uses objective indicators (e.g., 38, 39). Furthermore, grouping major indicators of social stratification in a single concept precludes the understanding of their independent effects on mortality (e.g., 9). Nevertheless, perceptions of inequality are interesting in their own right (because of the "availability heuristic" people tend to over-represent the proportion of individuals in their own strata) (40).

[4] Wilkinson makes a distinction between status and income when he describes Eastern Europe (e.g., 14, p. 126) where wages of manual workers could be higher than those of white-collar workers.

about one-fifth of the world's total population (46). (Wilkinson's terminology of "developed" and "developing" countries (development theory) implies that the latter will reach the living standard of the former, a hypothesis disputed by several rival theories (e.g., 47).) Wilkinson's rationale is that developed countries have passed through the epidemiologic transition from infectious diseases to noncommunicable diseases. This choice omits that some infectious diseases have re-emerged in developed countries (e.g., tuberculosis) (48) during the last decades, which have been marked by increases in income inequalities and poverty (49). In addition, "developing" regions suffer from noncommunicable diseases as well. The probability of death from noncommunicable diseases is higher in poor sub-Saharan countries than in wealthy countries (50). These data challenge a benevolent, evolutionary view of population health transitions and call for international models of social inequalities in health. The analysis of trends in the international distribution of income between the 1960s and the 1990s shows that between-country income inequality, rather than within-country, is the most important factor in world income inequality (51).

Several sociological theories have been proposed to explain world social inequalities: imperialism, dependency theory, world-system theory, and globalization (the latter being distinct from the rhetoric of "globalization" in which an increasingly competitive international economy renders futile the policymaking efforts of local governments (52)) (53–56). For example, world-system theory has provided evidence that becoming peripheral in the international division of labor produces social conflict through income inequality (57). The negative health effects of transfers of resources between empires and their colonized countries, between core and peripheral countries, and between debt-ridden countries and the International Monetary Fund have also been documented (e.g., 58–60). Nevertheless, the income inequality and social cohesion model ignores the impact of international economic relations on levels of income inequality within nations.

Class Relations and Income Inequality. Although income inequality, an indicator of social stratification, is a strong predictor of mortality and morbidity rates, a model of social inequalities in health should address the social mechanisms that generate income inequality in the first place (61). In Wilkinson's analysis it is the receipt of income that is important, not the way income was generated. In this way, the model linking income inequality, social cohesion, and health is based on how income is used to consume various social goods rather than on how income results from particular production relations (e.g., 14, pp. 191, 211).[5] In

[5] Absent from the income inequality and social cohesion model is any substantial reference to occupational health (i.e., the impact of the labor process on health at the point of production). Thus a main difference between "occupational hazards" and "labor process" approaches is that in the former, the connection to class relations is ignored, while occupational deaths, injuries, and illnesses are under-reported and understudied (62).

Wilkinson's framework, Bill Gates's class position is characterized more by his capacity to buy a Leonardo da Vinci masterpiece than by his being a founder, director, and major shareholder of Microsoft. (That high income predisposes to a sort of consumer pathology (14, p. 191) is far from evident, however; a recent survey of U.S. millionaires shows their patterns of consumption to be *relatively* restrained (63).) The "starting fact" for Wilkinson's model is that by some process (which he does not discuss) income is distributed unevenly and that this has consequences for health. Theories of social stratification and class analysis seek to explain how relational positions in a social system (social formation in neo-Marxian terminology) generate income inequalities (64–66).[6] Different positions in production relations (e.g., moneylender, landlord, manager, worker) generate various sources of income (e.g., much greater income can be generated from the position of manager than that of worker; see the Appendix at the end of the chapter for an example of a social system with some class, political, and cultural relations). Although any class location can receive low incomes (e.g., there are many poor business owners) (68), high income and wealth are overwhelmingly associated with capital ownership in capitalist economic systems (69).

Central to Marxian class analysis is the concept of exploitation that provides a social mechanism for explaining how income inequalities are generated. There are several non-Marxian (e.g., commonsense such as "taking unfair advantage of someone else's labor," Saint-Simonian, Lutheran, Lockean) and Marxian (e.g., neo-Marxist and classical) notions of exploitation. Among the most prominent neo-Marxist notions of exploitation we find Roemer's and Wright's. In brief, Roemer maintains that exploitation is generated by an unequal distribution of productive assets among rational actors (i.e., property relations). Following Roemer's 1982 theory (33), in a society divided into two groups, S and its complement S', S is exploited and S' is exploiting if S would be better off if it withdrew with its per capita share of productive, alienable assets; S' would be worse off if it withdrew with its per capita share of productive, alienable assets; and S' would be worse off if S withdrew from society with its own assets. Roemer (70) has since amended this definition in response to several criticisms (such as, his definition did not capture the relation of domination between exploiter and exploited and did not mention labor). Wright's definition of exploitation precisely includes these two factors (domination and labor). According to Wright (66), class

[6] For example, Robinson and Kelley's neo-Marxian model of the consequences of ownership and authority relations for income synthesizes production relations (ownership of the means of production) with authority relations. The basic form of their model specification is as follows (65):

$$Yi = Bo + B1Oi + B2Ai + ui$$

where Yi is earnings, O is a capitalist ownership variable (coded 1 for owners who hire labor and 0 otherwise), and A is an authority variable based on a scaling of supervisory rank (coded 0 for nonsupervisors, 1 for supervisors whose subordinates are nonsupervisors, and 2 for supervisors whose subordinates are also supervisors). See 67 for the health effects of the dimensional and categorical aspects of class relations.

exploitation occurs when: (*a*) the material welfare of a social group causally depends on the material deprivation of another; (*b*) the causal relation in (*a*) involves the asymmetrical exclusion of the exploited from access to certain productive resources, usually backed by force in the form of broadly defined property rights; and (*c*) the causal mechanism that translates exclusion in (*b*) into differential health and welfare involves the appropriation of the fruits of labor of the exploited by those who control the relevant productive resources (without implying that the value of what labor produces is exclusively determined by labor effort).

The "classical" or "traditional" view of exploitation[7] is of particular interest here because of the body of empirical tests to which it has been submitted (e.g., 72). "Classical" Marxism starts with a theory of value (the Labor Theory of Value) that leads to a theory of exploitation. In Marxian terms, class is defined as the process of producing, appropriating, and distributing surplus labor (73). Laborers perform a certain amount of labor that is sufficient to produce the goods and services that their current standard of living requires (necessary labor). Nevertheless, laborers perform more than this necessary labor (surplus labor), which might be retained by laborers or, alternatively, might be appropriated by non-laborers (exploitation). Exploitation thus occurs when the class process involves appropriation of the surplus labor of laborers by non-laborers (73). Thus, exploitation can be quantified through the ratio of s (surplus value), the size of the difference between the necessary labor time embodied in the commodities produced by workers, to v (variable capital) that is embodied in their wages. This rate of exploitation, s/v, is hypothesized to determine the rate of profit, $s/(c + v)$, where c is "constant capital," or the necessary labor time that went into producing factories, materials, and equipment used by labor in production.[8]

Class exploitation can be measured at different levels (such as individual, neighborhood, national). For example, an indicator of class exploitation (the ratio of the total value added in the manufacturing sector to wages and salaries in the manufacturing sector) at the national level has been used to predict violent rebellion (72). However, even if the association between a class-based measure of exploitation and mortality rates were weaker than with income inequality, it does not mean that the class-based measure lacks heuristic value. In fact, a measure of exploitation based on value added to wage ratios may be preferable because the rate of exploitation provides an explicit social mechanism, while income inequality does not.

[7] Although this notion of exploitation usually refers to Marx's version of the Labor Theory of Value, it also encompasses recent developments such as the "New Solution" to the transformation problem which deals with the quantitative relation between labor values and prices (71).

[8] The rate of profit is hypothesized to vary with the rate of exploitation and inversely with the "organic composition of capital" (c/v), or the ratio of "constant capital" to "variable capital": $s / (c + v) = s/v \,/\, (c + v)/v = s/v \,/\, (c/v) + (v/v) = s/v \,/\, (c/v) + 1$ = rate of surplus value/organic composition of capital + 1.

Various economic, political, and demographic explanations have been proposed to account for the extent and increases in income inequality. The economic explanations typically involve a variety of social class concepts that are implicitly Weberian or Marxian (explanations based on demographic factors and racial segregation have also been proposed (5, 74, 75)). For example, the increase of income inequality in the United States has been attributed to several factors, including: a shift toward a service sector economy that generates both high-wage and low-wage jobs, and declines in middle-wage jobs (76); the segmentation of the labor market (77); a steady increase in the demand for skilled workers relative to unskilled workers between and within industries (5, 78); the internationalization of financial markets and the relative decline in manufacturing jobs (79); and technological change and its consequences (e.g., computerization) (74). Most recently, Galbraith (80) has argued that U.S. income inequality results from U.S. government monetarist policies that have used high interest rates to control inflation while producing a series of recessions that led to high unemployment, which in turn resulted in wage inequality. Another set of explanations has emphasized political factors (e.g., class formation, the formation of class-based organizations acting in their economic and political interest) in the surge of income inequality. Among them we find: decline in union density (81–83); changes in fair labor practice rules (83); social policies such as cutbacks in income transfers (84); and political decisions such as changes in capital gain taxes and state corporate tax laws that promote an "investor capitalism" strategy of low wages and high capital return (83). Many authors provide models that integrate these political and economic factors (e.g., 75, 77). The income inequality and social cohesion model cannot deal with these explanations because it does not include measures of class structure (e.g., the set of class relations in a country) or political factors.

Marxian class-based explanations are preferable because they expose the social mechanisms of exploitation in a way that income distribution models cannot. In this way, Marxian class analysis of the labor process is even deeper than Weberian class analysis as the former links exchanges in the labor market and production through the concept of exploitation, while Weberian class analyses keep labor market exchanges and production separate (66, p. 34). Such a Weberian approach is evident in social epidemiology, where research into the health effects of work stress and work organization have been conceptualized as independent of social class (e.g., 85).

Social Cohesion

The Concept of Social Cohesion. Over and above income inequality, the construct of "social cohesion," as played out through social trust, reciprocity, and concern for the well-being of one's community, is the cornerstone of Wilkinson's model (14, p. 211). As with many psychosocial constructs, social cohesion is intuitively appealing, but it is difficult to define (86). Following the work of

Putnam (87) in Italy, Wilkinson defines social cohesion as participation in public affairs, civic responsibility, or involvement in public life (the social cohesion of the ex-communists in northern Italian regions). Social cohesion can be measured with indicators of voting participation, newspaper readership, or number of cultural voluntary associations (14, pp. 119–120). Somewhat curiously, although social cohesion should (by definition) deal with social relations, most of the aspects of social cohesion discussed by Wilkinson pertain to individual psychological attributes (such as emotions, stress, attributions, helplessness, motivation, self-perception, disrespect)[9] rather than indicators of relations per se. Moreover, lack of reference to labor unions created a "middle-class bias" in the measurement of social cohesion. Given its importance to the Wilkinson model of income inequality, it is unfortunate that he does not attempt a more rigorous definition of the construct of social cohesion, and settles for "the social nature of public life" (14, p. 146).

One way social cohesion could be defined would be the amount of individual participation in social groups in the community. Following this definition we suggest that social cohesion is not always good for the health of populations, contrary to what Wilkinson implies (i.e., more social cohesion produces better population health). We suggest that the relation between social cohesion and health is more likely to follow an inverted U shape. No participation, as in the many examples provided by Wilkinson, produces social isolation and its associated health hazards (e.g., suicide). On the other hand a society with no internal divisions into social groups, a uniform society with massive participation, will also have negative effects on health. (Actually, a society with no social group divisions will be like a collection of competitors (91).) Optimal social cohesion (i.e., without political coercion) will be more likely to happen at intermediate levels of participation (91).[10] Recently, Lynch and Kaplan (1) have noted that the hypothesis of social cohesion does not contemplate the fact that some of the most unhealthy societies in this century have been highly cohesive and that this

[9] Wilkinson explains people's belief in the universality of self-interest and the emotional basis of individualism as rooted in erroneous attributions about the causes of human behavior (market relations make people behave selfishly, and people perceive that behavior as human nature) (14, p. 145). To show that emotions are socially determined, Wilkinson presents an example from a social cognitive theory of emotion. This theory originated in the clinical observations of Gregorio Marañon, a clinician close to the Francoist (fascist) regime in Spain. In the early 1960s, U.S. psychologists Schachter and Singer (88) conducted an experiment showing that the arousal induced by adrenaline was experienced emotionally by experimental subjects in accordance with the emotion (joy or anger) displayed by a confederate with whom the subjects were sharing a room. But Wilkinson does not reveal that in the experiment, subjects who were told to expect being aroused could explain the arousal as an effect of the drug. Thus, contrary to what Wilkinson seems to believe, most emotions are not a matter of cognitive interpretation but are rooted in objective material contingencies over time (e.g., Pavlov; 89, 90).

[10] The collection of social groups is the social structure of a society. A measure of the degree of differentiation of a society will be the sum of all the differences between social groups A and B of the form $(A \cap \neg B) \cup (\neg A \cap B)$.

hypothesis runs the risk of idealizing a communal past that never existed. Some fascist societies, most notably Nazi Germany, were characterized by high levels of participation, as mobilization was used as a form of social control (92). Nazi culture was indeed characterized by the idea of a single, undivided, and total People's Community (93). Any beneficial effect of social cohesion on health (such as anti-smoking campaigns) was definitely offset by the many other consequences of Nazi mass participation. A recent example that social cohesion is not always desirable stems from research on the AIDS epidemic in the United States, where the subjective experience of integration into social networks among men at risk for AIDS was associated with distress rather than with its reduction, as the social integration hypothesis would predict (94).

As discussed earlier in regard to income inequality, Wilkinson's model does not contemplate the relation between class and social cohesion. For example, political sociologists using the resource mobilization model have shown that members of the middle class have more time and resources to devote to civic participation than do members of the working class (95). Furthermore, in spite of Wilkinson's claim that market economies undermine social cohesion, the capitalist class (wealthy owners of capital) has been described as particularly cohesive by political sociologists (e.g., forming "inner-circle" cliques) (96). This omission of the relationship between social class and social cohesion is vulnerable to methodological problems similar to those signaled for income inequality. However, Wilkinson is probably right that capitalist economies produce conditions of income inequality that have negative effects on interpersonal relations, but the most important point is that these negative effects will not be evenly distributed across the population. As with other aspects of capitalist political and economic relations, disease rates linked to interpersonal relations will be higher among the working class and, in particular, among its female and non-white segments.

Wilkinson argues that the relation between social cohesion and health reveals an anthropological disposition toward equality and social cohesion.[11] He builds his evidence through reviewing research conducted in boundary disciplines, such as anthropology, social psychology, behavioral neuroscience, political science, and history. However, Wilkinson's argument is not fully convincing. For example, many of the supposedly egalitarian primitive societies studied by anthropologists (such as hunter-gatherers) have some elements of gender and age hierarchies (97). Wilkinson also does not mention the controversy surrounding Power's ethological research on the alleged egalitarian nature of chimpanzee social organization (98, 99). Overall, the examples provided by Wilkinson cast doubt on the universality of competition in human societies, but they do not

[11]Wilkinson's appealing, but not entirely convincing, "left sociobiology" is reminiscent of Koprotkin's in the 19th century.

prove that cooperation is a natural state in all human societies. One aspect that Wilkinson does not highlight is that most cohesive and cooperative societies not only are more egalitarian but are characterized by non-capitalist modes of production (100).

Political Change, Class Formation, Social Cohesion, and Health. A significant characteristic of the "income inequality and social cohesion model" is the absence of politics as a determinant of population health. Even when reviewing the historical transformation of the Soviet Union, changes in population health are interpreted as the consequence of a breakdown in social cohesion, rather than changes in the mode of production (i.e., from state socialism to some form of capitalism) (14, pp. 121–130). Even taking into account that social inequalities in Russia had been building before privatization (101), during the two years after the failed coup of 1991 half of the country's assets were transferred from state to private hands (102). Also, during the early 1990s, Russian life expectancy dropped sharply (a five-year decline between 1990 and 1994) (103). It is reasonable to expect that these major changes in class relations might have had an influence on national mortality and morbidity rates over and above social cohesion (such as participation in civic activities, membership in cultural community organizations) (see 104). It seems parsimonious to suggest that the breakdown in social cohesion has been only one of several proximal mediators of the effects of political change on population health (105). The 20th century has provided several examples of significant changes in mortality and morbidity rates in countries that went through political revolutions (e.g., Cuba) (18, 106) or substantial changes in legislation brought about by elected governments (such as the United Kingdom (18) and Kerala (107)). Class formation played a pivotal role in many of these political transformations. For example, the political power achieved by the working class through worker mobilization was a key determinant in establishing European welfare states (108).

The Political Uses of Social Cohesion. Models that emphasize social cohesion as a potential determinant of population health have consequences for social and health policy (14, pp. 26–28). One is to downplay the beneficial role of medical care and social services in the determination of population health (e.g., 18, 109, 110). Although the advantageous effect of medical care on national mortality rates and life expectancy is smaller than that of other social factors, access to medical care is important in reducing mortality and morbidity rates and improving quality of life. In the United States, the contribution of medical care has been estimated to add 1.5 years of life for clinical preventive services and 3.5 to 4 years for curative services (111).

Wilkinson's major hypothesis places income inequality as a main determinant of social cohesion. Although reduction in income inequalities is a central piece of

Wilkinson's policy recommendations, his views on its implications for increasing social cohesion/health are not shared by current U.S. and U.K. administrations and their associated scholars (112). In the United States, scholars and government officials during the New Democrat administration, while deeply aware of income inequalities, stress the need for increasing community social cohesion as an *alternative* to reductions in income inequality, either through taxation or state transfers (24, 113–117). Parallel developments have been noted in the United Kingdom under New Labour's "Third Way" (118–122). Among the policies that have been proposed to build social cohesion in communities we find community policing (114); non-standard, "flexible" work arrangements (115); involvement in *local* politics (although former Secretary of Labor Robert Reich also recommends progressive income taxation and minimum health insurance for employees) (116); and charities, nongovernmental organizations, and moralistic government programs (24, 60, 120, 121).

Thus the consequence of an emphasis on the necessity for communities to be socially cohesive, combined with a downplay of measures aimed at reducing income inequality, makes communities ultimately responsible for their health (e.g., 117, 123). As U.S. deprived and segregated working-class communities often lack the political and economic resources that ensure the social cohesion of the middle class (95), the result is a "blaming the community" model (124) that can easily justify the need for more policing and other forms of government control of working-class communities (119). In the absence of detailed social mechanisms linked to class, gender, and race relations, it is easy to default to a community "responsibility" rhetoric that places the burden of reducing inequalities in health on the capacity of communities to be cohesive (e.g., 117). No model of income inequality and social cohesion that is conceived within a public health framework should be open to the interpretation that intervening to build social cohesion in communities is an "equal weight" alternative to more fundamental political and economic changes needed to alter income distribution itself. Indeed, it is worth pondering that the likely public health benefits of interventions designed to improve social cohesion will leave untouched more fundamental economic and political relations.

CONCLUSION

In spite of providing a large body of data on the association between economic inequality and health, the "income inequality and social cohesion" model lacks depth with regard to other sociological alternatives (such as class relations, class formation). The first determinant of population health in Wilkinson's model is defined by the distribution of income, while the second and most important determinant in this model is the theoretical construct of social cohesion that affects health through many different mechanisms, most of them psychological.

Wilkinson has made important contributions to our understanding of the determinants of population health through his focus on income inequality, but faithful to the Durkheimian tradition, his model shies away from the central issue of what produces economic inequality in the first place. Neo-Marxian (e.g., control over productive assets) and even neo-Weberian (e.g., labor market position) models provide social mechanisms that explain why income inequality occurs. Marxian models also make an explicit linkage between ill-health and how economic inequality is generated through exploitation within the labor process. In addition, exploitation implies a structural conflict among classes that limits the amount of social cohesion achievable through income redistribution alone. Neo-Marxian and neo-Weberian models thus have more potential to explain a wider range of social phenomena linked to ill-health than do neo-Durkheimian models of social integration. Social cohesion, the construct in Wilkinson's model, is itself the consequence of social relations (here more broadly defined as economic, political, and cultural relations) that are absent from the income inequality/social cohesion model. For example, gender discrimination in wages, political underrepresentation of minorities, or negative stereotypes about the abilities of nonprofessionals might limit the degree of cohesion within populations due to their impact on economic, political, and cultural relations. While Wilkinson's model does not lay out the social mechanisms that might determine social cohesion (economic, political, and cultural), this construct becomes key as a hypothesized mediator of the effects of income inequality.

We believe that the construct of "social cohesion" can easily be used to fit explanations that are the sociological equivalent of "blaming the victim," where communities, rather than individuals, are held accountable for "not coming together" or "being disorganized." For example, it is not unusual to hear members of both the Clinton and Blair administrations calling for more community cohesion at the same time that they are delivering economic policies that increase income inequality. More and better indicators of income inequality are not substitutes for an understanding of how social inequalities occur (such as class, gender, and race relations). Neither are constructs such as "social cohesion" likely to constitute an alternative explanation to political processes that historically have had a major impact on population health. Richard Wilkinson is to be congratulated for focusing attention on income inequality as a determinant of population health. His book has provided a basis for a continuing debate that could result in more comprehensive models that include how inequalities are generated in the first place and that more clearly define the social mechanisms through which economic inequalities affect population health.

Acknowledgments — We would like to thank Richard Wolff and Paul Cockshott for their input. This work was supported by DHHS grants U48/CCU310821 and OUO3528-01.

APPENDIX: EXAMPLE OF A SOCIAL SYSTEM

The following is an example of a social system. It does not pretend to include all class relations of any society (e.g., household class relations and gender and racial relations are not included). Similarly, the treatment of political and cultural relations is limited and could be substituted by many more elaborate conceptualizations. This formalization only attempts to provide a blueprint for the study of the income-generating class relations in societies as an alternative to single dimensional frameworks such as Wilkinson's.

SOCIAL SYSTEM

$$S = <p \cup q, Env, E \cup C \cup P>$$

where p and q are the components (persons); *Env* is the physical and material environment (state, firm, household); *E, C,* and *P* are economic, cultural, and political relations, respectively. (For example, singing a tune involves a cultural—artistic—relation; selling the CD involves an economic relation; and having a law prohibiting the use of certain sentences in the song involves a political relation.) Here we develop the example of class relations following the Marxian model of Resnick and Wolff (73), although other relational class frameworks could have been used, such as Wright's (125).

SOCIAL SUBSYSTEMS

Economic Subsystem

$$Es = <p_e^{1jk} \cup p_e^{2jk} \cup p_e^{3jk} \cup p_e^{4jk} \cup p_e^{5jk}, Env, E_{fcp,m,n} \cup E_{scp,m,n} \cup E_{a,m,n}>$$

Economic (Class and Non-Class) Positions of Persons

p_e^1 = *productive capitalist* (e.g., an industrial capitalist).[12] Anyone who makes his or her money expand in value by directly appropriating the surplus produced by productive workers; participates in the fundamental class process.

p_e^2 = *unproductive capitalist* (e.g., unproductive banker, landowner, wholesale trader, monopolist). Anyone who expands his or her value in any manner other than directly appropriating productive laborers' surpluses; participates in subsumed class or non-class economic processes. For example, a banker who lends at interest to a productive capitalist sees his value expand (because he gets back his principal plus interest), but such a banker does not

[12]The distinction between "productive" and "unproductive" labor follows Resnick and Wolff's (73) terminology (see 126, 127 for alternative positions on the productive/unproductive distinction).

appropriate any productive laborer's surplus. The industrial/productive capitalist to whom the banker lends distributes a portion of what she appropriates to the banker as interest (a subsumed class payment). If this banker also lends at interest to workers, his value expands: he is an "unproductive capitalist" whose interest receipts are not a subsumed class payment, but rather a non-class payment.

p_e^3 = *productive laborer* (e.g., productive miner, cook, construction worker, assembly line worker, computer engineer). Anyone who usually sells his or her labor power to industrial capitalists and produces surplus labor appropriated by productive capitalists; participates in the fundamental class process. Capitalism usually requires the sale of labor power as a commodity, but that does not make it always or necessarily the case. If, for example, some state agency allocated productive workers to various productive capitalists at assigned wages, they would still produce surplus appropriated by such productive capitalists notwithstanding the absence of a market in labor power (this has happened in wartime situations).

p_e^4 = *unproductive laborer* (e.g., unproductive bank teller, post office clerk, private household laborer, corporate lawyer, manager). Anyone who performs labor but does not perform surplus labor appropriated by a capitalist; participates in subsumed or non-class processes.

p_e^5 = *ancient laborer* (e.g., self-employed/"petit bourgeois" M.D., lawyer). A productive laborer who appropriates his or her own individual surplus; participates in the ancient class process.

q_e = *consumers* (recipients of economic production). These could be disaggregated into class positions.

Environment

Env (household, firm, state)

Economic (Class and Non-Class) Processes[13]

E_{fcp} = *fundamental class processes.* Economic process of production and appropriation of surplus labor that is embodied in a surplus product. Only productive capitalists and productive laborers participate in this process. The fundamental class process refers to performing surplus labor that is embodied in a surplus product. It is a different matter whether or not that surplus product acquires a "value" by passing through the non-class process of market exchange. In other words, surplus products may, but need not, acquire the additional status of surplus value depending on whether class processes occur in a society that also displays market exchange processes for the products of such surplus labor. When a worker

[13]In Resnick and Wolff's (73) theory, non-class processes are all economic processes other than fundamental and subsumed class processes, plus all cultural processes, plus all political processes.

sells labor power for a wage, that is an exchange process, not a class process. Hence we cannot infer whether a worker participates in a class process or how he or she participates from the fact that a commodity exchange process (i.e., labor power for money) has occurred.

E_{scp} = *subsumed class process*. Economic process of distribution of surplus labor. Productive capitalists are distributors in this process; unproductive capitalists and unproductive workers are recipients of this distributed surplus labor.

E_{ncp} = *non-class process*. All economic processes that are not directly related to the production, appropriation, or distribution of surplus labor. Unproductive capitalists and unproductive laborers participate in this process in which no surplus labor is being produced, appropriated, or distributed.

E_a = *ancient class process*. Economic process in which the laborer appropriates her or his own surplus labor. Only ancient laborers (i.e., self-employed, petit-bourgeois) participate in this process.

Cultural Subsystem

$$Cs = <p_c^{ij1} \cup p_c^{ij2} \cup q_c, Env, C_{art,1,m} \cup C_{sci,1,m} \cup C_{id,1,m}>$$

Cultural Positions of Persons

p_c^1 = person who performs new cultural activities (e.g., researcher, inventor, composer)

p_c^2 = person who does not produce new cultural activities (e.g., scholar, performer, interpreter, technician)

q_c = recipient of cultural activity (e.g., reader, public, audience)

Environment

Env (household, firm, state)

Cultural Processes[14]

C_{art} = artistic occupation

C_{sci} = scientific/technical occupation

C_{id} = ideological occupation

Political Subsystem

$$Ps = <p_p^{i1k} \cup p_p^{i2k} \cup p_p^{i3k} \cup q_p, Env, P_{rd,1,n} \cup P_{pd,1,n} \cup P_{d,1,n}>$$

[14]In Resnick and Wolff's (73) theory, all persons in a social system engage continuously in many sorts of cultural processes (via songs, speech, dance, prayer, etc.).

Political Positions of Persons
p_p^1 = subordinate, follows orders
p_p^2 = supervisor, gives orders
p_p^3 = does not give or receive orders
q_p = recipient of political relation

Environment
Env (household, firm, state)

Political Processes
P_{rd} = representative democracy (liberal democracy)
P_{pd} = participatory democracy (anarchism)
P_d = dictatorship, authoritarian relation (fascism)

Note: A biological subsystem could be included (e.g., including kinship relations). Persons are usually involved in more than one relation within subsystems, as indicated by subscripts and superscripts (e.g., a worker who owns a 401(k) plan) (68).

REFERENCES

1. Lynch, J., and Kaplan, G. A. Wither studies on the socioeconomic foundations of population health? *Am. J. Public Health* 87: 1409–1411, 1997.
2. Delzell, E. Beyond social class. *Epidemiology* 7: 1, 1996.
3. Shy, C. The failure of academic epidemiology: Witness for the prosecution. *Am. J. Epidemiol.* 145: 479–484, 1997.
4. Rothman, K. J., Adami, H.-O., and Trichopoulos, D. Should the mission of epidemiology include the eradication of poverty? *Lancet* 352: 810–813, 1998.
5. Danzinger, S., and Gottschalk, P. *Uneven Tides: Rising Inequality in America.* Russell Sage, New York, 1993.
6. Wolff, E. N. *Top Heavy: A Study of Wealth Inequality in America.* Twentieth Century Fund, New York, 1995.
7. Mechanic, D. Social research in health and the American sociopolitical context: The changing fortunes of medical sociology. *Soc. Sci. Med.* 36: 95–102, 1993.
8. Dooley, D., and Catalano, R. Recent effects on the psychological effects of unemployment. *J. Soc. Issues* 44: 1–12, 1988.
9. Rogot, E., et al. *A Mortality Study of 1.3 Million Persons.* NIH Pub. No. 92-3297. NHLBI, Bethesda, Md., 1992.
10. Navarro, V. Race or class versus race and class: Mortality differentials in the U.S. *Lancet* 336: 1238–1240, 1990.
11. Pappas, G., et al. The increasing disparity in mortality between socioeconomic groups in the US, 1960 and 1986. *N. Engl. J. Med.* 329: 103–109, 1993.
12. Davey Smith, G., Bartley, M., and Blane, D. The Black report on socioeconomic inequalities in health 10 years on. *BMJ* 301: 373–377, 1990.

13. Macintyre, S. The Black report and beyond: What are the issues? *Soc. Sci. Med.* 44: 723–745, 1997.
14. Wilkinson, R. G. *Unhealthy Societies.* Routledge, London, 1996.
15. Lynch, J. W., and Kaplan, G. A. Understanding how inequality in the distribution of income affects health. *J. Health Psychol.* 2: 297–314, 1997.
16. Durkheim, E. *Selected Writings.* Cambridge University Press, Cambridge, England, 1972.
17. Tyroler, H. A., and Cassel, J. Health consequences of culture change—II. The effect of urbanization on coronary heart mortality in rural residents. *J. Chron. Dis.* 17: 167–177, 1964.
18. Susser, M. Health as a human right: An epidemiologist's perspective on the public health. *Am. J. Public Health* 83: 418–426, 1993.
19. Dooley, D., and Catalano, R. The epidemiology of economic stress. *Am. J. Community Psychol.* 12: 387–409, 1984.
20. Kawachi, I., and Kennedy, B. P. The relationship of income inequality to mortality: Does the choice of indicator matter? *Soc. Sci. Med.* 45: 1121–1127, 1997.
21. Kawachi, I., et al. Social capital, income inequality, and mortality. *Am. J. Public Health* 87: 1491–1499, 1997.
22. Adler, N. E., et al. Socioeconomic inequalities in health. No easy solution. *JAMA* 269: 3140–3145, 1993.
23. McGinnis, M., and Foege, W. H. Actual causes of death in the United States. *JAMA* 270: 2207–2212, 1993.
24. Mead, L. M. *The New Paternalism: Supervisory Approaches to Poverty.* Brookings Institution, Washington, D.C., 1997.
25. Adler, N. E., et al. Socioeconomic status and health: The challenge of the gradient. *Am. Psychol.* 49: 15–24, 1994.
26. Lynch, J. W., et al. Income inequality and mortality in metropolitan areas of the United States. *Am. J. Public Health* 88: 1074–1080, 1998.
27. Muntaner, C., Nieto, J., and O'Campo, P. Additional clarification re: the Bell Curve: On race, social class, and epidemiologic research. *Am. J. Epidemiol.* 146(7): 607–608, 1997.
28. Wright, E. O. *Interrogating Inequality.* Verso, London, 1994.
29. Judge, K., Mulligan, J., and Benzeval, M. Income inequality and population health. *Soc. Sci. Med.* 46: 567–569, 1998.
30. Waldmann, R. J. Income distribution and mortality. *Q. J. Econ.* 107: 1283–1302, 1992.
31. Becker, G. S. *The Economic Approach to Human Behavior.* University of Chicago Press, Chicago, 1976.
32. Coleman, J. *Foundations of Social Theory.* Harvard University Press, Cambridge, Mass., 1990.
33. Roemer, J. E. *A General Theory of Exploitation and Class.* Harvard University Press, Cambridge, Mass., 1982.
34. Rosenberg, A. *Economics—Mathematical Politics or Science of Diminishing Returns?* University of Chicago Press, Chicago, 1992.
35. Green, D. P., and Shapiro, I. *Pathologies of Rational Choice Theory: A Critique of Applications in Political Science.* Yale University Press, New Haven, Conn., 1994.
36. Roberts, M. *Analytical Marxism: A Critique.* Verso, London, 1996.

37. Blau, P. On limitations of rational choice theory for sociology. *Am. Sociol.* 28: 16–21, 1997.
38. Krieger, N., Williams, D. R., and Moss, N. E. Measuring social class in US public health research. *Annu. Rev. Public Health* 18: 341–378, 1997.
39. O'Campo, P., et al. Neighborhood risk factors for low birthweight in Baltimore: A multilevel analysis. *Am. J. Public Health* 87: 1113–1118, 1997.
40. Wegener, B. Concepts and measurement of prestige. *Annu. Rev. Sociol.* 18: 253–280, 1992.
41. Gregorio, D. I., Walsh, S. J., and Paturzo, D. The effects of occupation-based social position on mortality in a large American cohort. *Am. J. Public Health* 87: 1472–1475, 1997.
42. Winkelstein, W. Determinants of worldwide health. *Am. J. Public Health* 82: 931–932, 1992.
43. World Health Organization. The state of the world's health. *J. Public Health Policy* 16: 440–451, 1995.
44. Benzeval, M., Judge, K., and Whitehead, M. *Tackling Social Inequalities in Health.* King's Fund, London, 1995.
45. Syme, S. L. To prevent disease: The need for a new approach. In *Health and Social Organization*, edited by D. Blane, E. Brunner, and R. G. Wilkinson. Routledge, London, 1996.
46. United Nations, Population Division. *World Population 1994.* New York, 1994.
47. Amin, S. *Re-reading the Postwar Period.* Monthly Review Press, New York, 1994.
48. From what will we die in 2020? *Lancet* 349: 1263, 1997.
49. McFate, K., Lawson, R., and Wilson, W. J. *Poverty, Inequality, and the Future of Social Policy.* Russell Sage, New York, 1994.
50. Murray, J. L., and Lopez, A. D. Mortality by cause for eight regions of the world: Global burden of disease study. *Lancet* 349: 1269–1276, 1997.
51. Korzeniewicz, R. P., and Moran, T. P. World-economic trends in the distribution of income, 1965–1992. *Am. J. Sociol.* 102: 1000–1039, 1997.
52. Navarro, V. *Neoliberalismo y Estado del Bienestar.* Ariel, Barcelona, 1997.
53. Magdoff, H. What is the meaning of imperialism? *Monthly Rev.* 43: 1–7, 1993.
54. Bornschier, V., and Chase-Dunn, C. *Transnational Corporations and Underdevelopment.* Praeger, New York, 1985.
55. Shannon, T. R. *An Introduction to the World-System Perspective.* Westview Press, Boulder, Colo., 1989.
56. Ross, R. J. S., and Trachte, K. C. *Global Capitalism.* State of New York University Press, Albany, 1990.
57. Moaddel, M. Political conflict in the world economy: A cross-national analysis of modernization and world system theories. *Am. Sociol. Rev.* 59: 276–303, 1994.
58. Navarro, V. *Imperialism, Health and Medicine.* Baywood, Amityville, N.Y., 1983.
59. Brand, H. The World Bank, the Monetary Fund, and poverty. *Int. J. Health Serv.* 24: 567–578, 1994.
60. Laurel, A. C., and Lopez Orellano, O. Market commodities and poor relief: The World Bank proposal for health. *Int. J. Health Serv.* 26: 1–18, 1996.
61. Muntaner, C., and Parsons, P. E. Income, stratification, class and health insurance. *Int. J. Health Serv.* 26: 655–671, 1996.

62. Leigh, J. P. Occupational injury and illness in the United States: Estimates, costs, morbidity, and mortality. *Arch. Intern. Med.* 157: 1557–1568, 1997.
63. Stanley, T. J., and Danko, W. D. *The Millionaire Next Door.* Longstreet Press, Atlanta, 1996.
64. Wright, E. O. *Class Structure and Income Determination.* Academic Press, New York, 1979.
65. Halaby, C. N., and Weakliem, D. L. Ownership and authority in the earnings function: Non-nested tests of alternative specifications. *Am. Sociol. Rev.* 58: 16–30, 1993.
66. Wright, E. O. *Class Counts. Comparative Studies in Class Analysis.* Cambridge University Press, New York, 1997.
67. Muntaner, C., et al. Social class, assets, organizational control and the prevalence of common psychiatric disorders. *Soc. Sci. Med.*, 1999, in press.
68. Muntaner, C., and Stormes, J. Social class and behavior. *Psychol. Rep.* 79: 379–382, 1996.
69. Edwards, R. C., Reich, M., and Weisskopf, T. E. *The Capitalist System.* Prentice Hall, Englewood Cliffs, N.J., 1986.
70. Roemer, J. E. *Egalitarian Perspectives.* Cambridge University Press, New York, 1994.
71. Rieu, D.-M. Reformulating the Quantitative Connection between Labor-value and Price. Paper presented at the Meeting of the Eastern Economic Association, Washington, D.C., April 3–6, 1997.
72. Boswell, T., and Dixon, W. J. Marx's theory of rebellion: A cross-national analysis of class exploitation, economic development, and violent revolt. *Am. Sociol. Rev.* 58: 681–702, 1993.
73. Resnick, R., and Wolff, R. *Knowledge and Class. A Marxian Critique of Political Economy.* Chicago University Press, Chicago, 1987.
74. Massey, D. The age of extremes: Concentrated affluence and poverty in the twenty-first century. *Demography* 33: 395–412, 1996.
75. Nielsen, F., and Alderson, A. S. Income inequality in U.S. counties, 1970–1990. *Am. Sociol. Rev.* 62: 12–33, 1998.
76. Morris, M., Bernhardt, A. D., and Handcock, M. S. Economic inequality. New methods for new trends. *Am. Sociol. Rev.* 59: 205–219, 1994.
77. Botwinick, H. *Persistent Inequalities: Wage Disparity under Capitalist Competition.* Princeton University Press, Princeton, N.J., 1993.
78. Levy, F., and Murnane, R. J. U.S. earning levels and earnings inequality: A review of recent trends and proposed explanations. *J. Econ. Lit.* 30: 1333–1381, 1992.
79. Westergaard, J. *Who Gets What? The Hardening of Class Inequality in the Late Twentieth Century.* Polity Press, Cambridge, Mass., 1995.
80. Galbraith, J. K. *Created Unequal: The Crisis in American Pay.* Free Press, New York, 1998.
81. Kalleberg, A. L., Wallace, M., and Althouser, R. P. Economic segmentation, worker power, and income inequality. *Am. J. Sociol.* 87: 651–673, 1981.
82. Leicht, K. T., Wallace, M., and Grant, D. S. Union presence, class, and individual earnings inequality. *Work Occup.* 20: 429–451, 1993.
83. Hout, M., Arum, R., and Voss, K. The political economy of inequality in the "age of extremes." *Demography* 33: 421–425, 1996.

84. Plotnick, R. D. Changes in poverty, income inequality, and the standard of living in the United States during the Reagan years. *Int. J. Health Serv.* 23: 347–358, 1993.
85. Karasek, R. A., and Theorell, T. *Healthy Work: Stress, Productivity and the Reconstruction of Working Life.* Basic Books, New York, 1990.
86. Muntaner, C., and O'Campo, P. A critical appraisal of the demand/control model of the psychosocial work environment: Epistemological, social, behavioral and class considerations. *Soc. Sci. Med.* 36: 1509–1517, 1993.
87. Putnam, R. D. *Making Democracy Work.* Princeton University Press, Princeton, N.J., 1993.
88. Schachter, S., and Singer, J. Cognitive, social, and physiological determinants of emotional state. *Psychol. Rev.* 69: 379–399, 1962.
89. Muntaner, C., et al. Placebo response to cocaine administration in humans: Effects of prior administration and verbal instructions. *Psychopharmacology* 99: 282–286, 1989.
90. Muntaner, C., et al. Cocaine intravenous infusions in humans: Dose-related cardiovascular and subjective effects. *Pharmacol. Biochem. Behav.* 34: 697–703, 1989.
91. Garcia Sucre, M., and Bunge, M. Differentiation, participation and cohesion. *Quality and Quantity* 10: 171–178, 1976.
92. Dahrendorf, R. Totalitarianism revisited. *Partisan Rev.* 55: 541–554, 1988.
93. Hobsbawm, E. *The Age of Extremes: A History of the World, 1914–1991.* Pantheon, New York, 1994.
94. O'Brien, K., et al. Social relationships of men at risk for AIDS. *Soc. Sci. Med.* 36: 1161–1167, 1993.
95. Morris, A. D., and Mueller, C. M. *Frontiers in Social Movement Theory.* Yale University Press, New Haven, Conn., 1992.
96. Kadushin, C. Friendship among the French financial elite. *Am. Sociol. Rev.* 60: 202–221, 1995.
97. Flanagan, J. G. Hierarchy in simple "egalitarian" societies. *Annu. Rev. Anthropol.* 18: 245–266, 1989.
98. Kemper, T. D. The Egalitarians—Human and Chimpanzee: An Anthropological View of Social Organization by Margaret Power. *Am. J. Sociol.* 97: 1757–1758, 1992.
99. White, F. The Egalitarians—Human and Chimpanzee: An Anthropological View of Social Organization (Margaret Power). *Am. Anthropol.* 95: 165, 1993.
100. Bonta, B. D. Cooperation and competition in peaceful societies. *Psychol. Bull.* 121: 299–320, 1997.
101. Palosuo, H., et al. Social patterning of ill health in Helsinki and Moscow. *Soc. Sci. Med.* 46: 1121–1136, 1998.
102. Burawoy, M. Review Essay: The Soviet descent into capitalism. *Am. J. Sociol.* 102: 1430–1444, 1997.
103. Notzon, F. C., et al. Causes of declining life expectancy in Russia. *JAMA* 279: 793–800, 1998.
104. Kohn, M. L., et al. Social structure and personality under conditions of radical social change: A comparative analysis of Poland and Ukraine. *Am. Sociol. Rev.* 62: 614–638, 1997.
105. Bobak, M., et al. Political changes and trends in cardiovascular risk factors in the Czech Republic, 1985–92. *J. Epidemiol. Community Health* 51: 272–277, 1997.

106. Navarro, V. Has socialism failed? An analysis of health indicators under capitalism and socialism. *Sci. Soc.* 57: 6–30, 1993.
107. Franke, R. W., and Chasin, B. H. Kerala state, India: Radical reform as development. *Monthly Rev.* 42: 1–23, 1991.
108. Hicks, A., Misra, J., and Ng, T. N. The programmatic emergence of the social security state. *Am. Sociol. Rev.* 60: 329–349, 1995.
109. Poland, B., et al. Wealth, equity and health care: A critique of a "population health" perspective on the determinants of health. *Soc. Sci. Med.* 46: 785–798, 1998.
110. Himmelstein, D., and Woolhandler, S. An American view. *Lancet* 352: 53–55, 1998.
111. Bunker, J. P., Frazier, H. S., and Mosteller, F. The role of medical care in determining health. In *Society and Health*, edited by B. C. Amick et al. Oxford University Press, New York, 1995.
112. Wilkinson, R. G. Our healthier nation. *Public Health Forum* 2(2): S1, 1998.
113. COSSA. Capitol Hill forum looks at income disparity. *COSSA Washington Update*, December 18, 1995, pp. 5–6.
114. COSSA. Kelling speaks at NIJ lecture; Sherman testifies before House. *COSSA Washington Update*, December 8, 1997, pp. 5–6.
115. Reich, R. B. Economia abierta y cohesion social. *El Pais DIGITAL*, January 16, 1998.
116. Reich, R. B. Broken faith. Why we need to renew the social compact. *The Nation*, February 16, 1998, pp. 11–17.
117. Stoto, M. A. *Sharing Responsibility for the Community's Health: A Synthesis of Reports from the Institute of Medicine*. National Academy Press, Washington, D.C., 1997.
118. Giddens, A. *Beyond Left and Right*. Stanford University Press, Stanford, Calif., 1994.
119. Wainwright, D. The political transformation of the health inequalities debate. *Crit. Soc. Policy* 16: 67–82, 1996.
120. The strangest Tory ever told. *The Economist*, May 2, 1998, pp. 14–15.
121. Beyond left and right. *The Economist*, May 2, 1998, pp. 52–53.
122. Jewkes, R., and Murcott, A. Community representatives: Representing the "community"? *Soc. Sci. Med.* 46: 843–858, 1998.
123. Reiss, A. J., and Roth, J. A. (eds.). *Understanding and Preventing Violence*. National Academy Press, Washington, D.C., 1993.
124. O'Campo, P. Personal communication.
125. Wright, E. O. *Classes*. Verso, London, 1985.
126. Laibman, D. *Value, Technical Change and Crisis*. M. E. Sharpe, New York, 1992.
127. Moseley, F. *The Falling Rate of Profit in the Post War United States Economy*. St. Martin's Press, New York, 1991.

CHAPTER 15

INCOME INEQUALITY, SOCIAL COHESION, AND HEALTH: CLARIFYING THE THEORY— A REPLY TO MUNTANER AND LYNCH

Richard G. Wilkinson

I am grateful to Carles Muntaner and John Lynch for their generous remarks in Chapter 14 and for raising several important points about the nature of the relationship between income distribution and population health (1). My view is, as they suggest, that population health is related to income distribution through the effects of income distribution on individual psychosocial welfare and on the quality of the social environment. As more recent evidence has allowed the picture to be substantially filled out, I will use most of this chapter to summarize what seem to be the most plausible processes linking income distribution to population mortality rates, before returning, at the end, to answer some specific criticisms raised by Muntaner and Lynch.

INEQUALITY AND THE SOCIAL ENVIRONMENT

My initial interest in social cohesion arose from a discussion (2) of the characteristics of a number of societies that were unusually egalitarian and unusually healthy. The impressionistic evidence then available suggested that all were unusually cohesive. Several of the examples discussed suggested not only a cross-sectional fit between the degree of equality, social cohesion, and health, but also that they changed together.

Since then, however, some striking quantitative evidence has become available that strongly confirms my initial impressions. Kawachi and colleagues (3) showed that measures of how much people trusted each other in each of the U.S. states were closely correlated both with mortality ($r = -0.8$) and with income inequality ($r = -0.7$). Path analysis suggested that the relationship between income inequality and mortality occurred almost wholly through measures of trust. The same paper also showed similar but weaker relationships with other measures of the social environment such as perceived fairness, helpfulness, and group membership.

In 1996, Kaplan and colleagues (4) reported a correlation of 0.7 between income inequality and homicide rates among the U.S. states. An earlier meta-analysis of some 34 studies had shown that the relationship between income inequality and both homicide and violent crime is robust (5). Indeed, the correlation has been reported in studies using international data—data from within countries other than the United States, and from within the United States—at both the state and lower levels of analysis. If homicide rates are indicative of the social environment, then the evidence suggests again that the relationship between income inequality and death rates from all other causes excluding homicide is mediated by the quality of the social environment (6).

Williams and coworkers (7) used the Minnesota Hostility Scale to measure hostility scores in random population samples in each of 10 U.S. cities. They found that the mean hostility scores for each city were strongly correlated with city mortality rates (r = 0.9). Using data on income inequality in the relevant Standard Metropolitan Areas (kindly supplied by John Lynch), I found that these same hostility scores were correlated with income inequality (r = 0.7).

These correlations are all remarkably powerful and suggest that income inequality is strongly and systematically related to the character of social relations and the nature of the social environment in a society. In their study of the regions of Italy, Putnam and colleagues (8) noted that their index of people's involvement in local community life was strongly correlated (r = –0.8) with income inequality. Talking about an egalitarian social ethos, rather than income distribution itself, they say, "Citizens in the more civic regions, like their leaders, have a pervasive distaste for hierarchical authority patterns"; and on the next page: "Equality is an essential feature of the civic community" (8, pp. 104, 105).

Although some of the data I have mentioned refer to U.S. state-level correlations, these kinds of relations cannot be dismissed as one of many possible, and perhaps meaningless, correlations that might crop up in U.S. state-level data alone. Rather, the evidence shows that strong relationships between income distribution and measures of the quality of social relations are very general. Not only has the relationship with homicide been found in numerous different settings internationally, but correlations are also shown in Putnam's work in Italy as well as in the qualitative evidence I discussed (2), which came from a number of different societies (Britain in the two World Wars, Roseto, Japan, and Eastern Europe during the 1970s and 1980s). The implication is that we are dealing with relationships that are widespread.

The evidence of such strong and widespread relations between income distribution and measures of the social environment is fundamentally important in its own right. Indeed, what it tells us about the impact of income inequality on the quality of life may be more important than what the association with mortality tells us about its impact on the length of life. In the past we probably thought of things like trust and hostility as individual psychological characteristics and would have assumed that average scores for whole towns would vary only as a result of sampling error, but we now know not only that there are systematic population differences in such psychosocial characteristics, but that these differences strongly correlate with structural variables such as income inequality. This contradicts our assumptions that psychosocial factors are essentially individualistic and demands that we do some fundamental rethinking if our politics are not to reflect outmoded prejudices.

Rather than imagining that the relationship between income inequality and mortality reflects the impact of just one of these measures of the social environment, we now see that numerous different measures of the social environment and of the quality of social relations all seem to be highly intercorrelated. The link between income distribution and mortality, then, is not the result simply of differences in trust or the nature of life on the streets alone, but almost certainly reflects highly intercorrelated characteristics of the nature of social relations throughout a society. So, rather than thinking of homicide rates simply as a measure of a bizarre and rare form of behavior without much connection to the ordinary life of the majority of a population, we should perhaps think of them in the light of Rose's (9) evidence on the distribution of different risk factors in populations. The statistical power of homicide as a social indicator is that it reflects one extreme of the distribution of social relations in society: where homicide rates are high, the whole distribution of social relations is shifted toward the more aggressive, conflictual end of the spectrum. That is, in the high homicide areas we would also expect to find lower levels of trust, higher levels of hostility, and presumably—if we had the data—higher rates of domestic conflict as well. But not only are different measures of social relations intercorrelated at the area and population level, they are also likely to be intercorrelated among individuals. For example, boys brought up in homes with high rates of domestic conflict are more likely to become violent adults (10). This would help explain why epidemiological studies have found, at both the ecological and the individual level, that measures of health are related to such a wide range of what seem to be very different measures of social affiliation. After all, some measures of social affiliation seem unlikely—*if taken at face value and on their own*—to exert the major influence on health that the statistical evidence suggests they do.

THE HEALTH IMPACT OF THE SOCIAL ENVIRONMENT

Although these relationships between income distribution and the social environment are exciting in themselves, the question here is whether they exert an important influence on mortality. Fortunately, it is not a difficult question. In the light of our growing knowledge of the determinants of population health, it would be very surprising if they did not. A strong tendency for an increase in social hierarchy (represented by wider income differences) to be closely accompanied by a move toward less supportive and more conflictual social relations is an extremely potent mix for health. *Social status* and *social relations* (at least in terms of "population-attributable risks") are probably the two most powerful known influences on population health. Two-, three-, or even four-fold mortality differences have often been reported between groups of high and low social status (11, 12). Reviews of the literature on health in relation to friendship, social support, and social involvement have shown that death rates may also be two to four times as high among those who are poorly socially integrated compared with those with more friends, more social support, or more community involvement (13, 14).

The statistical link between income distribution and health once lacked the underpinning of any evidence of the mechanism through which it operated, but that gap has now been amply filled. We now know that, as income differences widen, people suffer not only the health effects of increased relative deprivation and low social status but probably poorer social relations as well. Indeed, that the search for mechanism should have led to the discovery of evidence that the quality of social relations is so intimately linked to income distribution provides striking confirmation of causality in the link between income distribution and health. Although there are almost certainly other pathways serving to link income distribution and mortality, it is hard to imagine others of anything like the same power. (Remember that many of the state contributions to welfare that might be regarded as candidates, such as social security benefits and education, are direct or indirect influences on income. As such, their effects are already subsumed by the effects of income distribution rather than being rival explanations.)

VERTICAL AND HORIZONTAL RELATIONS

The next step toward understanding these relationships is to ask why income distribution is correlated with measures of social relations. Putnam and coworkers (8) refer to the egalitarian relations that they see as essential to the development of community life as "horizontal" relationships and contrast them with the "vertical" patron-client relations predominating in the less civic regions of Italy. Why social inequality and friendship should vary inversely in relation to each other and should have such powerful influences on health becomes clearer when we see that they are perhaps two sides of the same coin. Social status, rank, or pecking order is, after all, about power, coercion, and access to resources without regard for the needs of others. In contrast, friendship is about mutuality, reciprocity, sharing, and a recognition that the needs of others are needs for us. These are, in effect, the two opposite principles of social organization. Measures of income inequality and the quality of social relations, of the relative strength of vertical and horizontal relations, are measures of the extent to which the social order is based on power or mutuality, coercion or sociality, antagonism or cooperation, reciprocity or competition, order-giving and order-taking or a more inclusive pluralism.

To know the balance between these competing principles in our social environment is crucially important to each of us. Adopting the right behavioral strategy depends on an accurate assessment of the nature of the social environment. We need to know whether pro-social behavior will be reciprocated and rewarded, or whether it will merely be exploited and taken advantage of as a weakness; whether to fend for ourselves in competition with others, or whether making social investments in the welfare of others helps—through the principles of reciprocity—to guarantee our own welfare.

The quality of social relations varies not only between societies but also within societies. Within a country, we know that violence is more common in some areas than others, and we have also seen that there are substantial differences in hostility and trust between areas. But although these differences are related to income inequality, the social breakdown and conflict—outside revolutionary periods—are not primarily between rich and poor. Instead, they tend to be concentrated in the most deprived areas. The next issue therefore is to understand why higher levels of relative deprivation seem to be accompanied (at least in modern market societies) by a poorer social environment and higher levels of violence—particularly among the poor.

VIOLENCE, RESPECT, AND INEQUALITY

Let us look first at why violence is related to income distribution. In its association with income inequality, violence has much in common with other causes of death. Both are strongly associated with relative deprivation and both show the strongest associations when income inequality is measured over larger (more socially heterogeneous) areas such as the 50 U.S. states rather than over smaller counties, zip code areas, or tracts (5, 15, 16). An understanding of why violence is related to income inequality therefore seems likely to cast light on the relation between income distribution and mortality from other causes; indeed, attempts to explain the relationship with mortality that do not also suggest an explanation for the relationship with homicide seem unlikely to get to the core of the social processes involved.

In a recent paper (6), using state-level crime rates as indicators of the social environment, we found that controlling for homicide—unlike property crime—removed the association between income distribution and other causes of death (excluding homicide). This again suggested that the relationship between inequality and violence is likely to illuminate the relation between inequality and health. Turning to the literature on the causes of violent behavior, we found the dominant theme to be that violent incidents are sparked when people feel they are disrespected, put down, and humiliated.

As there is not space to discuss this literature properly here, readers are urged to read the summary in Wilkinson and colleagues (6). However, note that even after spending 25 years as a prison psychiatrist before becoming director of the Center for the Study of Violence at Harvard, Gilligan wrote, "I have yet to see a serious act of violence that was not provoked by the experience of feeling shamed and humiliated, disrespected and ridiculed, and that did not represent the attempt to prevent or undo this 'loss of face' " (17, p. 110). Based on his own experience of street violence, McCall makes much the same point in his autobiography: "the underlying issue was always respect. . . . That was explanation enough. . . . It was universally understood that if a dude got disrespected, he had to do what he had to do (18, p. 52).

Where people are denied access to the usual sources of respect—jobs, education, money—violence often may be an attempt to make people respect them. In the words of Scheff (19, p. 188):

> rage is used as a defence against a threat to self, that is, feeling shame, a feeling of vulnerability of the whole self. Anger can be a protective measure to guard against shame, which is experienced as an attack on self. As humiliation increases, rage and hostility increases proportionally to defend against loss of self-esteem. . . . hostility can be viewed as an attempt to ward off feelings of humiliation (shame) generated by inept, ineffectual moves, a sense of incompetence, insults, and a lack of power to defend against insults.

This psychological material may seem too individualistic to some, but the need is precisely to understand the links between individual and structural processes. Wider income differences clearly mean more people are denied access to economic sources of status, respect, and prestige and so are more likely to feel sensitive and vulnerable to being disrespected. It cannot be a mere coincidence that homicide is strongly related to income inequality and is triggered, at the individual level, by people feeling they are not respected.

SOCIAL STATUS AND HEALTH

If violence is related to income inequality because it is substantially about problems of low social status, lack of respect, loss of face, and feeling humiliated, what does this tell us about the relationship between income distribution and health? Can health be affected by these same issues of social status, respect, and implications of inferiority? Could those be the individual psychosocial stressors that give rise to the ecological relationships between social cohesion and population mortality rates?

Although in the past we tended to assume that the social gradient in health within each country was a reflection of the direct effects of the different material circumstances in which people live, epidemiology increasingly emphasizes the importance of psychosocial pathways. The relation between mortality and income inequality seems, in itself, to direct our attention to social status and relativities. That mortality rates among the 50 U.S. states are much more closely related to the income distribution than to the median income of each state (4) also suggests that income matters to health when it is a measure (and determinant) of social status. The same follows from the fact that income differences are related to health *within* countries and states—where they are related to social status—but are almost unrelated to the income differences *between* developed countries and states that have no significance for individual social status (20).

However, perhaps the most powerful evidence that social status itself may affect health comes from work on the physiological effects of low social status among non-human primates. Shively and colleagues (21) have shown that among captive macaque monkeys, low social status results in increases in atherosclerosis, worse LDL:HDL ratios, central obesity, and signs of depression. Because they could experimentally manipulate changes in social status while controlling diet and the environment, these researchers removed most other possible explanations for the physiological effects. It is hard to avoid the conclusion that these are the direct effects of low social status itself. Sapolsky (22), studying baboons in the wild, also concluded that low social status is potentially harmful to health, and pointed particularly to the evidence of raised basal cortisol levels and attenuated cortisol responses to experimental stressors.

In studies of both wild and captive animals, the link between low social status and its physiological effects seems to be the chronic social stress of low status itself. Because many of the same physiological risk factors found in the studies of non-human primates are also associated with low social status in humans (23), it strains plausibility to argue that the causal processes are totally different—all the more so since the patterns of raised basal cortisol levels and attenuated cortisol responses to experimental stressors, first identified by Sapolsky (24) among low-status baboons, have now been reported by Kristenson and colleagues (25) to be important contributors not only to health differences between men in a Swedish and a Lithuanian town but also to the social gradient within each town.

Having established the need to identify sources of chronic anxiety intimately related to low social status itself, we can now see that the role of disrespect, shame, and humiliation in the link between violence and income distribution may point to a key source of angst central to low social status. Such a suggestion fits well with the thesis of Sennett and Cobb's (26) *The Hidden Injuries of Class.*

EARLY CHILDHOOD

There is a third component of this picture. Although social relations and social status are perhaps the two most important of the well-established risk factors for population health, a third—which is rapidly emerging as a very powerful influence on health—is early childhood emotional development (27–32). Early emotional trauma, poor attachment, and domestic conflict seem to affect stress responses throughout life in much the same way as do low social status and lack of social support. And once again, the patterns do not seem to be confined to humans (22, 33).

It is interesting that we use much the same words to describe the consequences of poor emotional attachment in early life and the effects of low social status. In both cases we use terms such as insecurity, fear of inadequacy, lack of confidence, and "inferiority complex." There can be little doubt that personal insecurities rooted in early emotional development make people more vulnerable to the insecurities and feelings of inferiority associated with low social status. Although these two processes have very substantial literatures, they are kept hygienically compartmentalized in different subjects. Psychology has a vast literature on the importance of early childhood emotional development, but has largely ignored social stratification. In contrast, a central theme in sociology has always been social class and social stratification, but there is little sociological literature on early childhood development. To understand health, and to see how emotional insecurity from early childhood exacerbates status insecurities and anxieties in relation to the social hierarchy during adult life, we need to bring these literatures together.

The health impact of early emotional insecurity and of the insecurities and anxieties resulting from low social status, coupled with the links between income inequality, disrespect, and violence, all point clearly to issues of social comparison, fears of inadequacy, and feelings of inferiority as the central source of chronic anxiety likely to be related to low social status and greater income inequality.

The health effects of friendship and social affiliations fit into the same picture. Friends and wider social affiliations provide positive feedback, boosting one's confidence, sense of adequacy, and self-worth, contrasting sharply with the health effects of negative social contact (34) and feelings of rejection. Not only does friendship have these positive effects, but personal insecurity tends to make people less likely to initiate social contact and friendship. Lack of confidence necessarily increases fears of rejection.

SOCIAL COMPARISONS, SHAME, AND SOCIAL STATUS

The problem is that the social hierarchy presents itself as if it were a hierarchy of human adequacy, from the most capable and successful at the top down to the most inadequate failures at the bottom. Central to our existence as creatures whose behavior is almost wholly learned is that we learn by monitoring how we compare with others. Inevitably, the social comparisons involved are a frequent source of anxiety as we fear that we are less successful, less attractive, less intelligent, and socially inferior.

Scheff (19) describes shame as "*the* social emotion." He says, "shame involves painful feelings that are not identified as shame by the person experiencing them. Rather they are labelled with a wide variety of terms that serve to disguise the experience of shame: having low self-esteem, feeling foolish, stupid, ridiculous, inadequate, defective, incompetent, awkward, exposed, vulnerable, insecure, helpless" (35). He notes, "there has been a continuing suggestion in the literature that shame is the primary social emotion, generated by the virtually constant monitoring of the self in relation to others" (19). In part, this echoes both Goffman (36), who said that embarrassment plays a prominent role in every social encounter, and Darwin (37), who in a chapter on blushing (and its relation to shame) asserted that shame "depends in all cases on . . . a sensitive regard for the opinion, more particularly the depreciation of others." In the same vein, Gilbert (38) has suggested that "shame" is distantly related to an evolved "submission" response of subordinate animals to superiors in the social hierarchy.

To see the power that shame and social comparisons have to create anxiety related to social status, think of the processes, described by Bourdieu (39), by which our cultural and aesthetic choices are riddled with ways of expressing social distinctions, which seem designed to trip up the uninitiated and expose their social inferiority. Add to this the way in which wealth appears as a marker of ability and success, and poverty, of inadequacy and failure. On top of that, add the effects of educational differentials and qualifications that stand as markers of competence.

Issues of social status are of course fundamental to class society. In the late 18th century, Adam Smith said he thought the underlying motive for most economic activity and for our desire to better our living conditions was the pursuit of what he called "regard." In *The Theory of the Moral Sentiments* (40) he asked, "What is the end of avarice and ambition of the pursuit of wealth and power and pre-eminence? Is it to supply the necessities of nature?" He answers, no: "The wages of the meanest labor can supply them. What [then] are the advantages of which we would propose to gain, by that great purpose of human life, which we call bettering our condition?" And he answers, again, "To be observed, to be attended to, to be taken notice of with sympathy, complacency, approbation are all the advantages, which we can propose to derive from it" (40, p. 50).

Echoing Adam Smith, several modern economists have emphasized the importance of relative income and social status in driving current consumerism (41, 42). But, as Schor points out in her book *The Overspent American* (42), "We live with high levels of psychological denial about the connection between our buying habits and the social statements they make."

The picture I have presented of the pathway from income distribution to health is not meant to suggest that health depends on social cohesion simply in the sense of people getting on better with their neighbors. The strength of community life, local associations, and friendship patterns seems most likely to be statistically associated with health because they reflect, on the one hand, people's social ease and confidence or, on the other, the extent to which social contact provokes anxiety, negative social comparisons, feelings of inadequacy, and angst as people feel belittled and undermined by status hierarchies. From this point of view, social cohesion could almost be regarded as a societal epiphenomenon reflecting the underlying individual processes that affect health. Inevitably, the causes of health and illness must always boil down to individual exposure to risk, but the exposures themselves (who, and how many, are exposed to what) are almost always determined by societal processes. Social cohesion is likely to work both ways round: as an expression of individuals' underlying social confidence, but also as a social environment that feeds back to increase people's sense of confidence, trust in others, and inclusion.

Income inequality is more strongly related to health when measured across large areas (countries or states) than across smaller areas (counties or census tracts) because, at the most local level, residential segregation means that the important social heterogeneity across the social hierarchy is lost. People at the top and bottom of society are unlikely to congregate within the same small areas. What counts is our sense of where we are in the class hierarchy. As Emerson said, "'Tis very certain that each man carries in his eye the exact indication of his rank in the immense scale of men, and we are always learning to read it." Not only do we know the social connotations of the part of town in which we live, but we also know where we fit into the work hierarchy and can place ourselves in the hierarchy of cultural class distinctions in terms of dress, speech, interests, education, aesthetic taste, and so forth. There can be little doubt that a substantial part of the link between income distribution and health is related to the social gradient in health across the social hierarchy. Rather than revealing some new dimension of health, the pointers suggest that the income distribution relationship casts light on the reasons for the health inequalities (43).

ANSWERS TO SPECIFIC CRITICISMS

Class and Hierarchy

In Chapter 14, Muntaner and Lynch criticized me for leaving class out of my interpretation of the link between income inequality and health. But I regard income distribution as a reflection and determinant of the hierarchy of power and status of which social class is made. Rather than leaving out class, I suspect that one of the most valuable aspects of this work is that it pinpoints the real psychosocial damage that social class distinctions inflict. Whether or not we can decide and agree on criteria for dividing the status hierarchy into discrete classes is a secondary issue compared with the existence of hierarchical inequality, which is the stuff of which class inequality is made. There is clearly a gradient in income, power, and privilege, and clear differences and conflicts of interest between the bottom and the top, even if the number of separate strata and the divisions between them are less clear. Identifying class divisions was easy when we could point to clearly defined oppositions of interest—between freeman and slave, patrician and plebeian, lord and serf, bourgeois and proletarian. Although there are still deep oppositions of interests between rich and poor, powerful and powerless, exploiter and exploited, all these relationships are now graded continua. Nor does anything controlling the development of human societies say that there will always be distinct social classes clearly demarcated by different functional relations to the productive system. Even in the top 5 percent of incomes, most people are "middle-class" salaried employees, dependent mainly on selling their labor. On the other hand, 44 percent of American households now own capital investments and, if income from other forms of property were included, the proportion would be still higher; yet most of these people are simultaneously employees (44). However, despite wider share ownership, the bulk of capital is now controlled by institutions such as pension funds, insurance companies, banks, and building societies or mortgage companies. Power too is graded according to seniority in the workplace, and the vast majority of people are employees. Even senior managers, wielding many of the powers of employers, are themselves employees, while at the other end of the spectrum, people in comparatively junior roles may have the power to hire and fire more junior employees in their sections. This is why we need to think about the strength of power relations between order-givers and order-takers, between people in different social ranks *throughout* society, rather than imagining that we have the security of belonging to one or other discrete, but mutually opposed, class communities.

Given the difficulty of providing a qualitative criterion for demarcating classes, or even of defining a boundary that does not leave large numbers of people with one foot on each side, income is probably as good a basis as any on which to produce a hierarchical ordering. It clearly reflects differences in people's power to control resources and use positions self-interestedly. Even the definitions of exploitation that Muntaner and Lynch suggest are dependent on income and the distribution of the value of what is produced. Although the interests of rich and poor, powerful and powerless, are so often opposed, where the fault line between them lies will differ from one political issue to the next. People will divide at one point over questions of employee rights, at another over environmental protection, at another on issues about direct versus indirect taxation, and at yet another on legislation against racism. But running through all the particularistic class distinctions that characterize different societies at different stages of economic development is the common fact that they are social hierarchies based on an ordering of power, status, and command over resources. Indeed, it has been suggested that what human social hierarchies have in common with social ranking systems among non-human primates is that both are fundamentally about power over, or access to, resources (38).

Instead of ignoring class, my analysis attempts to go to the heart of how its "hidden injuries" pervade our lives; to understand why things such as dignity, humiliation, disrespect, dishonor, social rejection, and inferiority matter so much and why they map onto social status. Sticking to material health risks and pushing off the psychosocial as too subjective is not a solution. We need to see why these things infiltrate our perception so that even blood pressure responds according to whether we are interviewed by someone of higher or lower social status (45, 46). So, despite thinking that we cannot draw any neat lines between social classes (and certainly could not get good health data based on whatever distinctions we chose), we can look at health according to the underlying differences in status and power as they are expressed by income differences.

Whether people regard themselves as being in the same or different social classes depends primarily on shared experience and thus on whether or not there is a large hierarchical distance between them (47, 48). So when Muntaner and Lynch suggest that the central issue is relations between classes, to me that means relations up and down the social hierarchy. Thus, rather than ignoring class relations as they suggest, my analysis focuses on exactly what the most profound effects of interclass (i.e., hierarchical) relations really are.

Health in Centrally Planned Economies

Muntaner and Lynch also criticized me for ignoring the effects of the privatization of the productive system in my discussion of health trends in Eastern Europe. I should point out that, as the section heading made clear, my discussion (2) was explicitly confined to trends during the 1970s and 1980s—prior to the upheavals of 1989. The trends preceding 1989 are particularly informative because life expectancy deteriorated in a number of Eastern European countries despite continued economic growth and *before* large-scale privatization. The collapse after 1989 is less testing for theories of the determinants of health because few of them would *not* have led to predictions of rising mortality. Nevertheless, progress has been made in sorting out the main factors at work (49).

Implicit in Muntaner and Lynch's suggestion that I ignored privatization is the belief that state socialist societies tended (at least before about 1970) to be much healthier than the populations of other countries with similar living standards as a direct result of state control of the productive system and the dispossession of private capitalism. According to Muntaner and Lynch, such underlying class factors will affect health directly, so that the association between health and income distribution or social cohesion is partly an overstatement of the strength of the causal links. However, the key to the once good health ratings of communist societies (50) may have been the greater equality and the smaller status differentials among most of the population. Swift had this to say about status differentials in Eastern Europe (51, p. 274):

> the ideological glorification of manual work . . . is, or was, perhaps the most distinctive feature of stratification systems in Eastern Europe. Marxist theory, as filtered through into the official ideologies of societies . . . led manual work to be considered especially important, and non-manual work second-rate. This glorification manifested itself in the prestige system of those societies when compared with those of the West: all research converges on the finding that prestige judgments in the East with respect to the manual and non-manual division were out of line with the rest of the world. Miners, cleaning women, unskilled construction labourers all scored substantially above the standard international metric; government ministers, accountants, office clerks, and lawyers all scored substantially below.

Smaller status differences may have been an important contributor to the impressive early health performance of many centrally planned economies.

Clarifying a difference of views may risk polarizing them, but let me suggest a clarification of the central difference between Muntaner and Lynch's and my own view of class and income distribution. To oversimplify, Muntaner and Lynch believe that income distribution is determined by relations between classes, whereas I come closer to believing that income distribution determines class (or, rather, position in the hierarchy and social distance).

As a thought experiment, imagine a society in which, apart from social security benefits and pensions, all income received by private individuals is income from employment and everyone in the economically active age range is an employee. None of the productive system is owned by private individuals and all capital is institutional capital belonging to banks, pension funds, corporations, and so forth. Hence, there is no private income from capital, ownership, or rent. But the imagined society is just as market-oriented as our own; capital is still moved around by institutions in search of profit, and firms can only survive by selling the goods and services they produce. Lastly, imagine that the gradations of income and power among the employed population are the same as among the existing employed populations now.

What would this society be like? I believe it would feel much like our own and that the problems of hierarchy, of inequalities in income and power would feel very familiar. Human beings would suffer the same invidious ranking, with all the same connotations of success and failure, ability and inadequacy. The ideology and institutional power of more senior people would still have a predominant influence on the economy and government policy. People from minorities would still be discriminated against, while children from more privileged backgrounds would continue to enjoy easier access to better education, jobs, and higher incomes. Similarly, the oppositions of interest between rich and poor would be almost unchanged and health inequalities would look much as they do now. Given that our imaginary society rules out any possibility of different social classes distinguished on the basis of categorically different relations to the productive system, these intuitively plausible effects of inequality would have to be accepted as the social effects of inequality itself rather than of some set of class relations which Muntaner and Lynch say I ignore. If similar hierarchical effects are indeed plausible in the absence of categorical class divisions, then I am right to ignore them and to try instead to understand the social processes set in train by social ranking—the processes of discrimination, distinction, exclusion, the need to be valued and respected, and the influences we draw about ourselves and others from social position. From my perspective, Muntaner and Lynch's belief in class means that they fail to theorize the effects of hierarchy, but class without inequality would mean very little.

However, more important than this disagreement is how we should solve these problems—whether conceived of in hierarchical or in class terms. My view is that we should be moving toward forms of economic and industrial democracy—trying forms of worker cooperatives, elected directors, employee share ownership, or almost any other forms of democratic decision-making. As well as having many other merits, economic democracy would bring the major sources of income inequality under democratic control. I believe this would lead to a substantial narrowing of differentials which, unlike changes in taxes and benefits, could not easily be reversed according to the whims of successive governments.

Income Distribution as a Determinant of the Social Environment

Muntaner and Lynch were worried that the position I accord to psychosocial factors may lead public health policy-makers to try to improve social cohesion while ignoring income distribution. First, not only are few theories proof against misuse, but their being misused tells us nothing about their validity. Second, the current political interest in community, social capital, cohesion, communitarianism, stakeholding societies, and so forth, predates the public health interest in these matters and has a long history. What research on income distribution and health has begun to inject into this field is the strongest evidence yet available that social cohesion and such like are powerfully determined by income distribution. In this situation it is surely wrong to suggest that the public health input encourages policy-makers to ignore income distribution. Our role has been precisely the opposite—to show the importance of income distribution both to health and to the nature of civil society. Indeed, I regard the evidence that income distribution gives us a handle on the psychosocial welfare of populations as the most important single feature of these relationships. Instead of being seen as a diversion from tackling income inequality, the link with social cohesion might be regarded as helping to put greater equality back on the political agenda by making it more attractive.

The Causes of Widening Income Differences

As to my failure to discuss the causes of changes in income inequality, I did once address the causes—or at least possible remedies—for widening income differences. The second half of my first booklet on income distribution and health was devoted to an analysis of how to reform social security and taxation to reduce income differentials. However, I regarded this as a task requiring separate expertise; hence, that section of the booklet was written by my co-author, Allison Quick (52). Since then, I have treated my subject area as the socioeconomic causes of ill-health within developed countries. In an attempt to lay down boundaries and avoid an infinite regress into causes of causes, I simply stopped at saying that wider income differences carry health costs. Others could wrestle with the extremely complicated, but crucial, issues of how income distribution can be influenced by changing industrial structure, education policy, and class relations; by the prevailing ideology on management of the national economy and the relative priorities given to keeping inflation and unemployment low; by the power of trade unions and the influence of new technology; by the development of "winner take all" markets; and by the changing proportions of households with two earners or no earners or of households made up only of the elderly or of young families with children. Establishing convincingly the empirical causes of changes in income distribution clearly requires rather more than a bald assertion that it is simply a matter of changing class relations.

CONCLUSIONS

In practice, it may make rather littler difference whether a change in income distribution comes from an exogenous change in class relations or from some other possible influence on income distribution. The result will feed back to the social environment, affecting levels of social prejudice, social distinction, tendencies to exclusion, the exercise of power, and the creation of insecurity, and, finally, to the insidious tendency for some people to be made to appear as inadequate failures in contrast to the successful and wealthy. All these are assaults on people's psychosocial welfare and social confidence. It is the angst they create that seems likely to be the most common source of the chronic stress tending to raise basal cortisol levels. That measures of social cohesion are related to health cannot plausibly be because making a friendly remark to a neighbor or belonging to some voluntary association is in itself so good for health. It is much more likely to be because more friendly and cohesive societies thrive where people are not belittled, cowed, or made to feel inadequate by the prominence of the status and power hierarchy.

Rather than being vague about how these processes affect health, I have argued that they involve some of the most powerful influences on population health that we know of; that they are also able to explain the similar links between violence and inequality; and that the parallel physiological effects of social rank among monkeys rule out many other explanations. In contrast, Muntaner and Lynch's alternative is not clearly specified and has an element of circularity. Why pay attention to the rate of exploitation and define it in terms of income flows and the division of the social product unless income distribution is important? Why emphasize the importance of trade union membership as a part of the structure of class relations that may influence income distribution if you think income differences are not what counts? Why ignore factors other than class relations that contribute to income differentials? Why insist that class relations are more determining of income distribution than determined by it? To suggest that income distribution is wholly determined by antecedent class relations and that these relations are more powerful influences on health than their consequences, either for income distribution or for the psychosocial processes related to it which I have discussed, is a tortuous path to choose. Rather than clinging to this misconceived "materialism," why not address the structural determinants of the psychosocial welfare of modern populations and, instead of worrying about its subjectivity, realize that it is precisely because these things so dominate our subjectivity that they are so important?

I have suggested elsewhere (53) that there is a culture of inequality, in which social relations are more violent, more aggressive, and less supportive, in which male behavior is more macho—or laddish—and in which there is a tendency to scapegoat weaker or more vulnerable sections of society, including women and racial, ethnic, or religious minorities (54–56). These tendencies show the danger of ignoring the subjective impact of structural inequalities.

REFERENCES

1. Muntaner, C., and Lynch, J. Income inequality, social cohesion, and class relations: A critique of Wilkinson's neo-Durkheimian research program. *Int. J. Health Services* 29(1): 59–81, 1999.
2. Wilkinson, R. G. *Unhealthy Societies: The Afflictions of Inequality.* Routledge, London, 1996.
3. Kawachi, I., et al. Social capital, income inequality and mortality. *Am. J. Public Health* 87: 1491–1498, 1997.
4. Kaplan, G. A., et al. Inequality in income and mortality in the United States: Analysis of mortality and potential pathways. *BMJ* 312: 999–1003, 1996.
5. Hsieh, C. C., and Pugh, M. D. Poverty, income inequality, and violent crimes: A meta-analysis of recent aggregate data studies. *Criminal Justice Rev.* 18: 182–202, 1993.
6. Wilkinson, R. G., Kawachi, I., and Kennedy, B. Mortality, the social environment, crime and violence. *Sociol. Health Illness* 20(5): 578–597, 1998.
7. Williams, R. B., Feaganes, J., and Barefoot, J. C. Hostility and death rates in 10 US cities. *Psychosom. Med.* 57(1): 94, 1995.
8. Putnam, R. D., Leonardi, R., and Nanetti, R. Y. *Making Democracy Work: Civic Traditions in Modern Italy.* Princeton University Press, Princeton, N.J., 1993.

9. Rose, G. *The Strategy of Preventive Medicine.* Oxford University Press, Oxford, 1992.
10. James, O. *Juvenile Violence in a Winner-Loser Culture.* Free Association Books, London, 1995.
11. Drever, F., and Whitehead, M. *Health Inequalities.* Office for National Statistics: Decennial Supplement, Series DS No. 15. The Stationery Office, London, 1997.
12. Black, D., et al. Inequalities in health. In *The Black Report,* edited by P. Townsend and N. Davidson. Penguin Books, Harmondsworth, 1988.
13. House, J. S., Landis, K. R., and Umberson, D. Social relationships and health. *Science* 241: 540–545, 1988.
14. Berkman, L. F. The role of social relations in health promotion. *Psychosom. Res.* 57: 245–254, 1995.
15. Franzini, L., Ribble, J., and Spears, W. Correlations between mortality, median income, and income inequality vary by population size in Texas. In press.
16. Wilkinson, R. G. Income, inequality and social cohesion. *Am. J. Public Health* 87: 104–106, 1997.
17. Gilligan, J. *Violence: Our Deadly Epidemic and its Causes.* G. P. Putnam, New York, 1996.
18. McCall, N. *Makes Me Wanna Holler: A Young Black Man in America.* Random House, New York, 1994.
19. Scheff, T. J. *Microsociology: Discourse, Emotion and Social Structure.* University of Chicago Press, Chicago, 1990.
20. Wilkinson, R. G. Health inequalities: Relative or absolute material standards? *BMJ* 314: 591–595, 1997.
21. Shively, C. A., and Clarkson, T. B. Social status and coronary artery atherosclerosis in female monkeys. *Arterioscler. Thromb.* 14: 721–726, 1994.
22. Sapolsky, R. M. *Why Zebras Don't Get Ulcers: A Guide to Stress, Stress-Related Disease and Coping*, Ed. 2. W. H. Freeman, New York, 1998.
23. Brunner, E. Stress and the biology of inequality. *BMJ* 314: 1472–1476, 1997.
24. Sapolsky, R. M. Endocrinology alfresco: Psychoendocrine studies of wild baboons. *Recent Prog. Horm. Res.* 48: 437–468, 1993.
25. Kristenson, M., et al. Attenuated cortisol response to a standardised stress test in Lithuanian versus Swedish men: The LiVicordia Study. *Int. J. Behav. Med.* 5(1): 17–30, 1998.
26. Sennett, R., and Cobb, J. *The Hidden Injuries of Class.* Knopf, New York, 1973.
27. Hertzman, C., and Wiens, M. Child development and long-term outcomes: A population health perspective and summary of successful interventions. *Soc. Sci. Med.* 43: 1083–1095, 1996.
28. Fonagy, P. Early influences on development and social inequalities: An attachment theory perspective. In *The Social Determinants of Health,* edited by A. Tarlov. New Press, New York, 1999.
29. Montgomery, S. M., Bartley, M. J., and Wilkinson, R. G. Family conflict and slow growth. *Arch. Dis. Child.* 77: 326–330, 1997.
30. Lundberg, O. The impact of childhood living conditions on illness and mortality in adulthood. *Soc. Sci. Med.* 36: 1047–1052, 1993.

31. Chrousos, G. P., and Gold, P. W. Introduction. In *Stress: Basic Mechanisms and Clinical Implications,* edited by G. P. Chrousos, et al., p. 771. Annals of the New York Academy of Sciences, New York, 1995.
32. Suomi, S. J. Long-term effects of different early rearing experiences on social, emotional, and physiological development in non-human primates. In *Neurodevelopment and Adult Psychopathology,* edited by M. A. Keshavan and R. M. Murray, pp. 104–116. Cambridge University Press, England, 1997.
33. Meaney, M. J., et al. Effect of neonatal handling on age-related impairments associated with the hippocampus. *Science* 239: 766–768, 1988.
34. Rael, E. G. S., et al. Sickness absence in the Whitehall II Study: The role of social support and material problems. *J. Epidemiol. Community Health* 49: 474–481, 1995.
35. Scheff, T. J., Retzinger, S. M. and Ryan, M. T. Crime, violence, and self-esteem: Review and proposals. In *The Social Importance of Self-Esteem*, edited by A. M. Mecca, N. J. Smelser, and J. Vasconcellos, p. 181. University of California Press, Berkeley, 1989.
36. Goffman, E. *Interaction Ritual.* Anchor Doubleday, Garden City, N.Y., 1967.
37. Darwin, C. *The Expression of Emotion in Men and Animals.* John Murray, London, 1872.
38. Gilbert, P. *Depression: The Evolution of Powerlessness.* Erlbaum, Hove, 1992.
39. Bourdieu, P. *Distinction: A Social Critique of the Judgment of Taste.* Routledge, London, 1984.
40. Smith, A. *The Theory of the Moral Sentiments.* Liberty Classics, Indianapolis, 1982.
41. Frank, R. H. *Choosing the Right Pond: Human Behavior and the Quest for Status.* Oxford University Press, Oxford, 1985.
42. Schor, J. *The Overspent American: When Buying Becomes You.* Basic Books, New York 1998.
43. van Doorslaer, E., et al. Income-related inequalities in health: Some international comparisons. *J. Health Econ.* 16: 93–112, 1997.
44. Leland, J. Blessed by the bull. *Newsweek,* April 27, 1998, pp. 51–53.
45. Long, J. M., et al. The effect of status on blood pressure during verbal communication. *J. Behav. Med.* 5: 165–171, 1982.
46. Kleinke, C. L., and Williams, G. Effects of interviewer status, touch, and gender on cardiovascular reactivity. *J. Soc. Psychol.* 134(2): 247–249, 1994.
47. Stewart, A., Prandy, K., and Blackburn, R. M. *Social Stratification and Occupations.* Macmillan, London, 1980.
48. Prandy, K. The revised Cambridge scale of occupations. *Sociology* 24(4): 629–655, 1990.
49. Walberg, P., et al. Economic change, crime, and mortality crisis in Russia: Regional analysis. *BMJ* 317: 312–318, 1998.
50. Sen, A. Public action and the quality of life in developing countries. *Oxford Bull. Econ. Statistics* 43: 287–319, 1981.
51. Swift, A. The sociology of complex equality. In *Pluralism, Justice and Equality,* edited by D. Miller and M. Walzer. Oxford University Press, Oxford, 1995.
52. Quick, A., and Wilkinson, R. G. *Income and Health.* S.H.A., London, 1991.

53. Wilkinson, R. G. The culture of inequality. In *Income Inequality and Health: A Reader,* edited by I. Kawachi, B. Kennedy, and R. G. Wilkinson. New Press, New York, 1999, in press.
54. Kennedy, B. P., et al. (Dis)respect and black mortality. *Ethn. Dis.* 7: 207–214, 1997.
55. Kawachi, I., et al. Women's status and the health of women: A view from the States. *Soc. Sci. Med.,* 1999, in press.
56. Wilkinson, R. G., Kennedy, B., and Kawachi, I. Women's status and men's health in a culture of inequality. 1999, in press.

CHAPTER 16

THE SOCIAL CLASS DETERMINANTS OF INCOME INEQUALITY AND SOCIAL COHESION

Carles Muntaner, John Lynch,
and Gary L. Oates

I. FURTHER COMMENTS ON WILKINSON'S REPLY

What follows is several comments on Richard Wilkinson's reply in Chapter 15 to our discussion (Chapter 14) of his "income inequality and social cohesion" model (1–3). Wilkinson's reply spans a review of findings on income inequality and health, an expansion of his hypotheses on the relation between social cohesion and health, and a reply to some of our criticisms. Because Wilkinson does not respond to a number of issues we raised—for example, international dependency as determinant of national income inequality; the role of political factors as determinants of income inequality and population health; exploitation as explanation for income inequalities; the need for formal definitions of social cohesion, functional forms of its relation with health, and the exchange aspect of social cohesion (its potential negative effects on health); the social psychology and the ethology of social cohesion; the impact of income inequality among individuals in different class locations; the policy implications of current research programs on social cohesion; and the systemic approach to social inequality—we direct the reader to Chapter 14 and we concentrate here on Wilkinson's reply.

Thus, we provide new arguments for incorporating social class in models of social inequalities in health; we critically examine the support for the psychological hypotheses that Wilkinson proposes as proximal determinants of health; we challenge the notion that research on income inequalities per se generates support for reducing social inequalities; and we provide a philosophical framework that reveals some fundamental differences between the "income inequality/social cohesion" model and other models of social inequalities in

This chapter is in two sections: section I by Drs. Muntaner and Lynch; section II (beginning on p. 383) by Drs. Muntaner, Oates, and Lynch.

health. Because Wilkinson criticizes us for not providing data[1] in our analysis on the role of social class in his model ("a bald assertion that is simply a matter of changing class relations"), we provide empirical evidence in section II of this response. In section II we show that social cohesion is shaped by class relations, and that Wilkinson's measurement of social cohesion excludes working-class forms of collective action.

INEQUALITY UNEXPLAINED

Wilkinson's reformulation of his income inequality, social cohesion, and health model in Chapter 15 still does not explain the origins of income inequality. We proposed in Chapter 14 a series of economic and political determinants of income inequality, and we addressed the public health implications of placing this artificial boundary in the problem being analyzed. Thus, omission of economic and political variables that might have an impact on income inequality and population health may lead to biased estimates of the aggregate relationship between income inequality and mortality rates. The field of international studies, where social class and income inequality are considered predictors of democratization (rather than health), provides a precedent for the current debate in public health. Following Bollen and Jackman (5):

> This omission [of direct measures of class structure] creates grave problems in interpreting the coefficient estimate for income inequality. The omitted variables are probably correlated with both income inequality and political democracy, so the coefficient for income inequality is biased. . . . Thus, although the coefficient estimate for income inequality may indicate the operation of unspecified aspects of the class structure, the exclusion of direct measures of the class structure means that we cannot judge which particular classes play key roles in the process of democratization.

For example, even crude dichotomous class categories can account for 25 percent of earnings inequalities as measured by the Theil Index (6).

A second methodological problem originates in Wilkinson's interpretations of these macro correlations (3). Ecological correlations of income inequality and mortality or morbidity rates could emerge at the aggregate level even if income inequality per se had no impact on individual mortality or morbidity risk (7). Recently, though, with the incorporation of methods that take into account the clustering of individuals into larger social units (8, 9), Sobaader (10) and Kennedy and colleagues (11) have provided evidence that income inequality indeed has an effect on individual health risk. However, in these studies, the

[1] Epidemiologic pragmatism (e.g., as in "race" or "income" categories without hypotheses) defends itself against realism (a synthesis of rationalism and empiricism) with accusations of "lack of data." However, more data on "race inequalities in health" do not provide any explanation and precisely function as a deterrent of serious investigations on economic, political, and cultural racism (4).

strength of the association between income inequality is lower than typically reported by Wilkinson (3). This is in part due to the addition of aggregate (e.g., county poverty and absolute income) and individual level (e.g., income) covariates (10) and to the fact that the strength of the relation between income inequality and health depends on the level of aggregation (10). For example, the effect of census tract income inequality on individual risk of anxiety disorders can be weak because race and class segregation makes neighborhood incomes homogeneous (12).[2] This is an instance where knowledge of political and economic mechanisms, those that generate segregation above the neighborhood level, is necessary to choose the appropriate level of aggregation to test for income inequality effects.

On "Misconceived Materialism," "Outmoded Prejudices," and Other Red Scares

Wilkinson states that our example on the recent increases in mortality in the former Soviet Union implies an endorsement of the centrally planned economy that characterized that country before the "merchant capitalist" period of the 1990s. We find this inference unjustified. Our point is that a sudden change in the class structure (i.e., a political and economic change) had a major effect on the health of its population (14). We did not deal with the potential causes of declining population health since the mid-1960s, a phenomenon that we acknowledged, however. Increased exploitation, which as Wilkinson notes can exist in centrally planned economies (see Economic Subsystem in the Appendix to Chapter 14), could account for this decline. The political oppression of labor organizations in the Soviet Union, which Muntaner and Llorente (15) noted almost two decades ago, could also account for that trend. In fact, because Wilkinson's population health model calls for reducing income inequality but leaves intact class relations, it gives implicit support to any social system that reduces income inequalities regardless of its class structure (e.g., the Soviet Union's state socialism or the new example in Chapter 15). On the other hand, the implications of a class exploitation model (see Chapter 14) lead to the implicit rejection of both these social systems despite their relative success in reducing income inequality. With regard to what Wilkinson calls "misconceived materialism," our example of a class system (Chapter 14 Appendix) shows that there is no manual/nonmanual labor distinction. Neither do we have any "outmoded prejudice"[3] against psychosocial factors affecting health (16–18). The

[2] Multilevel analyses, though originally developed to estimate contextual effects, can be used to emphasize the effects of individual behavior on health (e.g., 13). In fact, survey methods, because they cannot measure the contextual nature of individual behavior itself, place the real limit on teasing apart "individual" and "social context" contributions to individual health.

[3] Wilkinson's preoccupation with novelty often makes him overlook previous research. See the section "Psychology in a Social Vacuum," below.

issue is that psychosocial factors need to be integrated with social relations rather than approached as isolated individual perceptions of relative inequality position (17; see below).

Social Class: Relational and Stratified

Wilkinson states that class is mostly determined by income differences, making class de facto an attitudinal response of individuals to their relative position in the distribution of income. This framework does not specify where income comes from, which is ultimately from production, as value is ultimately created from labor, not the other way around (19). Similarly, the thought experiment presented by Wilkinson (in Chapter 15) is unrealistic because he does not detail the relations of production in that society, only unequal distribution of incomes. As we showed in the Appendix to Chapter 14, a mere statement about lack of ownership (a legal criterion) does not describe the economic and political processes that take place in the production of goods and services.

Contrary to Wilkinson's interpretation, the class framework presented in Chapter 14 is not dichotomous (e.g., capitalist vs. worker) but integrates class relations within a continuum. Muntaner and his collaborators have conducted several studies that show associations between relational/stratified class indicators and health (e.g., wealthy capitalist, poor capitalist; large capitalist, small capitalist; worker, manager; supervisor, worker) (4, 17, 20–22). Wilkinson is correct when he points out that Boswell and Dixon's rate of surplus value uses income (23). However, theories of exploitation provide social mechanisms for the emergence of economic inequality beyond income (e.g., wealth) and yield multiple measures that are empirically distinct from income inequality (e.g., according to the role of business services, depreciation, or benefits and pension plans in the calculation of the rate of surplus value (24)). Therefore, the rate of surplus value is preferable to catch-all income inequality indicators that do not specify social mechanisms (24). Similarly, measures of "SES" (socioeconomic status) are strong predictors of health outcomes but explain little (17), while its component indicators (occupational stratification, income, educational credentials) are interrelated through different social mechanisms (e.g., status attainment, inter- or intra-generational mobility, age, labor markets, institutions) (eg., 25) and have unique effects on health (26).

PSYCHOLOGY IN A SOCIAL VACUUM: WILKINSON'S CULTURE OF INEQUALITY

Wilkinson's "culture of inequality" fulfills the urgent need for explaining the micro effects of social inequalities. This is yet another instance where class analysis provides a more encompassing framework than the "income inequality and social cohesion model." The task of class analysis is precisely to understand not only how macro structures (e.g., class relations at the national level) constrain micro processes (e.g., interpersonal behavior) but also how micro processes (e.g., interpersonal behavior) can affect macro structures (e.g., via collective action) (27).

Wilkinson is certainly correct in addressing the lack of research on the psychological effects of inequality. While there is a substantial scholarship on the psychology of racism and sexism, little research has been done on the effects of class ideology (i.e., classism). This asymmetry could reflect that in most wealthy democratic capitalist countries, income inequalities are perceived as legitimate while gender and race inequalities are not (4). Most work on the psychology of inequality and classism has been qualitative (28–32). Most of these ethnographies, as well as some recent empirical studies (33, 34), point to the relational aspects of classism (e.g., the educated upper middle class holding views of inferiority about the working class or its most deprived elements).

But it is not only the psychological effect (e.g., humiliation) associated with lower capacity to purchase goods and services that seems to matter. Thus, although Wilkinson uses Sennett and Cobb's classic *The Hidden Injuries of Class* (29) for his argument about the psychology of inequality, he fails to mention Sennett's new volume (30), which stresses the erosion of control over the labor process even among persons of *relatively high* income (e.g., the rise of nonstandard work arrangements, lack of control due to mechanization). Attitudes about the causes of social inequalities (i.e., classist ideology) are part of class relations. Those with relatively high incomes (e.g., capitalists, managers, and professionals) hold attitudes that justify social inequalities, cast in terms of reductionist biological hypotheses (e.g., the inheritance of intelligence) or idealist lay psychology (e.g., self, effort, morality, responsibility, will power) (32).

Wilkinson is correct in stressing the need to explain the social psychology of health inequalities—that is, psychological social psychology (i.e., the study of how society affects individual behavior and health)—as associations between social indicators and mortality rates presuppose individual-level mechanisms whereby social relations affect individual behavior and health. Nevertheless, Wilkinson's social psychology neglects precisely the impact of social (economic, political, and cultural) relations on individual behavior. His approach is similar to the U.S. interpersonal social psychology that was criticized by British psychology more than 20 years ago (35, 36). That approach to social psychology was abandoned because it focused on interpersonal behavior without analyzing the social relations that determine it.

In addition to social psychology, Wilkinson uses the literature on animal and human stress to summarize the evidence on the health effects of social inequalities. While these fields have shown substantial progress in recent years (e.g., Sapolsky's research on stress), Wilkinson's presentation of them as "novelty" does not acknowledge a long research tradition in the physiology of social hierarchies among primates (37) and in the study of human physiological psychology (e.g., the Swedish school that linked responses of the sympathetic–adrenal medullary system and the pituitary–adrenal cortical system to workplace stress (38)). These omissions might contribute to overstating the degree of progress that has been achieved with the "income inequality" approach and overlooking what is known about the health effects of hierarchies within the labor process (38).

We next review several hypotheses advanced by Wilkinson that have already been refuted decades ago in social psychology, or for which there is enough evidence to cast doubt on their alleged generality.

The Relatively Deprived as "Men of Respect": A New Version of the Frustration/Aggression Hypothesis

Disrespect is now claimed to account for the association between inequality, violence (i.e., lack of social cohesion), and health. But this sweeping generalization does not take into account the social relations where "disrespect" takes place. The history of a comparable violence hypothesis, the "frustration/aggression" hypothesis of the 1940s (39) can shed light on the plausibility of the "disrespect/violence" hypothesis. Once researchers started to take into account the social context of behavior (as in Bandura's Social Learning Theory), the frustration/aggression model was rejected (40). For example, frustration (or humiliation, or disrespect) under authoritarian social relations is not a good predictor of aggression (e.g., soldiers under instruction; a worker reprimanded by a supervisor in the workplace). Military and most forms of criminal aggression do not require being offended: actually, emotional arousal can interfere with effective aggression. Most aggression is instrumental; it is emitted because it has been rewarded in the past or under instructions that signal future rewards (41). For example, the pilot of a Lockheed F-117A Stealth Fighter that drops bombs over Iraq or Kosovo does not have to be upset, or frustrated, or feel any kind "disrespect" to emit aggressive behavior. The role of "disrespect" as a determinant of aggression changes in organizations according to economic, power, and cultural relations. Thus, inside mafia organizations, enforcing "respect" kept the cost of business transactions low, as there was no possibility of appealing to external law enforcement (42, 43). Once this culture of "disrespect" and violence proved unnecessary for the economic goals of the organization (due to technological change, among other factors), it drastically declined (44).

The notion that large income inequality undercuts community cohesion through its emotional effects (e.g., frustration, bitterness) was a popular hypothesis in political sociology (45). Wilkinson, like some political sociologists, conflates the idea of inequality with inequity (5), thus implying that the experience of inequality is perceived as unjust. However, inequality refers to the distribution of income while equity refers to the evaluation of people's relative position (5). From what is known in political sociology, there is no basis to expect that a high degree of income inequality will necessarily be seen as unjust or undermine the legitimacy of a society by itself and give rise to antisocial behavior as Wilkinson claims. For example, surveys conducted in wealthy capitalist countries indicate that inequality does not necessarily translate into perceptions of inequity and that populations can view inequality as legitimate (46). Moreover, a population's objective perception of inequality is made difficult by the availability heuristic, a social cognitive phenomenon that impels people to over-represent the proportion in their own social class (or income bracket), which constitutes the majority of those with whom they interact (47, 48). Although many other factors could be invoked (e.g., class, race and ethnic formation, media propaganda), these two social facts alone (i.e., the asymmetry between inequality and equity, and the availability heuristic) cast doubt on the soundness of this aspect of the psychosocial hypothesis proposed by Wilkinson.

The above argument does not mean that at the aggregate level we cannot find strong associations between income inequality and violence. Such a relation is complex, however, involving different types of inequality (e.g., exploitation, agrarian inequality) and types of violence (e.g., collective revolt, different sorts of crime, state-sanctioned violence) (23). What can be challenged is that such relationship, if found, is likely to originate from an individuals' perception of his or her position in the distribution of income.

The Relatively Deprived as French Existentialists:[4] *The Anxiety Hypothesis*

According to Wilkinson, anxiety is an important consequence of income inequality that affects individual health. Psychiatrists distinguish between medically treated anxiety disorders (e.g., the DSM-IV's panic disorder, obsessive compulsive disorder, specific phobia, social phobia) and psychological, everyday anxiety that is measured in a continuum (e.g., MMPIs MAS scale, Spielberger's State/trait scale). Psychological anxiety could be defined as conditioned fear or as an expectation that includes negative affect, resulting from perceptions of threat and inability to predict the outcomes of future situations (49). This distinction is relevant because it avoids medicalization and its potential iatrogenic consequences, among them labeling and stigma. In Chapter 15 Wilkinson seems to refer to this latter form of anxiety, less severe and more pervasive than psychiatric disorders.

Stressing the psychopathology of the relatively deprived is a common approach in mental health research (e.g., research on vulnerability to stress, lack of self-esteem, fatalism, (50)) that runs the risk of portraying the relatively poor as passive victims (e.g., Franz Fanon's notion of victimization; both current authors are also vulnerable to this criticism). This approach to psychopathology ignores the resiliency, endurance, and capacity for collective action among relatively

[4] The term "French existentialist" refers to the middle-class intellectual movement inspired by Jean Paul Sartre in post–World War II France that underscored the role of anxiety in everyday life.

deprived persons even when they face severe, uncontrollable events (e.g., homelessness, unemployment) (28).

Actually, evidence suggests that mild forms of everyday anxiety (uncertainty) seem to be a characteristic of the middle class, in particular among those who fear downward mobility (31, 51). On the other hand, anxiety *disorders* are more frequent among the working class: in a recent survey of East Baltimore, Muntaner and colleagues (17) have shown higher rates of anxiety disorders among those with absolute lower family incomes and those who *do not* derive income from property. Thus Wilkinson's culture of inequality hypothesis reflects a middle-class notion[5] of pervasive cognitive anxiety that, even if valid, would underestimate the severe psychiatric impact of social inequalities among the lowest strata of the income distribution.

The Relatively Deprived as Leisure Class: Do Persons with Relatively Low Income Work at All?

Another problem in Wilkinson's theory is that it overlooks the nonpsychological effects of income inequalities (e.g., environmental exposures, injuries, infectious diseases) (52–55). Given that production (occupational and environmental health) is considered one of the top determinants of population health (56, 57), it is surprising that in Wilkinson's model people do not work, they just receive paychecks. Wilkinson's hypothesis amounts to stating that the health of, for example, Appalachian nurse aides is determined by their perceptions of being at the lower end of the income distribution in their community (where, owing to class segregation, they seldom interact with higher-income persons) rather than by exposure to job strain, authoritarian management, and lack of health benefits. Nurse and health aides have some of the highest rates of musculoskeletal disorders, back injuries, and assaults on the job (58). But in Wilkinson's model, nowhere can we find a labor process that would expose aides to high demands (ten-hour shifts, understaffing resulting in high client loads, no lunch breaks), low control (lack of ergonomic standards, exposures to emotionally demanding interactions with dying clients, lack of supplies that would allow for proper care of the elderly), and indignity (such as older women being patronized by the young male MBAs who manage them). In particular, issues of lack of respect (the SEIU AFL-CIO's "Dignity Campaign") are framed in terms of lack of *respect at work*, not shameful or humiliating perceptions of relative deprivation or interpersonal interactions outside the labor process (59).

[5] Another aspect of this alleged "middle-class bias," namely in the definition of social cohesion as well as in recent articles on "collective efficacy" and "social capital," is addressed empirically in section II of this chapter.

Culture Is (also) about Social Relations

Thus, psychosocial explanations, although real and necessary, need to take into account social[6] relations (Chapter 14 Appendix) to give a deep account of how social inequalities affect health. Wilkinson could take advantage of what has been learned during the last decades to build realistic socio-psychological models of social inequalities in health that incorporate gender, race, and class relations (60). Just as the macro component of the model ("income inequality") overlooks economic, political, and cultural relations, its micro components (social cohesion, culture of inequality) do not spell out how social relations affect individual behavior (i.e., the task of contemporary psychological social psychology) (59) and health (60).

REGRETTABLE BUT TOLERABLE: REACTIONS TO INCOME INEQUALITY RESEARCH AMONG THE UPPER MIDDLE CLASSES

Sen[7] has recently lamented that unemployment is "regrettable but tolerable" in Europe but not in the United States, where the Protestant work ethic of individual responsibility and accountability considers lack of opportunity to help oneself socially unacceptable (62). The argument could be turned around with regard to income inequality, to suggest that in the United States income inequality is "regrettable but tolerable" as the American self-amelioration culture does not include any provision for equality of outcome (e.g., protecting against poverty and lack of health care). This seems to be true among the educated elites (33), precisely those academics and government officials who read research on income inequalities.

Contrary to Wilkinson's claim, it is doubtful that his research on income inequality has had a major impact on the understanding of social cohesion. Using

[6] In order to support the existence of social epidemiology as a research field, we need to establish the distinctiveness of social facts. Mortality and morbidity rates are *biosocial concepts,* as death is a biological fact while dying as a result of a city's contaminated water supply or war is a social fact—making epidemiology a biosocial science. *Social facts* occur above the level of the individual organism, in social systems. A social system is defined by an environment, animals of the same species, and the set of their relations or structure of their social system, and presumes biological processes (e.g., homicide implies biological death). But in epidemiology, "social factors" are seldom defined as social facts. Social facts have properties that are not shared by any individual in isolation. For example, although modern manufacturing plants might have many employees working under conditions of high autonomy, manufacturing a car is a social fact as no single individual in isolation can build a car. Similarly, in racial social systems, political exclusion such as barring non-whites from unions, economic discrimination such as whites receiving higher incomes, or blacks being exposed to ideologies claiming white superiority, are social facts associated with some biological or geographical element such as skin color or place of origin.

[7] Amartya Sen (often quoted by authors in the "income inequality and social cohesion" model) has a reputation as an advocate for reducing social inequalities that is probably exaggerated (61).

the MEDLINE database on articles in the health sciences, we found 76 articles on social cohesion and zero articles on income inequality and social cohesion between 1980 and 1989. In the 1990s, at the beginning of which Wilkinson published his most visible empirical articles, the corresponding figures were 170 and four. Even if these four articles on income inequality and social cohesion were published in journals having a large impact, it is unlikely that students of social cohesion have incorporated the notion that income inequality determines social cohesion. A more parsimonious view would be that these two research areas have little impact on each other. Some features of Wilkinson's model could account for this observation: (*a*) lack of explanations for the social origins of income inequalities and their link to interpersonal behaviors; and (*b*) overabundance of conjectures on individuals' perceptions of inequality and their associated breakdown in social cohesion as determinants of health inequalities.

An emphasis on the psychology of social cohesion rather than income inequality should be expected as people seek explanations (63), and Wilkinson provides only post-hoc psychological hypotheses on the breakdown of social cohesion. Thus readers appropriately emphasize that aspect of the model of which they can make some sense. For example, a political science journal states that "Richard Wilkinson and other academic authorities have concluded that inequalities of health and education are *not merely* the product of income differences" (64). Another publication summarizes Wilkinson's research as follows: "A leading figure in this work, says that what seems to matter are the *social meanings* attached to inferior living conditions . . . the quality of the social fabric *rather than* increases in average wealth" (65). Similarly, the *British Medical Journal*'s comment on Wilkinson's research states, "*as important* for health as income differentials is social capital—that is, features of social organization (civic participation, social trust) that facilitate cooperation for mutual benefit" (66). (Emphasis added in all three quotations.) A common feature of these interpretations of Wilkinson's research is that subjective appraisals and a loss of social cohesion are understood as independent of income inequalities, not as a consequence. Also consistent with our argument, it is significant to note in the last example that the author *does not* seem to consider income inequalities as part of "social organization." So why does Wilkinson shy away from class, gender, and race relations, repeating instead a known empirical association (67) and restricting explanations to mostly discredited psychological hypotheses (40)?

WHAT IT REALLY COMES DOWN TO: THEORETICAL DIFFERENCES HAVE POLITICAL IMPLICATIONS

Table 1 presents the two basic theoretical differences between models of social inequalities in health: whether inequality relations are binding or nonbinding

Table 1

Models of social inequalities in health according to kind of inequality relation proposed (binding or nonbinding) and their implicit values (equality or inequality)

	Kind of inequality relation	
Values	Binding ("unchangeable")	Nonbinding ("changeable")
Equality	Class, gender, and race	Income inequality and social cohesion
Inequality	Functionalism, sociobiology	Social cohesion

(e.g., a business owner implies a worker that works for her[8] vs. a ranking of income), and whether the model's implicit values do or do not promote the end of social inequalities in health. Thus, class analysis concurs with the income inequality and social cohesion model in the goal of ending social inequalities in health, but calls for a substitution of social relations that generate economic inequalities (e.g., eliminating "owner/worker" relations). The income inequality and social cohesion model would maintain those social relations and merely reduce income inequalities through some other unspecified mechanism (i.e., a nonbinding relation). Some varieties of class analysis (e.g., Marxian crisis theory) also predict that capitalism cannot survive with substantial redistributions of income (e.g., the rising "organic composition of capital" hypothesis (Chapter 14 footnote 8)). Moreover, it could be argued that the social cohesion model (Table 1) that informs most of New Democrat and New Labour "community" initiatives does not even aim at reducing social inequalities to improve population health through income redistribution (68).

Thus, both class analysis and income inequality approaches share egalitarian values that aim at eliminating social inequalities in health. However, Wilkinson's model avoids class, gender, and race relations, implying that the (psychological) effects of income *distribution* are the determinants of health inequalities and that there is nothing harmful about the way income inequalities are *produced*—which is the focus of the class approach to health inequalities. As opposed to class-based, social democratic policies, the emphasis of Wilkinson's model on social cohesion is reminiscent of Christian democratic public policies in Europe, one of the main traditions of European welfare states (69). Christian democratic social policies have produced a smaller reduction in economic inequality than have

[8] This dichotomy is a short-cut simplification for an elaborate map of class processes and locations (see Chapter 14).

social democratic policies (e.g., pension systems). This was achieved by transferring social responsibility to families and communities (i.e., social cohesiveness) while weakening the power of class-based labor movements (69).

CONCLUSION

In a period of unprecedented international economic inequalities, not even concealed by members of the emerging transnational capitalist class (70, 71), it is even more important that researchers do not shy away from uncomfortable explanations, even at the risk of negative consequences (72, 73). This is not an easy task. Particularly in Europe and the United States, the individualist ethic of Protestant liberalism among the elitist upper middle class (32) provides justification for adopting positions that avoid or disregard conflict (e.g., unfulfilled expectations of "making a difference" or "being a winner" (74). (There is a substantial amount of theoretical and empirical scholarship on this topic (e.g., 32).) Nevertheless, given the evidence reviewed here and in Chapter 14, the impact of class relations on income inequality and population health should not be ignored (5). A basic disregard for the class, gender, and race relations that generate income inequality (empirical studies have been conducted for more than 20 years (75–80)) has implications for social policy. For example, scholars that are supportive of Wilkinson's model (81) seem to believe that organizing conferences of enlightened consumer advocates and philanthropic billionaires (e.g., Ralph Nader, Bill Gates, Warren Buffet) might be a sound strategy to reduce income inequalities (82). From a class analysis perspective this proposition seems *extremely* naive and ineffective as it reflects a lack of understanding of the conflict of interests underlying class relations.

It is not our goal to diminish the leading contribution of Wilkinson's income inequality studies to the advancement of social epidemiology in the last decades of this century. However, important as they might be to update and monitor social inequalities in health, associations between income inequality and health had been documented earlier (67, 83–85), and deeper models that incorporate political and economic determinants of income inequality have been advanced (see Chapter 14). In a period of conservative hegemony, it could be argued that going back to simple models that do not address how the workings of capitalism affect health provides the sole venue under which health inequalities can be studied. Models such as the "income inequality and social cohesion" model provide a pragmatic and safe middle ground where left, liberal, and conservative researchers eschew the social mechanisms that generate income inequalities, thus avoiding the issue of whether eliminating health inequalities requires fundamental policies (e.g., replacing managed care with a national health insurance) or reformist policies (giving tax breaks so the relatively deprived can afford some managed care) (Table 1, right column). Nevertheless, the aim of science is still to provide the best possible explanations without attention to the powers that be.

Unless social epidemiologists are willing to take intellectual risks (4) their discipline is unlikely to provide any serious insight into how social systems generate health inequalities.

REFERENCES (SECTION I)

1. Wilkinson, R. G. Income inequality, social cohesion, and health: Clarifying the theory—a reply to Muntaner and Lynch. *Int. J. Health Serv.* 29: 525–543, 1999.
2. Muntaner, C., and Lynch, J. Income inequality, social cohesion, and class relations: A critique of Wilkinson's neo-Durkheimian research program. *Int. J. Health Serv.* 29: 59–82, 1999.
3. Wilkinson, R. G. *Unhealthy Societies: The Afflictions of Inequality.* Routledge, London, 1996
4. Muntaner, C. Social mechanisms, race and social epidemiology. *Am. J. Epidemiol.* 150: 121–126, 1999.
5. Bollen, K. A., and Jackman, R. W. Income inequality and democratization revisited: Comment on Muller. *Am. Sociol. Rev.* 60: 983–989, 1995.
6. Beck, S. H. The decomposition of inequality by class and by occupation. *Sociol. Q.* 32: 139–150, 1991.
7. Gravelle, H. How much of the relation between population mortality and unequal distribution of income is a statistical artefact? *BMJ* 316: 382–385, 1998.
8. O'Campo, P., et al. Violence by male partners against women during the childbearing year: A contextual analysis. *Am. J. Public Health* 85: 1092–1097, 1995.
9. Diez-Roux, A. V., et al. Neighborhood environment and coronary heart disease. *Am. J. Epidemiol.* 146(1): 48–63, 1997.
10. Sobaader, J. Effects of Income Inequality on Morbidity. Ph.D. dissertation, Boston University, 1998.
11. Kennedy, B. P., et al. Income distribution, socioeconomic status, and self-rated health in the United States: Multilevel analysis. *BMJ* 317: 917–921, 1998.
12. Muntaner, C. Neighbourhood Unemployment, Social Cohesion and Anxiety Disorders: Multilevel Analysis. Seminar on Social Inequalities, Department of Mental Hygiene, The Johns Hopkins School of Public Health, Baltimore, December 16, 1998.
13. Sampson, R. J., Raudenbush, S. W., and Earls, F. Neighborhoods and violent crime: A multilevel study of collective efficacy. *Science* 277(5328): 918–924, 1997.
14. Health in Russia is broken, but who is to fix it? *Lancet* 353: 337, 1999.
15. Muntaner, C., and Llorente, M. Aggression: An avoidable achievement. *Mientras Tanto* 13: 69-81, 1984.
16. Lynch, J. W., Kaplan, G. A., and Salonen, J. T. Why do poor people behave poorly? Variations in adult health behaviour and psychosocial characteristics, by stage of the socioeconomic life course. *Soc. Sci. Med.* 44: 809–820, 1997.
17. Muntaner, C., et al. Social class, assets, organizational control and the prevalence of common groups psychiatric disorders: Results from two U.S. epidemiologic surveys. *Soc. Sci. Med.* 47 (12): 243–253, 1998.
18. Lynch, J. W. Socioeconomic factors in the behavioral and psychosocial epidemiology of cardiovascular disease. In *Integrating Behavioral and Social Sciences with Public*

Health, edited by N. Schneiderman, et al. APA Press, Washington, D.C., 1999, in press.
19. Shaikh, A., and Tonak, E. A. *Measuring the Wealth of Nations: The Political Economy of National Accounts.* Cambridge University Press, Cambridge, England, 1994.
20. Muntaner, C., et al. Psychotic inpatients' social class and their first admission to state or private psychiatric Baltimore hospitals. *Am. J. Public Health* 84(2): 287–289, 1994.
21. Muntaner, C., and Parsons, P. E. Income, social stratification, class, and private health insurance. *Int. J. Health Serv.* 26(4): 655–671, 1996.
22. Muntaner, C., et al. Arrest among psychotic inpatients: Assessing the relationship to diagnosis, gender, number of admissions and social class. *Soc. Psychiatry Psychiatr. Epidemiol.* 33(6): 274–282, 1998.
23. Boswell, T., and Dixon, W. J. Marx's theory of rebellion: A cross-national analysis of class exploitation, economic development, and violent revolt. *Am. Sociol. Rev.* 58: 681–702, 1993.
24. Amsden, A. H. An international comparison of the rate of surplus value in the manufacturing industry. *Cambridge J. Econ.* 5(3):229–249, 1981.
25. Wong, R. S.-K. Multidimensional influences of family environment in education: The case of Socialist Czechoslovakia. *Sociol. Educ.* 71: 1–22, 1998.
26. Sorlie, P., Backlund, E., and Keller, J. U.S. mortality by economic, demographic and social characteristics: The National Longitudinal Mortality Study. *Am. J. Public Health* 85(7): 949–956, 1995.
27. Wright, E. O. The conceptual status of class structure in class analysis. In *Bringing Class Back In*, edited by S. G. McNall, R. F. Levine, and R. Fantasia. Westview Press, Boulder, Colo., 1991.
28. Liebow, E. *Tell Them Who I Am: The Lives of Homeless Women.* Free Press, New York, 1994.
29. Sennett, R., and Cobb, J. *The Hidden Injuries of Class.* Knopf, New York, 1973.
30. Sennett, R. *The Corrosion of Character: The Personal Consequences of Work in the New Capitalism.* Norton, New York, 1998.
31. Newman, K. *Falling From Grace*. Free Press, New York, 1988.
32. Lamont, M. *Money, Morals, and Manners: The Culture of the French and the American Upper Middle Class.* University of Chicago Press, Chicago, 1992.
33. Phelan, J., et al. Education, social liberalism, and economic conservatism: Attitudes toward homeless people. *Am. Sociol. Rev.* 60: 126–140, 1995.
34. Phelan, J., et al. The stigma of homelessness: The impact of the label "homeless" on attitudes toward poor persons. *Soc. Psychol. Q.* 60(4): 323–337, 1997.
35. Tajfel, H. *The Social Psychology of Minorities.* Minority Rights Group, London, 1978.
36. Tajfel, H. *Introducing Social Psychology.* Penguin Books, Harmondsworth, England, 1978.
37. Rodriguez Delgado, J. M. *Brain Control and Aggression.* Harper and Row, Hagerstown, Md., 1970.
38. Frankenhauser, M. A biopsychosocial approach to work life issues. In *The Psychosocial Work Environment: Work Organization, Democratization and Health,* edited by J. V. Johnson and G. Johansson, pp. 49–60. Baywood, Amityville, N.Y., 1991.

39. Dollard, J. *Frustration and Aggression.* Kegan Paul, Trench, Trubner, London, 1944.
40. Bandura, A. *Aggression: A Social Learning Analysis.* Prentice Hall, Englewood Cliffs, N.J., 1973.
41. Muntaner, C., Llorente, M., and Nagoshi, C. Instructional control, interpersonal aggression and the type A behaviour pattern. *Aggressive Behav.* 15: 161–170, 1989.
42. Maas, P. *Underboss: Sammy the Bull Gravano's Story of Life in the Mafia.* Harper-Perennial, New York, 1997.
43. Fighting organised crime requires understanding how it works. *Economist.* February 10, 1996.
44. Organised crime: Streamlined for success. *Economist.* October 11, 1997.
45. Lipset, S. M. *Political Man: The Social Bases of Politics.* Double Day, New York, 1959.
46. Kelley, J., and Evans, M. D. R. Class and class conflict in six western nations. *Am. Sociol. Rev.* 60(2): 157–178, 1995.
47. Wegener, B. Concepts and measurement of prestige. *Annu. Rev. Sociol.* 18: 253–280, 1992.
48. Kelley, J., and Evans, M. D. R. The legitimation of inequality: Occupational earnings in nine nations. *Am. J. Sociol.* 99(1): 75–125, 1993.
49. Barlow, D. H. *Anxiety and its Disorders.* Guilford, Press, New York, 1988.
50. Muntaner, C., Eaton, W. W., and Diala, C. Socioeconomic inequalities in mental health. *Health,* 1999, in press.
51. U.S. Department of Labor. *Report on the American Workforce.* U.S. Government Printing Office, Washington, D.C., 1994.
52. Blane, D., Montgomery, S. M., and Berney, D. R. Social class differences in lifetime exposure to environmental hazards. *Sociol. Health Illness* 20: 532, 1998.
53. Boer, J. T., et al. Is there environmental racism? The demographics of hazardous waste in L.A. county. *Soc. Sci. Q.* 4: 793–810, 1997.
54. Caraher, M., et al. Access to healthy foods. Part 1. Barriers to accessing healthy foods: Differential by gender, social class, income and mode of transport. *Health Educ. J.* 57(3): 191–201, 1998.
55. O'Campo, P., et al. Neighbourhood risk factors for low birth weight in Baltimore: A multilevel analysis. *Am. J. Public Health* 87: 1113–1118, 1997.
56. Doll, R. A. Health and the environment in the 1990s. *Am. J. Public Health* 82: 933–941, 1992.
57. Leight, et al. Occupational injury and illness in the United States. *Arch. Intern. Med.* 157: 1557–1568, 1997.
58. Meyer, J., and Muntaner, C. Injuries in home health care workers: An analysis of occupational morbidity from a state compensation database. *Am. J. Ind. Med.* 35: 295–301, 1999.
59. Chau-Kiu, C. Variation in structuralist and individualist explanations among classes in Hong Kong. *Sociol. Spectrum* 19: 93–118, 1999.
60. Kohn, M. L., and Schooler, C. *Work and Personality: A Study in the Impact of Social Stratification.* Ablex, N.J., 1983.
61. Uses and misuses of Amartya Sen. *Economist,* January 9, 1999.

62. Sen, A. Inequality, unemployment, and contemporary Europe. *Int. Labour Rev.* 136: 155–172, 1997.
63. Nisbett, R. E., and Ross, L. *Human Inference: Strategies and Shortcomings of Social Judgement.* Prentice Hall, Englewood Cliffs, N.J., 1980.
64. Warning: Inequality kills (editorial). *New Statesman* 127(2214): 4, 1998.
65. Eckersley, R. Is life really getting better? *Futurist* 33: 23–27, 1999.
66. Stewart Brown, S. Emotional well-being and its relation to health. *BMJ* 317: 1608–1610, 1998.
67. Rodgers, G. B. Income inequality and life expectancy. *Popul. Stud.* 33: 343–351, 1979.
68. Britain; Crossing the Rubicon on welfare. *Economist,* March 6, 1999.
69. Navarro, V. The political economy of the welfare state in developed capitalist countries. *Int. J. Health Serv.* 29: 59–82, 1999.
70. Soros, G. *The Crisis of Global Capitalism: Open Society Endangered.* Little Brown, London, 1998.
71. Soros, G. The capitalist threat. *Atlantic Monthly* 279: 45–58, 1997.
72. Waitzkin, H. Is our work dangerous? Should it be? *J. Health Soc. Behav.* 39: 7–17, 1998.
73. Navarro, V. A historical review (1965–1997) of studies on class, health, and quality of life: A personal account. *Int. J. Health Serv.* 28: 389–406, 1998.
74. Muntaner, C. Teaching social inequalities in health: Barriers and opportunities. *Scand. J. Public Health* 18:1–5, 1999.
75. Mount, R. I., and Bennett, R. E. Economic and social factors in income inequality: Race and sex discrimination and status as elements in wage differentials. *Am. J. Sociol. Econ.* 34(2): 161–174, 1975.
76. Wright, E. O., and Perrone, L. Marxist class categories and income inequality. *Am. Sociol. Rev.* 42: 32–55, 1977.
77. Wright, E. O. Race, class and income inequality. *Am. J. Sociol.* 83: 1368–1397, 1978.
78. Robinson, R. V., and Kelley, J. Class as conceived by Marx and Dahrendorf: Effects on income inequality and politics in the United States and Great Britain. *Am. Sociol. Rev.* 44:38–58, 1979.
79. Gorin, Z. Effect of type of property relations on income inequality: Evidence from research. *Human Factor* 13: 69–89, 1976.
80. Hill, R. C. Unionization and racial income inequality in the Metropolis. *Am. Sociol. Rev.* 39:507–522, 1974.
81. Inequality Meets Epidemiology: The Career of Richard Wilkinson. Available from http://www.inequality.org/wilk.html.
82. Ralph Nader Appeals to Bill Gates to Join with Warren Buffett in Convening a World Conference of Billionaires and Multi-billionaires to Discuss Disparities in National and Global Wealth. Available from http://www.inequality.org/nader.html.
83. Messner, S. F. Regional differences in the economic correlates of the urban homicide rate. *Criminology* 21: 477–488, 1983.
84. Flegg, A. T. The role of inequality of income in the determination of birth rates. *Popul. Stud.* 33: 457–477, 1979.
85. Lynch, J. W., and Kaplan, G. A. Understanding how inequality in the distribution of income affects health. *J. Health Psychol.* 2: 297–314, 1997.

II. PRESENTATION OF AN ALTERNATIVE MODEL

The psychosocial construct of social cohesion, broadly understood as social behaviors indicating trust, reciprocity, and concern for the well-being of the members of one's community, is the key determinant of health in Wilkinson's model (1, p. 211). More specifically, Wilkinson defines social cohesion as participation in public affairs, civic responsibility, or involvement in public life. Thus, social cohesion can be measured with indicators of voting participation, newspaper readership, or number of cultural voluntary associations (1, pp. 119–120). In our previous analysis (2), we critically examined Wilkinson's notion of social cohesion and we proposed some alternatives (see Chapter 14). Here we concentrate on two components of that critique, namely that (*a*) social class determines the type of social cohesion emerging in communities, and (*b*) Wilkinson's proposed indicators exclude or minimize forms of social cohesion emerging from working-class communities, thus resulting in lack of content validity (3).

While social cohesion should by definition refer to social relations, several elements of social cohesion examined by Wilkinson (1) concern individual psychology (e.g., emotions, stress, attributions, helplessness, motivation, self-perception, disrespect). We focus here on the sociological aspects of Wilkinson's notion of social cohesion and define social cohesion as the amount of individual participation in social groups in the community (see Chapter 14). Indicators of membership in civil organizations, a central measure of social cohesion used in Wilkinson's research program (3), would correspond to this definition. But in order for a psychometric measure to have content validity it must include a representative sample of indicators of the construct it is supposed to measure (4). Thus, measures of social cohesion based on organization membership exclude or minimize forms of group participation that are characteristic of working-class communities, such as informal help networks, gift giving, or union membership (5, 6). This omission is relevant to social epidemiology because working-class forms of cohesion can affect the health of communities through collective political action (e.g., research on collective control) (7).

In political sociology, research within the resource mobilization framework has revealed that members of the middle class have more time and resources to devote to civic participation than members of the working class (8–10). Therefore we expect that the forms of civic social activism tapped by Wilkinson's indicators will be positively associated with "non-working-class" locations and negatively associated with working-class location. Next, because group participation antecedes collective political participation (e.g., voting, strikes) (6, 10), we hypothesize that Wilkinson's forms of organization membership will mediate the association between middle-class and political participation while union membership will be the mediator of political participation for working-class locations. In testing these hypotheses we take into account the role of potential confounders such as expected efficacy of individual political action, income, and education.

The Need to Account for Individual Political Efficacy

The need to adjust for individual expectations of political efficacy stems from a long-standing body of work in political sociology and from recent developments in class analysis: namely, from the search for ways of explaining collective action using methodological individualism, in particular through rational action models of individual behavior (e.g., 11–14). Rational action, in its methodological individualist version used by rational choice Marxists,[9] is a descriptive theory of human behavior which develops from several strong assumptions, such as expected utility maximization, autonomy, and cognitive proficiency (see 17–22). Rational choice, or instrumental rationality, has been defined as a set of rules for choosing among alternatives. Available alternatives are first evaluated by multiplying certainty and utility, and the alternative yielding the maximum value is then selected (23).[10] Przeworksi (11) provides a typical example of the application of instrumental rationality to the question of class and political participation—arguing that major social transformations will not be attempted by powerful movements under capitalism because they are costly to rational workers. That is, organizations of rational workers will consent to capitalism when this strategy is best for the material interest of individual rational workers (12).

The relationship between class and political participation is thus explained by the expected political efficacy of individual workers (26). Political efficacy, the belief in one's ability to influence the political environment, is a significant psychological predictor of political participation (27–30) and has also been related to an individual's location in the social structure (29–33). Efficacy should therefore be considered a potential mediator of the relation between social class and political participation. Different definitions of political efficacy tend to focus on the expected effectiveness of one's political behavior. For example, Almond and Verba (34) consider efficacy "subjective competence," while Gamson's (35) definition stresses "individuals' perception of their ability to influence." Such definitions of political efficacy establish a correspondence with individual rationality, since rational actors are guided by efficacy concerns (36). Inasmuch

[9] Rational choice is far from exhausted by methodological individualism, nor do rational choice advocates such as Coleman (15) or Burt (16) neglect the relevance of social structure.

[10] Although influential in class analysis (e.g., 13, 14), the empirical support for models based on rationality varies greatly across social and behavioral sciences (24). For example, while rational choice economists often assume that individuals tend to maximize expected utility (i.e., the assumption that there is an objective individual "utility" or self-interest which the subject optimizes), some behavioral psychologists have conducted experimental research supporting at least one alternative behavioral equilibrium in which individuals do not maximize expected utilities but distribute their behavior to obtain an average return across different options (25).

as the rational choice framework stresses the notion of an optimal relationship between means and ends, political action can thus be seen as the rational course of action for efficacious individuals. Besides the link that students of political participation have drawn between political efficacy and individual rationality, political efficacy has exemplified the paradigm of methodological individualism in political sociology since the early 1960s (e.g., 37). The belief that individual political action does or can have an impact upon the political process is a psychological variable (34, 37). As a consequence, models relying on political efficacy as the main determinant of political participation qualify as methodological individualism.

Thus, by adjusting for individual expectations of political efficacy we can claim that the effects of social cohesion (organization or union membership) are indeed social (i.e., cannot be reduced to individual behavior) (e.g., 38).

Hypotheses

According to the preceding examination of theoretical and empirical amendments to the construct of social cohesion and its relation to social class, we formulate two hypotheses on the relation between class, organization membership, union membership, and political participation.

Hypothesis 1. Capitalist, managerial, or professional ("non-working-class") class location will be positively associated with organization membership, while working-class location will be positively associated with union membership, even after accounting for the effects of income and education.

Hypothesis 2. Organization membership and union membership will mediate the relationship between social class and political participation even after accounting for the effect of individual expectations of political efficacy, income, and education on political participation.

METHODS

We used data from the American portion (N = 1,719) of the Political Action I survey (39) and from a sub-sample (N = 523) of the American portion of the Political Action II survey (40). The sub-sample is comprised of respondents to the Political Action I survey who were re-interviewed seven years later as part of the Political Action II project.[11] These data are particularly appropriate for our study because they facilitate the operation of class in a manner that measures the presence or absence of control over the means of production (i.e., capitalist,

[11]The American portion of the Political Action I survey was conducted between June and September of 1974, and the American portion of the Political Action II survey was conducted between May and September of 1981. Both surveys are based on multi-stage area probability samples of households.

managerial, and professional class ("non-working-class") vs. working-class positions) and include multiple indicators of social cohesion (i.e., organization and union membership) as well as different forms of political participation (i.e., conventional and protest).

We used two structural equation models (SEM) with latent variables (41) to determine the relative mediating roles of organization and union membership and their relation to social class. These models combine structural equation and factor modeling, and they directly adjust for the fact that latent variables are imprecisely measured (42). The preliminary model, depicted in Figure 1, is based on cross-sectional data from the Political Action I survey. The exogenous variables are the dichotomous *social class* indicator (working-class location versus non-working-class location) and the two control variables, *income* and *education*. The explanatory variables are social cohesion (*membership in civic organizations* and *union membership*), and individual perceptions of *political efficacy,* and the two ultimate dependent variables are *conventional participation* and *legal protesting*.[12] Four of the variables included in this model—organization membership, political efficacy, conventional participation, and legal protesting—are latent variables, and a complete description of their indicators is provided in the Appendix at the end of the chapter (loadings for these indicators are listed in Table 4). The 1974–1981 period covered by our analyses was chosen because it covers moments of singular political participation (conventional and protest) in the United States, with special significance for health policy (44).

A preliminary analysis of the Political Action I data allowed us to take advantage of a large sample size (N = 1,719) to test our hypothesis on the association between social class and different forms of social cohesion (organization and union membership). The preliminary model presented in Figure 1 does not allow for the possibility that perceptions of political efficacy and social cohesion (membership in civic organizations or unions) occupy different temporal planes. A politically efficacious individual might, for example, be predisposed to join an organization or union out of the belief that his or her presence will be beneficial to it. On the other hand, the experience of belonging to an influential organization or union may boost an individual's sense of political efficacy. Thus any effect that organization membership exerts on participation in the preliminary model could nonetheless be attributable to political efficacy—since it may be the case that efficacy influences organization or union membership. Similarly, if organization

[12]Political sociologists study different realms of political participation—pointing out that individuals who engage in unconventional activities might not engage in conventional activities, and vice versa. Thus studies that examine a single realm risk mislabeling as nonparticipants individuals who may in fact be active. We should expect that organization and union membership have a stronger relationship to political participation for the more demanding forms of political participation (e.g., protest) (43).

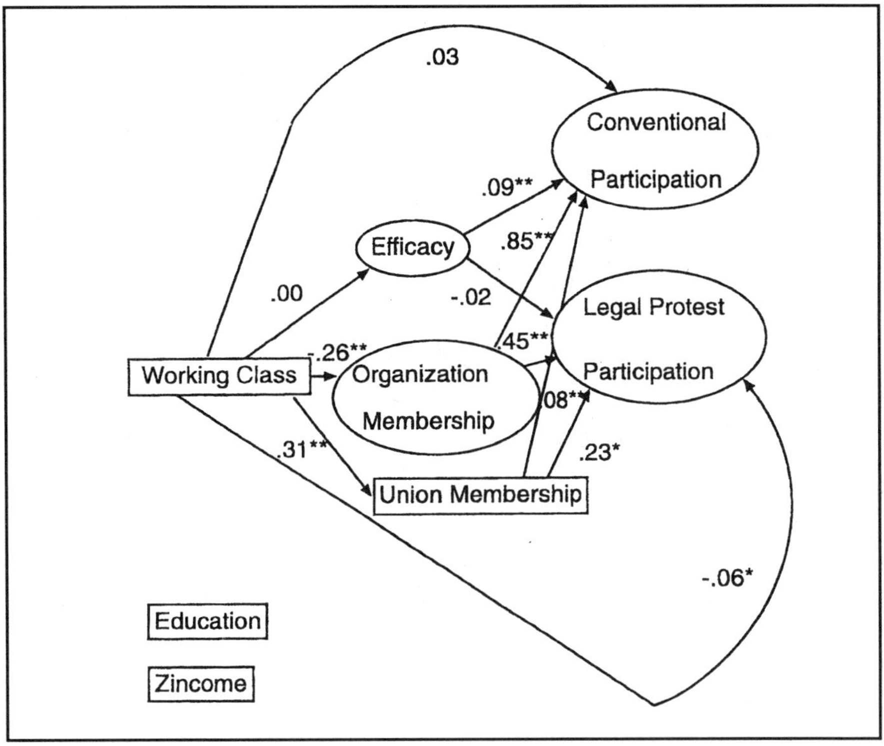

Figure 1. Coefficients from the preliminary "recursive" structural equation model of the relationship between class, political efficacy, organization membership, and political participation in the United States. ** $P < .01$; * $P < .05$. (Zincome = Z of family income; see Appendix.)

or union membership actually influences political efficacy, the former could be the ultimate source of any observed political efficacy effect on participation.

The second model, presented in Figure 2, is designed to remove the effects of political efficacy and organization or union membership on participation of any reciprocal relationship between the two variables. It utilizes panel data from the sample of Americans who were interviewed in 1974 and again in 1981. Measures of working-class membership, income, and education are included at time 1 (1974) only, while conventional and legal protest participation are measured exclusively at time 2 (1981).

The Political Action I survey provided class indicators that closely approximate neo-Marxian categories based on the notion of control over productive assets (45, Appendix). Studies comparing neo-Marxian and neo-Weberian indicators of class position tend to produce similar results for broad class categories (46). Our results on the relationship between class, organization membership, union membership,

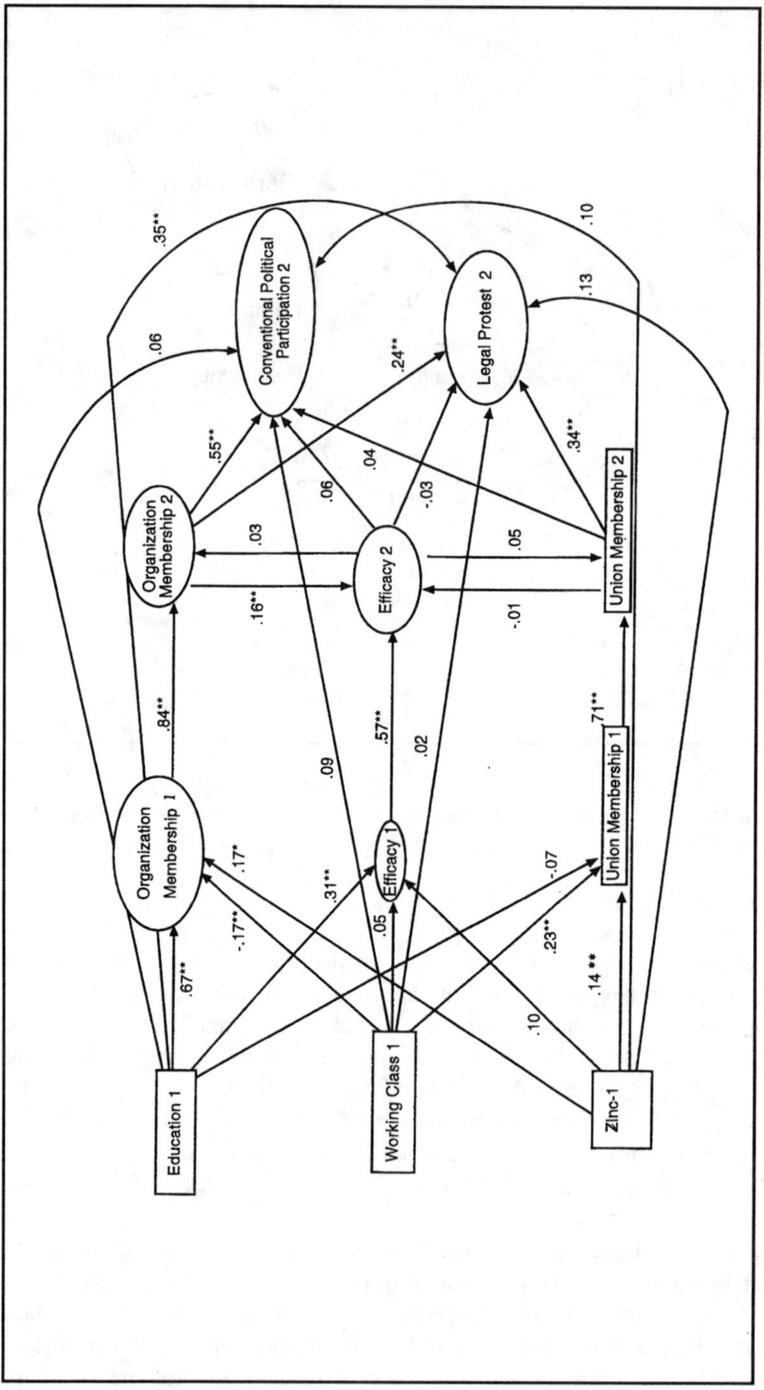

Figure 2. Coefficients from the reciprocal effects model of the relationship between class, political efficacy, organization membership, and political participation in the United States. $^{**}P < .01$; $^{*}P < .05$. *Note:* 1 indicates time 1 (1974); 2 indicates time 2 (1981). (ZInc = Z of family income; see Appendix.)

and political participation were not substantially affected by alternative specifications that omit indicators of income and education from the model.

Organization membership, union membership, and political efficacy were measured at both time 1 and time 2, with direct paths from the time 2 measures to the two forms of participation. Social class, income, and education, the three exogenous variables in the model, also exert direct effects on the two participation variables. There are also paths from the three exogenous variables to the time 1 measures of organization membership, union membership, and political efficacy. Each of the time 1 organization membership, union membership, and political efficacy measures in turn influences the corresponding measure at time 2. Reciprocal relationships are specified between political efficacy and each of the two forms of social cohesion (organization membership and union membership). Identification is obtained by using the time 1 measures of organization membership, union membership, and political efficacy as instruments for their time 2 counterparts and by excluding cross-lagged effects from the model.[13] The Root Mean Square Error of Approximation (RMSEA) (47) was used to assess the similarity between the observed and the estimated variance-covariance matrices (goodness-of-fit). As opposed to the chi-squared statistic, the RMSEA does not have the strong assumption that the model holds exactly in the population, while it takes into account the error of approximation in the population and the precision of the fit measure itself (41). Values of .05 or less indicate a close fit, and values of up to .08 represent close approximations in the population.

RESULTS

Findings from both preliminary and reciprocal effects models are consistent with the proposition that organization membership and union membership are associated with "non-working-class" (i.e., capitalist, manager, and professional locations) and working-class locations, respectively, and that both forms of social cohesion are mediators of the social class–political participation relationship.

The preliminary model (which predicts membership in organizations and unions and two forms of political participation) provides the first hint as to the association between class, organization membership, and union membership (Table 2). (Loadings for indicators of the latent variables included in the preliminary model (political efficacy, organization and union membership, conventional participation, and legal protesting) are presented in Table 4 in the Appendix.) Membership in organizations is associated with "non-working-class" location

[13]The absence of cross-lagged effects means that each observed contemporaneous effect in the reciprocal effects portion of the model actually represents the sum of two effects: the excluded cross-lagged effect and the "true" contemporaneous effect. Thus the observed effect of efficacy at time 2 on organization membership at time 2, for example, is in fact the sum of the (unmodeled) path from political efficacy at time 1 to organization membership at time 2 and the true path from efficacy at time 2 to organization membership at time 2.

Table 2

Estimates for preliminary model, United States, 1974,[a] standardized coefficients

	Political efficacy	Organization membership	Union membership	Conventional participation	Legal protest
Working class	.00	–.26**	.31**	.03	–.06*
Political efficacy	—	—	—	.09**	–.02
Organization membership	—	—	—	.85**	.45**
Union membership	—	—	—	.08**	.23**
Z of family income	.11**	.20**	.20**	.08**	.01
Education	.25**	.01	.01	–.18**	.18**

[a]RMSEA < .05; N = 1,256.
***P* < .01; **P* < .05.

and exerts a strong positive effect on conventional activism and legal protesting (particularly the former).[14] The second social cohesion variable, union membership, also facilitates conventional and legal protest activism but is associated with working-class location. Individual expectations of political efficacy induce conventional participation (although to a seemingly lower degree than do organization membership and union membership), but fail to significantly influence legal protesting.

Political participation remains more a function of social cohesion than of expectations of political efficacy even after the reciprocal relationships between efficacy and the two social cohesion variables (organization membership and union membership) are controlled for (Table 3 displays the results from the reciprocal effects model). (Loadings for indicators of the latent variables included in the reciprocal effects model (the time 1 and time 2 measures of political efficacy and organization and union membership, and the time 2 measures of

[14]The surprisingly negative path from education to conventional participation is apparently attributable to linear dependency between education and organization membership. The correlation between these variables is .66. The education effect on conventional participation becomes .28 (*P* < .01) when the equation is estimated without organization membership as a predictor. This collinearity also appears to inflate (slightly) the path from organization membership to conventional participation. Without education in the model, this path becomes .79 (*P* < .01).

Table 3

Estimates for reciprocal effects model, United States,[a] standardized coefficients

	Political efficacy		Organization membership		Union membership		Conventional participation	Legal protest
	T1	T2	T1	T2	T1	T2	T2	T2
Working class, T1	.05	—	–.17**	—	.23**	—	.09	.02
Political efficacy, T1	—	.57**	—	—	—	—	—	—
Political efficacy, T2	—	—	—	.03	—	.05	.06	–.03
Organization membership T1	—	—	—	.84**[b]	—	—	—	—
Organization membership, T2	—	.16**	—	—	—	—	.55**	.24**
Union membership, T1	—	—	—	—	—	.71**	—	—
Union membership, T2	—	–.01	—	—	—	—	.04	.34**
Z of family income, T1	.10	—	.17*	—	.14**	—	.10[†]	.13[†]
Education, T1	.31**	—	.67**	—	–.07	—	.06	.35**

[a]RMSEA < .05; N = 327; $\chi^2 = 870.78$; $df = 626$.

[b]The errors between organization membership at time 1 (T1) and time 2 (T2) were allowed to correlate. This yielded a significant ($P < .01$) correlation of .45.

**$P < .01$; *$P < .05$; [†]$P < .10$.

conventional participation and legal protesting) are presented in Table 4 in the Appendix.) The impact of organization and union membership on the two modes of participation remains significantly positive, with conventional participation again being especially responsive to both forms of social cohesion. The positive effect of union membership now becomes confined to the protest realm, after being also significant for conventional participation in the preliminary model. Individual expectations of political efficacy, a stimulant of conventional activism but not of protesting in the preliminary model, now becomes statistically irrelevant to both forms of participation.

The reciprocal effects portion of the model (i.e., the observed effects of the time 2 measures of individual political efficacy and organization membership on each other and of efficacy and union membership on each other) offers some insight into the diminished predictive power of individual expectations of political efficacy (vis-à-vis its effects in the preliminary model). Thus, findings indicate that organization membership (significantly) stimulates efficacy (.16), but that the reverse effect is nonsignificant (.03).[15] Thus it is social cohesion (organization and union membership), rather than political efficacy, that apparently assumes temporal precedence in any causal relationship between these two variables and is more appropriately deemed the ultimate source of effects exerted by both variables on participation.[16]

Findings presented in Tables 2 and 3 also address the question of whether political efficacy and social cohesion (membership in organizations or unions) are rooted in the class structure (the class effects can be examined by inspecting either of these tables). Organization membership is a significant function of social class, rendered less likely by working-class position. Conversely, the likelihood of union membership, the second social cohesion variable, is enhanced by working-class position. As to the question of which variable—efficacy or social cohesion (membership in civic organizations or unions)—is more strongly influenced by social class, the answer appears to be social cohesion. The effect of class on organization membership is appreciably higher than the corresponding effect on efficacy, and the class effect on efficacy trails the class effect on union membership as well.

DISCUSSION

Results support our two hypotheses and thereby are consistent with the conclusion that measures of social cohesion used in the "income inequality and social cohesion" research program lack content validity because they exclude forms of social cohesion emerging from working-class locations (union membership). Thus, not measuring unionization and other forms of working-class solidarity might result in a characterization of these communities as not socially cohesive and attribute their population health experience to this alleged collective liability (see reference 1 and Chapter 14 for examples of community disintegration). The often unintended consequence of such erroneous characterization could be to justify punitive moralistic (e.g., welfare reform) or oppressive (e.g., community policing) policies, as currently implemented in Britain and the United States (48, 49).

[15]Given the model's design, we cannot say precisely when each of these effects occurs, since each observed contemporaneous effect actually represents the sum of the unmodeled cross-lagged effect and the true contemporaneous effect. For example, the observed effect of organization membership at time 2 on efficacy at time 2 is the sum of the (unmodeled) effect of organization membership at time 1 on efficacy at time 2 and the "actual" effect of organization membership at time 2 on efficacy at time 2.

[16]Apparently it is organization membership that spurs the relationship between social cohesion and political efficacy, as efficacy and union membership are seemingly statistically irrelevant to each other (the path from political efficacy to union membership and its reverse being a nonsignificant .05 and –.01, respectively).

Results also support the hypothesis that social cohesion is a mediator of the relation between class and political participation, itself an indicator of social cohesion that has important implications for the health of nations (44). Unions mediate the association for the working class while other types of organizations mediate it for other classes (i.e., capitalist, managerial, and professional classes, the surplus appropriating and receiving classes; see Chapter 14).

In the liberal democratic capitalist country examined, social cohesion (i.e., membership in organizations and unions) is shown to be a stronger predictor of political participation than is individual expectation of political efficacy. The predictive power of organization and union membership remains apparent even after controlling for the reciprocal relationship between organization membership, union membership, and political efficacy. However, in spite of the good fit of the model, a relatively small sample in the analysis of reciprocal effects cautions against strong inferences and recommends replication of these results with larger samples.

The observed tendency for social cohesion to be strongly influenced by class location supports the argument that its role as mediator of a class-health relationship should be examined in models of social inequalities in health (see Chapter 14). In addition, the pronounced explanatory role of organization and union membership in our models indicates that the mechanisms by which civil organizations and unions may effect their influence need to be empirically ascertained.[17] Singular attention to indicators of civic organizations and unions in our study represents a limited depiction of the social psychological mechanisms through which class influences social cohesion—the encompassing nature of organization membership and its likely association with many such mechanisms notwithstanding (50, 51). Network analyses focusing on norms of fairness and rationality (e.g., 36) or links to friends and associates (52) and on social learning theory, which emphasizes processes of modeling, instructional control, and contingencies of reinforcement (20), might both be of assistance in capturing social cohesion more precisely. Variables reflecting these perspectives were not analyzed owing to the absence of suitable indicators.

Our study also has implications for the limits of methodological individualism in social epidemiology. Given that the findings point to the centrality of collective action, viewing methodological individualism as a constraint on social explanation appears to be unwarranted (53). Thus, the strength of the association between

[17]Although our study does not address the issue, several authors have argued that "non-rational" factors such as emotions, norms, and commitment—all of which are linked to membership in groups—might be important mediators of the relationship between class and political participation (20, 23, 36, 43). For example, results from Weakliem and Heath (38) suggest that social contact (face-to-face discussions of political topics) was the most parsimonious mechanism mediating the relationship between class and party choice. A more explicitly "rational" alternative (reading about political issues in newspapers) was included in the list of options examined.

social cohesion (organization and union membership) and political participation, as opposed to the weaker effects of individual efficacy, suggests that exclusive reliance on properties of individuals might offer an incomplete explanation of the relationship between class and health as well (54, 55).[18]

Overall, our study provides empirical evidence for the limitations of current measures of social cohesion and highlights the role of social class as a determinant of social cohesion. Models of social inequalities in health, such as Wilkinson's income inequality and social cohesion model, should amend the measurement of social cohesion by adding forms of social participation that characterize working-class communities (e.g., union membership, informal forms of cooperation) and add social class as a determinant of social cohesion.

Acknowledgments — We thank Mel Kohn, Elliot Liebow, Stanley Presser, John Roemer, Carrie Schoenbach, Carmi Schooler, George Davey-Smith, and Erik Wright for their ideas or comments at different stages of this study. This work was supported by funds from NIH and CDC, project numbers Z01 MH02610-04, Z01 MH02610-05, U48/CCU310821, and the Benedict Foundation (Dr. Muntaner).

APPENDIX: DESCRIPTION OF INDICATORS BY LATENT VARIABLE

Conventional Participation

	"How often do you
OFFICIAL	. . . contact public officials or politicians?"
MEETING	. . . attend a political meeting or rally?"
DISCUSS	. . . discuss politics with people?"
CONVINCE	. . . try to convince friends to vote the same as you?"
CAMPAIGN	. . . spend time working for a political party or candidate?"
WORK	. . . work with other people in this community to try to solve some local problem?"
VOTED	"Did you vote in the [last general] election?"

[18]The inclusion of education and income as control variables provides a partial test of the non-economic control over the labor process (Wright's "lived experience" (56, 57)) and political (58) consequences of class locations. Some class theories have considered education in the definition of class locations (e.g., skills/credentials (14)), and according to Roemer's neo-Marxist definition of class, there is a deductive correspondence between class location and income (13). Nevertheless, other contemporary theories of class that are thought to be closer to Marx's own conceptualization in Volume III of *Capital* have provided some evidence that challenges this hypothesis (e.g., 59). Controlling for these variables could be understood as an approximation to partial out the economic effects of class locations (i.e., the differential distribution of the social surplus) on political participation. Class effects are thus presumably grossly reflective of political and cultural consequences of control over the means of production.

The first six indicators are accompanied by the response categories 4 = often; 3 = sometimes; 2 = seldom; 1 = never. The seventh (VOTED) is a dichotomy: 1 = yes; 0 = no.

Legal Protest

BOYCOTT	"Joining in boycotts"
DEMO	"Attending lawful demonstrations"
PETITION	"Signing a petition"
STRIKE	"Joining in wildcat strikes"

Political Efficacy

NOSAY	"People like me have no say in what the government does."
DONTCARE	"I don't think public officials care much about what people like me think."
LOSETIE	"Generally speaking, people we elect to congress lose touch with the people pretty quickly."
NOTOPIN	"Parties are only interested in people's votes, but not their opinions."

Accompanying response categories are 1 = strongly agree; 2 = agree; 3 = disagree; 4 = strongly disagree.

Organization Membership

POLORG	"political party"
POLORG2	"other political organizations"
CIVICORG	"civic groups"
RELIGORG	"church or religious organizations"
RACEORG	"racial or ethnic organizations"
INTGPORG	"special interest groups or hobbies"
PROFORG	"professional associations"

For each item, membership is coded 1 and non-membership, 0.

Union Membership

Membership is coded 1; non-membership, 0.

Class

1 = Working class—employees who fall within none of the four middle- and upper-class occupation categories (see below)

0 = Middle and upper class—a combination of the following occupational categories:

capitalists: self-employed and supervising at least one person
self-employed: self-employed and supervising no one
supervisors: employed individuals who supervise others
professional/managerial: non-supervisory employed individuals who hold/held jobs classified as such by the International Labor Organization.

Note: Classifications are based on respondents current or last job. Respondents who had never held a paid job were excluded from the analysis.

Table 4

Factor loadings[a,b] for each indicator in the four latent variables of the model: conventional participation, legal protest, political efficacy, and organization membership

	Preliminary model	Reciprocal effects model	
		Time 1	Time 2
Conventional Participation			
MEETING	.79	—	.72
OFFICIAL	.77	—	.71
CAMPAIGN	.82	—	.69
WORK	.65	—	.64
DISCUSS	.57	—	.55
CONVINCE	.56	—	.41
VOTED	.51	—	.36
Legal Protest			
BOYCOTT	.81	—	.51
DEMO	.79	—	.54
PETITION	.73	—	.48
Political Efficacy			
DONTCARE	.85	.76	.82
NOTOPIN	.80	.81	.75
LOSETIE	.77	.77	.64
NOSAY	.58	.58	.61
Organization Membership			
POLORG	.54	.42	.43
POLORG2	.52	.22	.26
PROFORG	.78	.50	.65
INTGPORG	.48	.30	.29
CIVICORG	.72	.35	.42
RACEORG	.64	.12	.16

[a] $P < .01$ or $< .05$ for each loading; — signals the dependent variables in the non-recursive models.
[b] Loadings suggest that latent variables are successfully measured with loadings exceeding .35 in the overwhelming majority of cases.

Control Variables

Z of family income	Standardized (gross yearly) family income in dollars
Education	Respondent's education in years

Construction of the Latent Variables

Latent variables were computed by summing the product of each item by its weight. Weights were obtained by dividing the factor score regression coefficient associated with each item by the sum of all factor scores (for items in each scale) coefficients. Each weight represents the indicator's proportional contribution to the overall scale. The indicators of conventional participation do not all have identical metrics, and so were standardized prior to being combined.

Loadings for indicators of the latent variables included in the preliminary and reciprocal effects models are listed in Table 4.

REFERENCES (SECTION II)

1. Wilkinson, R. G. *Unhealthy Societies: The Afflictions of Inequality.* Routledge, London, 1996.
2. Muntaner, C., and Lynch, J. Income inequality, social cohesion, and class relations: A critique of Wilkinson's neo-Durkheimian research program. *Int. J. Health Serv.* 29: 59–82, 1999.
3. Kawachi, I., et al. Social capital, income inequality, and mortality. *Am. J. Public Health* 87: 1491–1499, 1997.
4. Anastasi, A. *Psychological Testing.* Macmillan, New York, 1982.
5. Fantasia, R. *Cultures of Solidarity: Consciousness, Action and Contemporary American Workers.* University of California press, Berkeley, 1988.
6. McNall, S. G., Levine, R., and Fantasia, R. *Bringing Class Back In: Contemporary and Historical Perspectives.* Westview Press, Boulder, Colo., 1991.
7. Johnson, J. V., and Johansson, G. *The Psychosocial Work Environment: Work Organization, Democratization and Health.* Baywood, Amityville, N.Y., 1991.
8. Verba, S. K., Lehman Schlozman, K., and Brady, H. E. *Voice and Equality: Civic Voluntarism in American Politics.* Harvard University Press, Cambridge, Mass., 1995.
9. Wallace, M., and Jenkins, J. C. The new class, postindustrialism, and neocorporatism: Three images of social protest in western democracies. In *The Politics of Social Protest: Comparative Perspectives on States and Social Movements,* edited by J. C. Jenkins and B. Klandermans, pp. 96–137. University of Minnesota Press, Minneapolis, 1995.
10. Morris, A. D., and Mueller, C. M. *Frontiers in Social Movement Theory.* Yale University Press, New Haven, 1992.
11. Przeworski, A. *Capitalism and Social Democracy.* Cambridge University Press, New York, 1985.
12. Przeworski, A. Class, production and politics: A reply to Burawoy. *Socialist Rev.* 2: 87–111, 1989.

13. Roemer, J. *A General Theory of Exploitation and Class.* Harvard University Press, Cambridge, Mass., 1982.
14. Wright, E. O. *Classes.* Verso, London, 1985.
15. Coleman, J. *Foundations of Social Theory.* Harvard University Press, Cambridge, Mass., 1990.
16. Burt, R. S. *Toward a Structural Theory of Action.* Academic Press, New York, 1982.
17. Becker, G. S. *The Economic Approach to Human Behavior.* University of Chicago Press, Chicago, 1976.
18. Elster, J. *Solomonic Judgments: Studies in the Limitations of Rationality.* Cambridge University Press, New York, 1989.
19. Cook, K. S., and Levi, M. *The Limits of Rationality.* University of Chicago Press, Chicago, 1990.
20. Macy, M. W. Learning theory and the logic of critical mass. *Am. Sociol. Rev.* 55: 809–826, 1990.
21. Rosenberg, A. *Economics—Mathematical Politics or Science of Diminishing Returns?* University of Chicago Press, Chicago, 1992.
22. Zey, M. *Decision Making: Alternatives to Rational Choice Models.* Sage, Newbury Park, Calif., 1992.
23. Esser, H. How "rational" is the choice of "rational choice"? *Rationality and Society* 5: 408–414, 1993.
24. Petersen, T. On the promise of game theory in sociology. *Contemp. Sociol.* 23: 498–502, 1994.
25. Herrnstein, R. J., and Prelec, D. Melioration. In *Choice Over Time,* edited by G. Lowenstein and J. Elster. Rusell Sage Foundation, New York, 1992.
26. Goldstone, J. A., and Opps, K. D. Rationality, revolution, and 1989 in Eastern Europe. *Rationality and Society* 6(1): 5–7, 1994.
27. Bobo, L., and Gilliam, F. Race, sociopolitical participation, and black empowerment. *Am. Polit. Sci. Rev.* 84: 377–393, 1990.
28. Guterbock, T. M., and London, B. Race, political orientation, and participation: An empirical analysis of four competing theories. *Am. Sociol. Rev.* 48: 439–453, 1983.
29. Paulsen, R. D. Education, social class and participation in collective action. *Sociol. Educ.* 64: 96–110, 1991.
30. Sherkat, D. E., and Blocker, T. J. The political development of the sixties' activists: Identifying the influence of class, gender, and socialization on protest participation. *Social Forces* 72: 821–842, 1994.
31. Finkel, S. Reciprocal effects of participation and political efficacy: A panel analysis. *Am. J. Polit. Sci.* 29: 891–913, 1985.
32. Herring, C. *Splitting the Middle: Political Alienation, Acquiescence, and Activism Among America's Middle Layers.* Praeger, New York, 1989.
33. Neal, A. G., and Seeman, M. Organizations and powerlessness: Test of the mediation hypothesis. *Am. Sociol. Rev.* 29: 16–26, 1964.
34. Almond, G., and Verba, S. *The Civic Culture.* Little Brown, Boston, 1963.
35. Gamson, W. A. *Power and Discontent.* Dorsey Press, Homewood, Ill., 1968.
36. Gould, R. Collective action and network structure. *Am. Sociol. Rev.* 58(2): 182–196, 1993.

37. Campbell, A., Gurin, G. and Miller, E. *The Voter Decides*. Row Peterson, Evanston, Ill., 1960.
38. Weakliem, D. L., and Heath A. F. Rational choice and class voting. *Rationality and Society* 6(2): 243–270, 1994.
39. Zentral Archive Fuer Empirische Socialforschung. *Political Action: An Eight Nation Study—1974*. Political Action, Cologne, Germany, 1974.
40. Zentral Archive Fuer Empirische Socialforschung. *Political Action: An Eight Nation Study—1981*. Political Action II, Cologne, Germany, 1981.
41. Joreskog, K. G., and Sorbom, D. *Lisrel 8 User's Reference Guide*. Scientific Software International, Chicago, 1993.
42. Oates, G. L. Self-esteem enhancement through fertility? Socioeconomic prospects, gender and mutual influence. *Am. Sociol. Rev.* 62: 965–973, 1997.
43. Oliver, P. E., and Marwell, G. Mobilizing technologies for collective action. In *Frontiers in Social Movement Theory,* edited by A. D. Morris and C. McClurg Mueller, pp. 251–272. Yale University Press, New Haven, 1992.
44. Navarro, V. *The Politics of Health Policy*. Baywood, Amityville, N.Y., 1994.
45. Wright, E. O. *Class Counts: Comparative Studies in Class Analysis*. Cambridge University Press, New York, 1997.
46. Marshall, G., et al. *Classes in Modern Britain*. Hutchinson, London, 1988.
47. Browne, M. W., and Cudeck, R. Alternative ways of assessing mode fit. In *Testing Structural Equations Models,* edited by K. A. Bollen and J. S. Long. Sage, Newbury Park, Calif. 1993.
48. Fox Piven, F., and Cloward, R. A. *The Breaking of the American Social Compact*. Vintage Books, New York, 1999.
49. Crossing the Rubicon on welfare. *Economist*, March 6, 1999, pp. 53–54.
50. Cress, D. M., and Snow, D. A. Resources, benefactors, and the viability of homeless SMOs. *Am. Sociol. Rev.* 61: 1089–1109, 1996.
51. McCarthy, J. D., and Wolfson, M. Resource mobilization by local social movement organizations. *Am. Sociol. Rev.* 61: 1070–1088, 1996.
52. Opp, K.-D. and Gern, C. Dissident groups, personal networks, and spontaneous cooperation: The East German revolution of 1989. *Am. Sociol. Rev.* 58: 659–680, 1993.
53. Schwartz, J. Functional explanation of metaphysical individualism. *Sci. Society* 17: 181–203, 1993.
54. Muntaner, C., and O'Campo, P. A critical appraisal of the demand control model of the psychosocial work environment: Epistemological, social, behavioral and class considerations. *Soc. Sci. Med.* 36: 1509–1517, 1993.
55. Diez-Roux, A. V. Bringing context back into epidemiology: Variables and fallacies in multilevel analysis. *Am. J. Public Health* 88(2): 216–222, 1998.
56. Burawoy, M. *The Politics of Production*. Verso, London, 1985.
57. Wright, E. O. Rethinking, once again, the concept of class structure. In *The Debate on Classes,* edited by E. O. Wright, et al. pp. 269–348. Verso, London, 1989.
58. Wright, E. O. Typologies, scales and class analysis: A comment on Hallaby and Weakliem. *Am. Sociol. Rev.* 58: 35–36, 1993.
59. Muntaner, C., and Stormes, J. Social class and behavior. *Psychol. Rep.* 79: 379–382, 1996.

PART VI
Analysis of Proposed Solutions: The Importance of the Political Context

CHAPTER 17

THE POLITICAL CONTEXT OF SOCIAL INEQUALITIES AND HEALTH

Vicente Navarro and Leiyu Shi

INTRODUCTION: THE IMPORTANCE OF POLITICS

A very important development in the social science and health literature over the last ten years has been a focus on how social inequalities are affecting the health of populations. (See Kawachi and colleagues (1) for an extensive review of the literature in this area and Navarro (2) for a description of how these types of studies have not always been so "popular"; see Chapter 1.) In this growing area of research, however, a subject rarely studied is the impact on social inequalities and health of political forces (such as political movements and parties) and the public policies they follow when in government. Indeed, a review of the latest literature on the relationship between social inequalities and health shows the dearth of references that either include or focus on political variables and their impact on health (1). This lack of attention to the importance of political variables also appears in the growing field of research on comparative international studies of health status. The state of Kerala in India, for example, has been widely studied, showing the relationship between its impressive reduction of inequalities in the last 40 years and improvements in the health status of its population. With very few exceptions (3, 4; see below), however, these reductions in social inequalities and improvements in health have rarely been traced to the public policies carried out by the state's governing party, the Indian Communist Party, which has governed in Kerala for the longest period during those 40 years.

Similarly, we have seen several studies that refer admiringly to the developments occurring in the northeastern regions of Italy in the last 40 years, with active popular participation in the governance of these regions paralleling active policies of reducing social inequalities and discouraging hierarchical relations. These studies are silent, however, on a critical element: all those regions were governed by the Italian Communist Party, which was to a large degree responsible for such policies. (An example here is the otherwise excellent book by Richard Wilkinson (5).)

Some studies have included political variables to explain variations in health status, tracing the variations to different political configurations. Cereseto and Waitzkin (4) have analyzed the health status and quality of life in capitalist countries and in countries they define as socialist. And Navarro (3) has analyzed changes in the health status of populations during the 20th century, comparing the performance of countries at similar levels of development under different political regimes. But these are exceptions. For the most part, the abundant literature on health status and health inequalities does not include many studies on the importance of political variants in shaping social inequalities and population health.

This chapter aims at correcting this deficit. Its objective is to show the importance of political parties, and the policies they implement when in government, in determining the level of equalities or inequalities in a society and in explaining the level of health of its population. We also analyze the mechanisms by which these political influences take place and their social and health consequences in advanced countries of the Organization for Economic Cooperation and Development (OECD). Data for this study are largely from *OECD Health Data Set 98* (6), an interactive database comprising systematically collated data on key aspects of the health care systems of the 29 OECD member countries within their general demographic, economic, and social contexts. Also used are data on political, economic, and social variables derived from the Comparative Welfare State Data Set assembled by Evelyn Huber, Charles Ragin, and John D. Stephens (7); data on household income and wage differentials are extracted from the *OECD Data Set 1997* (8) and the U.S. Bureau of Labor Statistics (9).

THE MAJOR POLITICAL REGIMES IN DEVELOPED CAPITALIST COUNTRIES

To show the importance of political forces in explaining social phenomena, including the level of inequalities and the health and well-being of populations, we have grouped the major developed capitalist countries according to the dominant type of political force that governed them during the time when their welfare states were established (from the end of World War II to the 1980s): *social democratic, Christian democratic* (or conservative parties within the Christian tradition), *liberal,* and *fascist* (the typology is adapted from Huber and Stephens (10; see also 11) (see Chapter 4). The assignment of a country to a particular political tradition is based on the political orientation of parties that governed either alone or as the major partner in a coalition for the greatest proportion of the time between 1945 and 1980. This period (1945–1980) was selected because, for most OECD countries, these were the years when welfare states were established and fully developed. It was in these expansive years, the golden years of capitalism, that the major characteristics of welfare states were shaped.

The Social Democratic Tradition

In the first group—the social democracies—we include those countries (Sweden, Finland, Norway, Denmark, and Austria) that have been governed by social democratic parties (either alone or as the major party in a coalition) for the majority of years during the period 1945–1980 (see Chapter 4, Table 5). As that table shows, the social democratic parties governed for an average of 23.5 years in these countries during that period. In this group of countries, the labor movements and their socialist parties have been very strong, while the capitalist classes and the political parties they have chosen to represent their interests have been weak and usually fragmented (see 10 for an explanation of this situation). The table also shows how these countries have been characterized by high union density (percentage of the working population enrolled in unions), high social security expenditures (as percentage of GDP), high taxation (as percentage of GDP), and high public employment in health services, education, and welfare (as percentage of the working-age population). They have the most extensive welfare states.

Table 1 shows that (on average) the social democratic countries also had the largest public expenditures in health care during the period 1960–1990, followed by the Christian democratic countries. The liberal countries and the ex-fascist countries had, in general, the lowest public expenditures on health in that same period. And the data in Table 2 show that (on average) the social democratic countries covered almost the entire population with a public medical care program; this coverage was lower (on average) in Christian democratic countries and even lower in liberal countries. The coverage in the ex-fascist countries, although low (during the fascist dictatorships, the lowest in all countries studied in this chapter), increased significantly during the democratic periods to a high level, primarily because of the social democratic governance during these periods.

The social democratic parties governing these countries were also characterized by their implementation of (*a*) *full-employment policies,* which explains their low unemployment (the lowest in these OECD countries during the period 1945–1980) (see the unemployment data in Chapter 4, Table 6), and (*b*) *universalistic social policies,* aimed at covering the whole population. Table 2 shows, for example, how health care benefits coverage includes the entire population.

Such policies have used the social services of the welfare state (health, education, and family supportive services such as child care and domiciliary services) as a means of creating employment and facilitating the integration of women into the labor force—which explains the high rate of female employment (see Chapter 4, Table 5) in these countries. The social democratic countries have had a very large percentage of the adult population working in the labor market, a consequence of the high rate of women's participation in the labor force, in particular in the social services of the welfare state. The exception here is Austria, where a Catholic tradition emphasizing the family (rather than the state) as the primary

Table 1

Public expenditures on health, 1960–1990, percent of GDP[a]

	1960	1970	1980	1990
Social democratic political economies				
Austria	3.0	3.4	5.3	5.3
Sweden	3.2	6.1	8.7	7.9
Denmark	3.2	5.2	7.7	7.1
Norway	2.3	4.1	5.9	6.5
Finland	2.1	4.2	5.1	6.5
Mean	2.8	4.6	6.5	6.7
Christian democratic political economies				
Belgium	2.3	5.0	5.5	6.9
Germany	3.2	4.6	7.0	6.7
Netherlands	1.3	5.0	5.9	6.1
France	2.4	4.3	6.0	6.6
Italy	3.0	4.5	5.6	6.3
Switzerland	1.9	3.1	4.6	5.7
Mean	2.4	4.4	5.8	6.4
Liberal Anglo-Saxon political economies				
United Kingdom	3.3	3.9	5.0	5.1
Ireland	2.9	4.3	7.1	4.9
United States	1.3	2.7	3.9	5.1
Canada	2.3	5.0	5.5	6.9
Mean	2.4	3.9	5.3	5.5
Former fascist dictatorships				
Spain	—	2.4	4.4	5.7
Portugal	—	—	—	—
Greece	—	—	3.1	3.5
Mean	—	2.4	3.8	4.6

[a]Source: reference 6.

provider of services to children and the elderly has kept women out of the labor force. This also accounts for the very low percentage—4 percent—of the working-age population in Austria employed in the social services of the welfare state, compared with 20 percent in Sweden, 18 percent in Denmark, and 15 percent in Norway. There is a clear relationship between the size of these sectors and the percentage of women in the labor force. This explains why the percentage of the

Table 2

Total public medical care coverage, 1960–1996, percent of population[a]

	1960	1970	1980	1990	1996
Social democratic political economies					
Austria	78.0	91.0	99.0	99.0	99.0
Sweden	100.0	100.0	100.0	100.0	100.0
Denmark	95.0	100.0	100.0	100.0	100.0
Norway	100.0	100.0	100.0	100.0	100.0
Finland	55.0	100.0	100.0	100.0	100.0
Mean	85.6	98.2	99.8	99.8	99.8
Christian democratic political economies					
Belgium	58.0	97.8	99.0	97.3	99.0
Germany	85.0	88.0	91.0	92.2	92.2
Netherlands	71.0	86.0	74.6	70.7	72.0
France	76.3	95.7	99.3	99.5	99.5
Italy	87.0	93.0	100.0	100.0	100.0
Switzerland	74.0	89.0	96.5	99.5	100.0
Mean	75.0	91.6	93.4	93.2	93.8
Liberal Anglo-Saxon political economies					
United Kingdom	100.0	100.0	100.0	100.0	100.0
Ireland	85.0	85.0	100.0	100.0	100.0
United States	20.0	40.0	42.0	44.0	45.0
Canada	71.0	100.0	100.0	100.0	100.0
Mean	69.0	81.3	85.5	86.0	86.3
Former fascist dictatorships					
Spain	54	61	99	99.8	99.8
Portugal	18	40	100	100	100
Greece	30	55	100	100	100
Mean	34	52	99.7	99.9	99.9

[a]Source: reference 6.

working-age population employed in the social services of the welfare state and the percentage of women who are working are lower in Christian democratic countries (6.2 percent and 46 percent, respectively), and much lower in ex-fascist countries (2.6 percent and 26 percent), than in social democratic countries (13.2 percent and 65.2 percent). It is also the social democratic countries that have smaller inequalities in household income (Table 3), larger supportive services for

Table 3

Household income and poverty[a]

	Household income inequality relative to national median incomes, ratio 90th to 10th percentile, 1990–91	Poverty rate, % population	
		Total	Children
Social democratic political economies			
Sweden	2.78	6.7	3
Denmark	2.86	7.5	5.1
Norway	2.80	6.6	4.9
Finland	2.75	6.2	2.7
Mean	2.79	6.75	3.92
Christian democratic political economies			
France	3.48	7.5	7.4
Germany	3.21	7.6	8.6
Belgium	2.79	5.5	4.4
Netherlands	3.05	6.7	8.3
Italy	3.14	6.5	10.5
Mean	3.14	6.7	7.84
Liberal Anglo-Saxon political economies			
United States	5.78	19.1	24.9
Canada	3.90	11.7	15.3
United Kingdom	4.67	14.6	18.5
Ireland	4.18	11.1	13.8
Mean	4.63	14.25	18.1
Former fascist dictatorships			
Spain	4.4	10.4	12.8

[a]Sources: For household income inequalities: Mishel, L., Bernstein, L., and Schmitt, J. International comparisons. In *State of Working America 1998–1999.* Cornell University Press, Ithaca, N.Y., 1999; for poverty rate: Smeeding, T. M. *Financial Poverty in Developed Countries: The Evidence from L.I.S.* Working Paper No. 155. Luxembourg Income Study, 1997.

families (such as child care services and domiciliary services for the elderly and disabled), and lower poverty rates for the overall population and for children (Table 3).

Why do the social democratic countries have the lowest household income inequalities? To answer this question, we need to understand the primary reasons for income inequalities in a country: (*a*) the percentage of national income that goes to capital versus labor, (*b*) the wage disparities within labor, and (*c*) the redistributive effect of state interventions—that is, changes in disposable income of households and individuals as a result of adding transfers from the state and subtracting income paid in taxes and fees to the state. The social democratic countries have (*a*) the lowest percentage of national income derived from capital and the highest derived from labor; profits derived from ownership of capital have historically tended to be the lowest among the countries under study (Table 4); (*b*) the lowest wage disparities within the labor force (Table 4); and (*c*) the highest redistributive effect of the state (Chapter 4, Table 5).

It is important to note that although mean wage differentials in social democratic countries (2.24 in 1990) were lower than those in Christian democratic countries (2.56 in 1990), they were not much different (Table 4). The mean household income inequalities in social democratic countries (2.79 in 1990–91), however, were much lower than those in Christian democratic countries (3.14) as a result of the much more favorable treatment of capital and lower redistributive effect of the state in the Christian democratic countries (Table 3).

We should also mention that while income derived from capital was lower in social democratic countries than in Christian democratic countries (Table 4), the rate of investment, measured by gross fixed capital formation as percentage of GDP (Table 4), and economic growth (Chapter 4, Table 6), were higher than in the Christian democratic and liberal countries. Only during the years 1989–1995 was the rate of economic growth of the social democratic countries lower, on average, than that of the Christian democratic and liberal countries. These empirical data question the assumption made by the Christian democratic and liberal parties that public policies favoring income derived from capital and high-income groups are required to stimulate investment and economic growth. The data presented here show otherwise. Rather than inequalities being a requirement for growth (as classical economics maintains), the *reduction* of such inequalities has been a precondition for economic efficiency and economic growth (Navarro (12) expands on this point) (see Chapter 2). *These social democratic countries have also been the countries with the lowest infant mortality rates* (Table 5) *during the period 1960–1996.*

It is not our purpose here to analyze the pathways by which reduction of income inequalities affects infant mortality rates. But our data show that the political forces that have been more successful in reducing income inequalities, such as the social democratic parties, have also been more successful in reducing infant mortality rates. The policies in the social democratic countries resulted from the strength of the labor movements, which, in alliance with other sectors and classes (rural farmers in Northern Europe and the middle class in Austria), have been the major force behind the reduction of inequalities and, consequently, the declines in infant mortality rates. We should stress that even in countries, such as Italy, that have not been governed by social democratic forces, those regions of

Table 4

Total profits, wage inequalities, and gross fixed capital formation, 1960–1989[a]

	Operative surplus (corporate profits, including state enterprises) and profits from unincorporated businesses (including earnings of self-employed persons), % of national income			Wage inequality[b]		Gross fixed capital formation, % of GDP		
	1960–73	1974–79	1980–89	1980	1990	1960–73	1974–79	1980–89
Social democratic political economies								
Sweden	21	15	17	2.04	2.21	23	21	19
Norway	27	20	27	2.06	—	28	33	25
Denmark	30	24	24	2.14	2.18	24	22	17
Finland	32	24	22	2.46	2.34	25	27	24
Austria	30	23	24	—	—	27	26	24
Mean	28.1	21.4	22.8	2.17	2.24	25.6	25.9	21.8

Christian democratic political economies								
Belgium	34	25	29	—	2.07	22	22	18
Netherlands	32	25	29	—	2.59	24	21	20
Germany	30	23	23	2.69	2.32	25	21	21
France	32	25	24	3.24	3.06	24	24	20
Italy	41	28	40	2.94	2.80	25	24	21
Switzerland	31	38	23	—	—	28	23	25
Mean	33.3	27	28	2.95	2.56	24.4	22.4	20.8
Liberal Anglo-Saxon political economies								
Canada	26	25	26	4.01	4.20	22	24	21
Ireland	31	30	33	—	—	20	26	20
Great Britain	21	24	20	2.79	3.37	18	19	17
United States	25	32	21	3.65	4.43	18	19	17
Mean	25.7	27.8	25	3.48	4.00	19.4	21.9	18.8

[a]Source: Adapted from reference 10, Table 4.
[b]Ratio of earnings of the 90th percentile of workers to those of the 10th percentile of workers.

Table 5

Infant mortality (deaths per 1,000 live births), 1960–1996[a]

	1960	1970	1980	1990	1996
Social democratic political economies					
Austria	37.5	25.9	14.3	7.8	5.1
Sweden	16.6	11.0	6.9	6.0	4.0
Denmark	21.5	14.2	8.4	7.5	5.2
Norway	18.9	12.7	8.1	7.0	4.0
Finland	21.0	13.2	7.6	5.6	4.0
Mean	23.1	15.4	9.1	6.8	4.5
Christian democratic political economies					
Belgium	31.2	21.1	12.1	8.0	6.0
Germany	33.8	23.6	12.6	7.0	5.0
Netherlands	17.9	12.7	8.6	7.1	5.2
France	27.4	18.2	10.0	7.3	4.9
Italy	43.9	29.6	14.6	8.2	5.8
Switzerland	21.1	15.1	9.1	6.8	4.7
Mean	29.2	20.1	11.2	7.4	5.3
Liberal Anglo-Saxon political economies					
United Kingdom	22.5	18.5	12.1	7.9	6.1
Ireland	29.3	19.5	11.1	8.2	5.5
United States	26.0	20.0	12.6	9.2	7.8
Canada	27.3	18.8	10.4	6.8	6.0
Mean	26.3	19.2	11.6	8.0	6.4
Former fascist dictatorships					
Spain	43.7	26.3	12.3	7.6	5.0
Portugal	77.5	55.1	24.3	11.0	6.9
Greece	40.1	29.6	17.9	9.7	7.3
Mean	53.8	37.0	18.2	9.4	6.4

[a]Source: reference 6.

the country that have been governed by parties following social democratic policies of reducing inequalities and creating employment, such as the former Italian Communist Party (today the Left Democratic Party), have had lesser inequalities and better mortality indicators than other regions. The regions of northern Italy—Tuscany and Piedmont, for example—mentioned in Richard Wilkinson's book *Unhealthy Societies* (5) were governed by Communist parties following social democratic policies. Explaining the reduction of mortality rates in these countries (or regions) in terms of specific interventions such as higher popular participation in civil and political societies or other types of interventions is insufficient. Rather, mortality reductions result from a larger set of related interventions guided by a political party or parties (socialist, social democratic, communist, labor, or whatever name is used to define these labor-oriented social democratic parties) that generate and reproduce a culture of solidarity and opportunity. Attempts to disaggregate these collective responses into their different components ignore the Hegelian dictum that the totality is more than the sum of its parts. *These data seem to allow the conclusion, therefore, that to reduce income inequalities and infant mortality, it is advisable to support labor-based social democratic parties.*

The Christian Democratic Tradition

In this group we include countries that from 1945 to 1980 were governed for long periods by conservative parties based in the Christian tradition—parties that define themselves as Christian democratic and those that, while not defining themselves in this way, consider themselves based in the Christian tradition. These countries (Belgium, the Netherlands, Germany, France, Italy, and Switzerland) form the least homogeneous group of all the countries considered here—a consequence of Christian democratic parties sometimes having to govern in coalition with other parties, including social democrats (as in Belgium, Germany, and the Netherlands). But despite the party alliances and coalitions in these countries, the conservative parties of Christian tradition were either the dominant forces in the coalitions or the parties governing for greater lengths of time in the 1945–1980 period (see Chapter 4, Table 5), and this is what explains their common characteristics.

First, the Christian democratic countries rely primarily on the family for the provision of social services to the elderly, the disabled, and children. Families in these societies have been burdened with caring work that in the social democracies is the responsibility of the state and in the liberal countries the responsibility of the market. This extra burden on the family in Christian democratic countries explains the very low rate of women's participation in the labor force (Chapter 4, Table 5): only 46 percent of women participate in the labor market, compared with 65.2 percent in social democratic and 52.8 percent in liberal countries. Only the former fascist countries (Spain, Greece, and Portugal) have a lower percentage of women in the labor force (26 percent). In the Christian democratic countries, class inequalities have been compounded by large gender inequalities, including gender inequalities in health. Spain's government commission on inequalities in health (the Spanish equivalent of the U.K. Black Commission) found, for example, that in the 30- to 50-year age group, women have twice as many stress-related conditions as men (13). In fact, women in this group suffer more stress-related conditions that any other group in Spain. Table 4 in Chapter 4 shows, for example, the number of hours that women work at home in Spain and Italy, versus those in Denmark, Sweden, and the United States. Women in southern European countries work much longer hours than those in northern Europe.

The second characteristic shared by the Christian democratic countries is the heavy reliance of families' standard of living on the salary and pension of the male breadwinner, considered the head of the family. This explains the enormous importance given by the labor movements of these countries to both maintaining and expanding wages and expanding social transfers (in particular, pensions) as a way of assuring families' standard of living. Thus these countries have large social transfers and underdeveloped social services. As Table 5 in Chapter 4 shows, the average level of social expenditures in the Christian democratic countries (21.6 percent of GDP) was lower than that in the social democratic countries (23.2 percent of GDP), although much higher than that in the liberal countries (15.2 percent of GDP). The same table also shows that only 6.2 percent of the working-age population was employed in services in the Christian democratic countries, compared with 13.2 percent in the social democracies. And the Christian democratic countries have lower public expenditures on health (Table 1) and a lower degree of health benefits coverage than the social democratic countries, although higher than in the liberal countries.

The relatively large social expenditures in the Christian democratic countries have required relatively large fiscal revenues (41.8 percent of GDP), lower than in the social democratic countries (48.8 percent of GDP) but much higher than in the liberal countries (36.5 percent of GDP).

The labor movement in the Christian democratic countries has been weaker than that in the social democratic countries, which explains the following situations. *First, income derived from capital represented a much larger percentage of the national accounts than in the social democratic countries* (Table 4). *Second, unemployment was higher than in the social democratic countries for most of the years 1960–1995* (Chapter 4, Table 6). *Third, wage disparities were larger than in the social democratic countries* (Table 4). *And fourth, the redistributive effect of the state was lower than in the social democratic countries* (Chapter 4, Table 5). *Poverty in general and among children was also greater in Christian democratic than in social democratic countries* (Table 3). *These are the causes of the greater household income inequalities* (Table 3) *and higher infant mortality* (Table 5) *in the Christian democratic countries.*

Former Fascist Dictatorships in Southern European Countries (1945–1975)

In this group of countries (Spain, Greece, and Portugal), fascist regimes governed for the entire 1945–1980 period or for most of that time. These were class dictatorships against the working and popular classes. There has been interest recently in defining such regimes as *caudillistas,* regimes based on the personal power of a *caudillo* or clan, rejecting their class character (see 14 for a critique of this position). However, an analysis of the nature of the state in these three countries during that period, of its repressive nature and its social and fiscal policies, reveals its class character. Fascism was a class response by the land-based oligarchies and other sectors of capital, including financial capital, to the threat posed by the growing power of the working class, expressed through democratic institutions—which those dictatorships disrupted. The class character of the fascist regimes was clearly evident in (*a*) the highly repressive nature of the states, a repression directed primarily at the working class; (*b*) the most regressive fiscal policies in existence in Europe at that time; and (*c*) the underdeveloped welfare states. In Spain in 1960, for example, public expenditures on health and education amounted to only 60 percent of the spending on the armed police forces (15). And in 1980, social expenditures in Spain (9 percent of GDP) were much lower than those in the Christian democratic countries (21.6 percent of GDP). During the fascist periods, the public medical care expenditures and the level of public medical care coverage were the lowest among the countries under study. And the percentage of the working population employed in services (2.6 percent) was much lower than in the Christian democratic (6.2 percent) and social democratic (13.2 percent) countries.

It was in the former fascist countries that labor was weakest. While much has been done since the democracies have been established (primarily by social democratic parties) to correct the underdevelopment of the welfare states and to reduce the large income inequalities, these countries still have the greatest income inequalities in the European Union. This results from the very large percentage represented by capital in the national accounts, the very large wage disparities, and the small redistributive effect of the state. These countries were heavily influenced by Catholic teachings that relied on women for the care of family members. They did not have supportive services for families, and poverty among children was very high. They also had high infant mortality rates during the 1945–1980 period, when they were governed by fascist regimes for the longest times. In all these countries, during the democratic periods, income inequalities have been reduced, the welfare state expanded, women's participation in the labor force expanded, and infant mortality reduced.

The Liberal Countries

This group (the United States, Canada, Ireland, and Great Britain) consists of the Anglo-Saxon countries where labor has been particularly weak and the capitalist class particularly strong. With the partial exception of Great Britain, social democratic parties have never governed at the national level (the United States and Canada) or, if they have, have done so for only short periods. These countries have been governed for the most part by parties clearly committed to a full expression of market forces, with as little interference from the state as possible. Some readers may be surprised that we have included Great Britain in this group, since the Labour Party governed for as long as 14 years in the period 1960–1980. We have done so—following the Huber and Stephens (10) typology—because Great Britain has more similarity with this group of countries than with the Christian democratic or social democratic countries. The British welfare state, for example, is not fully universal or comprehensive—with the exception of the National Health Service (which Churchill called the jewel in the British crown)—and has a relatively low level of social expenditures. Canada also has a universal national health program. Both countries, however, share with the other liberal countries the residual and assistential nature of the welfare state. *Benefits are provided based on proven financial need (means-tested programs) rather than on citizenship alone (as in social democracies) or on workers' rights (as in the Christian democracies).* The liberal countries also have, after the ex-fascist countries, the lowest public expenditures on health care (Table 1) and (with the exception of Britain and Canada) the lowest coverage by public medical care.

In all these liberal countries, social transfers by the welfare state are supplemented by benefits acquired through the labor market through collective bargaining, with public social expenditures concentrated on the needy (need being defined by political-administrative criteria). Welfare functions are assigned to the private sector, with the state covering only the minimum. Wages tend to be low, requiring involvement of all family members in the labor force; this explains the large percentage of employed women in the liberal countries (with the exception of Ireland, whose Catholic tradition emphasizes a reliance on the family and which thus has a lower percentage of women in the labor force). The integration of women into the labor force in the liberal countries is facilitated by an extensive, privatized personal and social services sector, the size of which is made possible by very low wages and low social protection—characteristics responsible for the marked social polarization in these societies.

In the liberal countries, the market reigns supreme. Capital has the strongest influence, labor the weakest. Inequalities are largest in these countries. Income derived from capital is the largest, wage disparities the most accentuated, and the state the least redistributive (only the fascist states were less redistributive). Tables 3 and 5 show how the liberal countries have the largest income differentials and the lowest rates of improvement in infant mortality rates. This group includes the country (of those included in the study) with the highest infant mortality—the United States (Table 5).

CONCLUSION

The empirical information provided in this study allows several conclusions. First, political variables such as the political party in government (either alone or as a majority partner in a coalition) for longer periods of time are important in influencing a country's level of income inequalities and social inequalities and its health indicators such as infant mortality. Second, these political forces represent the interests of classes and other social forces with different interests in redistributive policies. Third, the labor movements and the social democratic parties that have governed as a majority for long periods since World War II have generally been the most committed to redistributive policies, contributing to better health indicators such as lower infant mortality rates. Fourth, and conversely, in countries with weaker labor movements and social democratic parties and stronger capitalist classes, such as the liberal Anglo-Saxon countries, there has been a weaker commitment to redistributive policies and worse health indicators. Finally, the Christian democratic parties (or conservative parties rooted in the Christian tradition) have made a compromise, with redistributive policies that are weaker than those in the social democracies but stronger than those in the liberal countries. The Christian democratic parties have emphasized the key role of the family rather than the state (as in the social democratic tradition) or the market (as in the liberal tradition) in the care of children and the elderly, overburdening families (especially women) with these tasks.

Our conclusions need to be qualified of course. This is an introductory study. We hope it will stimulate some much needed research on the relationship between political forces and health. For instance, it would be interesting to use the typology presented here to analyze countries that, for specific periods, do not seem to fit the type; such atypicality calls for an expansion of the study to better explore its causes. Also, further study is required on the possible impact of a "dose-response" effect of the length of time a particular party was in power—that is, a possibly more direct causal relationship between time in government, either alone or in coalition, and reduction of inequalities and improvements in health. Also requiring further study are "mixed cases" in which the balance of forces within government may have had different effects on redistributive policies. Belgium and the Netherlands, for example, with conservative governments of the Christian tradition during most of the period 1945–1980, still have had large social democratic parties. This explains, in part, their different redistributive intensity within the conservative and Christian democratic tradition compared with other countries in the same group. Comparative policy studies, such as the one reported here, also need to be complemented by more traditional and equally informative case studies analyzing experiences and making evaluations country by country. These further areas of investigation could overcome some of the limitations of the present study, which cannot be resolved at this aggregate multi-country level.

We believe, however, that this study offers more than just pointers on the road to understanding the complex and highly sensitive (and extremely relevant) work on the relationship between politics, policy, and health. None other than Rudolph Virchow, one of the founders of public health, wrote that politics is "public health in the most profound sense" (quoted in 16).

The empirical information provided here already suggests we can conclude that, for those wishing to optimize the health of populations by reducing social and income inequalities, it seems advisable to support political forces such as the labor movement and social democratic parties, which have traditionally supported larger, more successful redistributive policies than have the Christian democratic or liberal parties.

Note — This chapter is adapted from an article published in *Social Science and Medicine,* in press, 2000.

REFERENCES

1. Kawachi, I., Wilkinson, R. G. and Kennedy, B. P. (eds.). *Income Distribution and Health: A Reader.* New Press, New York, 1999.
2. Navarro, V. A historical review (1965–1997) of studies on class, health, and quality of life: A personal account. *Int. J. Health Serv.* 28(3): 389–406, 1998.
3. Navarro, V. Has socialism failed? Health indicators under capitalism and socialism. *Science and Society* 57(1), 1993.
4. Cereseto, S., and Waitzkin, H. Capitalism, socialism, and the physical quality of life. *Int. J. Health Serv.* 16(4): 643, 1986.
5. Wilkinson, R. G. *Unhealthy Societies: The Afflictions of Inequality.* Routledge, London, 1996.
6. OECD Health Policy Unit. *OECD Health Data Set 98.* Paris, 1998.
7. Huber, E., Ragin, C., and Stephens, J. D. Comparative Welfare State Data Set, 1998. Available from: www.unc.edu/~jcsteph/
8. OECD. *OECD Data Set 1997: OECD Main Economic Indicators: Historical Statistics 1960–1997.* Paris, 1998.
9. U.S. Bureau of Labor Statistics. *Bureau of Labor Statistics Data.* U.S. Department of Labor, Washington, D.C., yearly.
10. Huber, E., and Stephens, J. D. Internationalization and the social democratic model: Crisis and future prospects. *Comp. Polit. Stud.* 13(3): 353–397, 1998.
11. Navarro, V. The political economy of the welfare state in developed capitalist countries. *Int. J. Health Serv.* 29(1): 1–50, 1999.
12. Navarro, V. Neoliberalism, "globalization," unemployment, inequalities, and the welfare state. *Int. J. Health Serv.* 28(4): 607–682, 1998.
13. Navarro, V., and Benach, J. *Health Inequalities in Spain* (in Spanish). Ministry of Health and Consumer Affairs, Madrid, 1996.
14. Pearson, L. *Franco.* Grijalbo, 1998.
15. United Nations Development Program. *Historical Series.* New York, 1992.
16. Taylor, R., and Rieger, A. Medicine as social science: Rudolph Virchow on the typhus epidemic in Upper Silesia. *Int. J. Health Serv.* 15(3): 547, 1985.

CHAPTER 18

IS THERE A THIRD WAY? A RESPONSE TO GIDDENS'S *THE THIRD WAY*

Vicente Navarro

Let me start this talk by introducing myself and telling you how I encountered the Third Way. As some of you may know, I divide my time between teaching public policy at The Johns Hopkins University in Baltimore and teaching political and social sciences at the Pompeu Fabra University in Barcelona, Spain. In Spain I am also Senior Advisor to Jose Borrell, who was elected by an overwhelming majority of the membership of the Socialist Party (PSOE) to be the Party's presidential candidate.

In this highly contested primary, the candidate Joaquin Almunia, put forward by Felipe Gonzalez (past President of the 1982–1996 Socialist governments and past Secretary General of the Socialist Party), was soundly defeated by the growing restlessness at the grassroots level with the experience of the 1982–1996 Socialist governments and the direction of the Socialist Party under Felipe Gonzalez. The Socialist governments had faced three general strikes—an unprecedented number—against their labor market policies. When Borrell decided to challenge the Gonzalez leadership, the "conventional wisdom" in Spanish political circles was that he did not have a chance. Borrell had been Minister of Public Works in the last Socialist government and the most critical voice within the Party against Gonzalez's policies. Despite the conventional wisdom, however, Borrell won overwhelmingly in the primary. And a new enthusiasm quickly spread to the rest of the Party and to the country.

For a while it appeared that Borrell could easily win the next election, scheduled for sometime in 2000, to be fought against Jose Maria Aznar, President of the Conservative party (the Popular Party), whose roots are in a party (Alianza Popular) funded by Manuel Fraja, a Minister of the Interior during the Franco regime. Aznar has never dissociated himself from Franco's regime. He once criticized the city of Guernica—the Basque town destroyed by Nazi air raids—for having changed the name of its main square from Caudillo Franco Square (the name given to the main squares of all Spanish towns) to Liberty Square. More recently, however, Aznar has been trying to move to the center, emphasizing his Christian democratic commitments. (The Spanish Church, incidentally, most of whose bishops were appointed by Franco, is very much to the right of the European ecclesiastic spectrum.) He was elected this year, 1999, as President of the Christian Democratic International. For this move to the center, Aznar has counted very heavily on Tony Blair, who has been quite receptive to Aznar's approaches. The Spanish media (most of which are center right or plain right) actually promote Blair as the most important European leader, one having great foresight, and they contrast New Labour with the Spanish Socialist Party (and in particular with Borrell), which they describe "as stuck in the past, holding steady to outdated dogma."

How did I come across Blair's Third Way? One night I received an urgent call from Borrell's office. They had found out that in a few days Aznar and Blair were going to publish a joint article in the Spanish and European press putting forward their proposal for resolving the unemployment problem in Europe, focusing primarily on the need to add further flexibility to the labor markets. Spain, incidentally, already has the largest percentage of temporary workers in the OECD—34 percent of the entire labor force works in temporary jobs—and the highest percentage of workers (after the United States) who are afraid of losing their jobs—68 percent of all workers, including those with fixed contracts. A series of calls to 10 Downing Street in London stopped publication of the joint article, but Blair and Aznar subsequently published individual articles, separate articles but published together, outlining a joint proposal on how to resolve the unemployment problem in Europe.

As you can guess, considerable tension arose between the Spanish Socialist Party and New Labour. To ease that tension, Peter Mandelson and Anthony Giddens—two of the primary intellectual forces behind the Third Way—visited Borrell in Spain, and Blair invited Borrell to London to try to smooth things over. Blair asked Borrell to write an introduction to the Spanish translation of Giddens's new book, *The Third Way,* and Borrell's office asked me—as one of his senior advisors—to prepare a draft for this introduction. This is how I came to read *The Third Way* for the first time. It reminded me very much of a document written several years ago by Al From, leader of the U.S. Democratic Leadership Council (DLC), when I had to face the DLC during the 1988 Democratic Presidential primaries. I was then Jesse Jackson's senior advisor and his personal representative in the Democratic Platform Committee. I could see how the leadership of the Democratic party had been shaken when Jackson, quite unexpectedly, received 40 percent of the delegates in the 1988 Democratic Party Convention in Atlanta. Clinton, Gore, and Gephardt raised hell and heaven to stop the prospect of a left represented by Jackson, and they established the DLC—in which From played a critical and leading role. From spoke about establishing a "third way" between the government-oriented tradition of the "old" Democratic Party and the market fundamentalism of the Republican Party.

Anyone who had closely followed the public policy proposals put forward by the Democratic Party and its leaders (Carter in 1980; Mondale in 1984; and Dukakis in 1988) would have found it difficult to define the Democratic Party as a government-oriented party. President Carter (described by the *New York Times* as the most conservative Democratic President ever) considerably reduced the size of the federal government, and candidates Mondale and Dukakis competed with President Reagan—and President Bush—in who would reduce government the most. All of them became "radical" centrists, abandoning all intention of using the state as a redistributive instrument of wealth and income in the United States. As Caspar Weinberger, Secretary of Defense under President Reagan, ironically stated at a conference at Washington University in August 1983: "The Democrats are trying to forget their past. They are in a situation of state denial. We Republicans are not. We are far more interventionist than the Democrats are. We have the most active industrial policy in the world today, through our Defense Department." To describe President Carter and candidates Mondale and Dukakis as New Dealers or government-oriented politicians required considerable imagination, of which From seemed to have plenty.

The Labour Party in Great Britain, however, was much to the left of the U.S. Democratic party. I could therefore see, at least intellectually, how a third alternative between the Labour Party and the Conservative Party of Margaret Thatcher could be envisioned. This is why I started reading *The Third Way* with interest, ready to see its merits. Actually, I was looking forward to finding in it something new and perhaps even valuable for the left or left of center. I was disappointed, however. It reminded me too much of the DLC.

You can understand why, after reading the book, I declined the invitation to write the introduction to the Spanish version of *The Third Way.* My introduction, had Borrell's office accepted the draft, would not have helped to ease the tensions between Blair and Borrell. It might have made them worse. I chose instead to write an introduction to Oskar Lafontaine's new book (written with his collaborator Christa Müller) *The Challenges of Globalization,* whose relevance to Europe and Spain (and, I should add, the United States) is much greater than that of *The Third Way.*

Let me now analyze *The Third Way* in response to your kind invitation to do so.

GIDDENS'S *THE THIRD WAY*

I want to clarify at the outset that, in spite of my personal experience with the Third Way on both sides of the Atlantic, I will try to be fair to the British version. I want to stress, right away, that it is not my intention to trash it. Far from it: I want to analyze it with the sense of balance and thoughtfulness that the Third Way deserves. There is indeed a great need for discussion and debate on where social democracy should be headed, to which the Third Way could have contributed. And I have chosen Anthony Giddens's book *The Third Way: The*

Renewal of Social Democracy (1) as the main reference point for my analysis and critique because I consider it the most elaborate description of what the Third Way intends to be. The book has received great acclaim, including from some publications known for their animosity to progressive positions. For example, the editorial pages of the *Financial Times* presented Giddens's book as highly relevant for Europe as well as for the United Kingdom. Actually, Giddens himself does not claim that *The Third Way* is relevant only to the United Kingdom. If that were the case, I would have left its evaluation to British commentators. But both Giddens and Blair (and their supporters in the European press) claim that their proposals are applicable to Europe and indeed even to the United States. They both call for the Third Way to replace the old social democratic parties, which they consider "dead" or "irrelevant"—harsh words that both have used to define social democracy. Even though Giddens's book carries the subtitle *The Renewal of Social Democracy*, he writes in the preface that "New Labour represents a break with old Labor . . . a similar sort of break that has been made by virtually all continental Social Democratic parties" (1, p. viii). Giddens speaks of a break rather than reform. The birth of a new social democracy seems to require the death of the old.

It is important to state from the very beginning that for Giddens to be able to present the Third Way as an intermediate position between what he defines as "classical social democracy" and neoliberalism, he has to stereotype each position so much that neither is recognizable. I don't deny that the Third Way could indeed be an intermediate position between what Giddens and Blair call labor and neoliberalism in Great Britain, but it is profoundly unfair—to the point of being plain false—that Giddens's classifications of "social democracy" and "neoliberalism" are assigned to those political traditions in Europe. Actually, Giddens shows a remarkable ignorance about the major political traditions in Western Europe: social democracy, conservatism, and liberalism.

Let me be specific. Already in the first chapter, when Giddens defines the two alternatives—the social democratic tradition and the neoliberal tradition—that the Third Way is supposed to transcend, he erroneously characterizes both positions. For example, he writes that "social democracy has been characterized by reliance on protectionism, by state ownership of the means of production, by keynesianism, by demand management, by confined roles for markets and by state dominance of the economy." But this definition ignores the enormous diversity among the forms of European social democracy. Actually, the best-known and oldest experiences in social democracy in Europe—in the northern European social democratic countries—have not followed Keynesian policies, have not based their economic policies on manipulation of demand, have followed the most anti-protectionist policies in Europe, and have had state-owned sectors that were among the smallest in the European Union. During the periods of social democratic governance in these countries—Sweden, Norway, Denmark, and Finland—their economies have been the most open in the OECD (with exports representing the largest percentage of their GDP); their economic policies have been primarily aimed at shaping supply rather than demand forces; their public deficits have been among the smallest in the OECD (reaching surpluses in many years during the period 1960–1990); and their state-owned sector in production has been quite small, and in none of them (except Norway) has that sector expanded during the social democratic years. And these have been the social democratic countries par excellence! Other social democratic parties in Europe have governed for shorter periods of time and have been greatly constrained by strong conservative and liberal parties with which, on many occasions, they have had to govern in coalition. But even in Germany, where the Social Democratic Party has traditionally followed demand-oriented economic policies, the conservative parties expanded the state sector more than did the social democrats. The same thing happened with the Socialist Party in France. Even during the expansionist period in the first two years of the first Mitterrand government, the state domain of the economy barely increased. It was the conservative De Gaulle, rather than Mitterrand or Jospin, who expanded the state sector. And in Spain, the state sector was reduced considerably during the socialist years.

Let me clarify that I am not calling these policies good or bad. I am just setting straight the record of social democracy in Europe. For a superb presentation of the northern social democratic experience, I recommend the article by Huber and Stephens, "Internationalization and the Social Democratic Model" (2). And for an excellent review of the social democratic experience, I would suggest you read the encyclopedic work of Wolfgang Merkell, unfortunately never translated into English. For those of you who read German, you might like to read his original *Ende der Sozial Democratic,* translated into Spanish as *¿Final de la Social Democracia?* (3). You may also find my analysis of the economic and social policies of social democracy (and Christian democracy and liberalism) entitled "The Political Economy of the Welfare State in Developed Capitalist Countries" (4) of some interest (see Chapter 4). All these publications provide plenty of evidence that Giddens's representation of European social democracy is plain wrong.

A similar misrepresentation appears in Giddens's characterization of the neoliberal tradition. He puts in the same box—neoliberalism—two distinct positions: the conservative and liberal. This political aggregation explains why he concludes that neoliberalism is in trouble today "because of the conflict in its ranks between conservatism on the one hand and market fundamentalism on the other" (1, p. 15). But in Europe, conservative parties have not been market fundamentalists. Christian democracy, for example, is not anti-statist. Quite to the contrary! French, Italian, and German conservative governments have been highly statist. The market fundamentalists in Europe have been the liberal parties, which for the most part have been quite small, though not insignificant. Here again, Giddens extrapolates from the British experience, assuming it is representative of the European experience. It is not! In Europe, the two alternatives he poses, social democracy and neoliberalism, do not have the characteristics he assigns to them. The Third Way aims at being something between the Conservative and Labour Parties in Great Britain, maybe along Liberal Party lines. But in continental Europe the political terrain is far more complicated, far richer, and I would say far more interesting. Actually, what Giddens deems "new" is in reality not so new in Europe. This explains the cool reception that *The Third Way* has received among many European social democrats. There is more than a touch of Christian democracy in what *The Third Way* calls for, with a sprinkling of Liberal Party.

Let me elaborate by analyzing Giddens's understanding of (*a*) the relationship between the state and civil society, (*b*) the family and its relationship to the welfare state, and (*c*) exclusion and inclusion in our societies.

Welfare State or Welfare Society

Regarding the first point, Giddens's position is similar to the Christian democratic position that establishes an inverse relationship between the welfare state and civil society, such that the expansion of one means the reduction of the other. As added evidence for this conflict, Giddens refers to the Soviet Union's experience, where the state asphyxiated and killed civil society. He calls, as does the Christian democratic tradition, for replacement of the welfare state by the welfare society, with organizations in civil society unhindered by the state—which does not interfere in the richness that only civil society can develop. There is no evidence, however, that in Western democracies the expansion of the welfare state intrinsically impoverishes civil society. Quite to the contrary. Goran Therborn, in his exhaustive study of the social organization of Europe, concludes that the northern European social democracies, with their more structured political societies and larger state funding for social and community purposes, have also had richer civil societies (as measured by the number of organizations in the non-state sectors) (5).

Giddens also makes general comments about the richness of civil life in the United States, where the welfare state is clearly underdeveloped. But I don't know of any comparative study that has looked at the richness of civil society on the two sides of the Atlantic. The only knowledge that I have is from my own experience. In Barcelona, I live in a working-class neighborhood (la Sagrera) in a city governed by left-wing parties (socialist, ex-communist, and green parties). In Baltimore, I live in an academic community, close to a working-class community (Hampden) that I know well. In Barcelona, there is an enormously rich civil society. During the weekends, for example, in the main squares and parks, youths play soccer, basketball, and all forms of sports. The neighborhood parks are full of civil activities, and the elderly play petane. In Baltimore, in Hampden, the number of activities is much lower and neighborhood life is much more limited. I am sure Baltimore's very few civil associations are recorded on paper (since they have tax advantages), while those in Barcelona are most likely unrecorded. It would be unthinkable for the elderly groups in Barcelona to register as Petanca La Sagrera Club. They would certainly act as a club, but I am quite sure that the need to register has not even occurred to them. I am sure, however, that the elders' association in Hampden is registered. Thus there may be more registered associations in Baltimore than in Barcelona, but, in practice, my experience suggests that there is a richer civil society in the latter than in the former. It is sufficient to look at the festivities held on the major holidays in Barcelona and the major festivities in Baltimore. There is no comparison.

A similar experience has been described for the communist-led regions of Northern Italy, where the old Italian Communist Party, now the Party of the Democratic Left, has greatly stimulated and enriched civil society while expanding public responsibilities in the city and regional governments. The dichotomy and conflict between welfare state and welfare society described in Giddens's *The Third Way* is false: one enriches rather than impoverishes the other.

The Family and the Welfare State

Another Christian democratic position reproduced by Giddens is his vision of the relationship between the family and the welfare state. He defines as an old social democratic position what is actually an old Christian democratic position. He assumes that the old social democracy based its welfare state on contributions made by the male worker who was supported by a wife staying at home. But this reliance of welfare state funding (1, p. 16) on the male breadwinner has been traditional in the Christian democratic countries, not the social democracies. Reliance of the welfare state on labor market contributions has characterized conservative governments based in the Christian tradition since the time of Bismarck. Traditional social democracy instead has funded its welfare state through general funds, as an entitlement of all citizens, not only of workers and their families. While criticizing this Christian democratic tradition (which he erroneously defines as social democratic), Giddens does not quite break with it. Indeed, while critical of the "traditional family" model, he is skeptical about the new forms of family that are replacing the old, calling for the principle of responsibility of parents toward their children and children toward their parents. While there would be broad agreement on the need to emphasize the two-way responsibility between parents and children, he extends this responsibility to the funding of services for the elderly by their own children, rather than by the state—a position characteristic of Christian democratic social policy. In the social democratic tradition, it is the state that has had the responsibility of helping families, through child care services and domiciliary services. This has allowed the integration of women into the labor force. Moreover, in the social democratic tradition, children are not expected to pay for the institutional care of their parents as Giddens proposes. In fact, it is the Christian democratic tradition that calls for children's financial support for the institutional care of their parents. In the social democratic tradition, the liberation of women and enrichment of the family—the key cell in civil society—require a massive expansion of social services of the welfare state. Giddens instead speaks about the unhealthy dependency created by the welfare state, and criticizes the Swedish welfare state as excessive.

In this critique of Sweden, Giddens relies on the work of Assan Lindbeck, one of the most liberal Swedish economists, whose work has been widely criticized by socialist scholars such as Walter Korpi and others as lacking rigor in its utilization of Swedish data. Korpi (6) has convincingly shown, for example, that Lindbeck's conclusions on the crisis of the Swedish welfare state and its supposed excessiveness are based on faulty data and sloppy work. Yet the majority of the international press—and Giddens with it—continues to cite Lindbeck's work without ever referring to Korpi, whose credibility in the scientific community is much higher than Lindbeck's. A point worth noting here is the recent resignation of Lindbeck from the Nobel Prize Committee in charge of selecting awardees of the Nobel Prize for Economics. This resignation was the indirect result of a worldwide protest about the continuous bias toward neoliberal economics in awarding the Nobel Prize.

Actually, a neoliberal touch also appears in some of Giddens's comments on pensions. Few would disagree with his remark that elderly persons should be seen as a resource and should be encouraged to be active participants in society. But his critical remarks about pensions creating dependency, and the need for the elderly to be responsible to society and do their share, offer a somewhat distorted image of pensioners. Most elderly people would be poor (and unemployed) if they did not have their pensions. In Great Britain, even after pensions, one in four elderly persons is poor. One should be very cautious in calling for elders to join the labor market again, unless this is voluntary, is not based on economic need, and can be enjoyable.

Exclusion and Inclusion in the Third Way

Finally, the Christian democratic tradition appears in the main objective of *The Third Way*. We can ask: having abandoned socialism, what is the Third Way's objective? According to Giddens and Blair, the objective is to avoid exclusion and facilitate inclusion. But whose exclusion and whose inclusion? Giddens speaks about the exclusion of the rich (a voluntary exclusion), who isolate themselves from society and develop their own services. Their exclusion impoverishes the public sphere because they do not need public services and thus do not add pressure for their improvement. Society loses from their exclusion. Giddens, while defining the problem, does not propose how to resolve this exclusion of the rich.

The other exclusion that concerns Giddens is the exclusion of the unskilled, of the vulnerable, who are outside the labor market and cannot get good jobs. To integrate this sector of the population, *The Third Way* proposes education plus community services such as child care, health care, transport, and continuing education to help people find good jobs. Here, *The Third Way* is not proposing anything new. The social democrats in northern Europe have traditionally provided massive training programs with supportive services, as have the German Christian democratic and social democratic parties. Even Giddens's call for responsibility—by which he means that the unemployed must try hard to integrate into the labor force lest they lose their benefits—is not new. In Sweden and Denmark, for example, the unemployed have to take a job at the end of the training program, or risk losing support if they refuse.

WHAT IS NEW ABOUT THE THIRD WAY?

Given these points, we might ask Giddens what is new about the Third Way. It may be new in the United Kingdom, but it is quite old in Europe and, I would say, in the United States. According to British professor of social policy Robert Walker (7), New Labour proposals for welfare are less advanced than the Wisconsin anti-poverty program. But even more important, we need to ask: what has the Third Way to offer to the majority of people who are not excluded (who are not rich or poor), the 80 percent of the population? It is here that *The Third Way* is remarkably silent, except for a generic call for an equality of opportunities. What differentiates this position from a liberal position with a social conscience, or a Christian democratic position? Actually, many Christian democrats in Europe consider themselves to the left of Blair. This explains why the social democrats in Europe have felt quite uneasy, to say the least, with the Third Way. Lionel Jospin, whom Giddens erroneously and self-servingly defined in a recent article in the *New Statesman* (8) as a "Third Wayer," has been quite critical of the Third Way. France's Minister of Employment and Vice President of the Socialist Government, Martine Aubry, recently referred to the Third Way as "lamentable." And one of the most influential voices, until recently, in today's European social democracies, Oskar Lafontaine, Germany's past Minister of Finance and ex-General Secretary of the German Social Democratic Party, has written a book that calls for changing the Stability Pact (which condemns Europe to a policy of austerity); changing the independence of the European Central Bank; regulating the international mobility of financial capital; and stimulating national and international demand—all policies opposed by Blair's Third Way. The resignation of Lafontaine has strengthened Blair—but it is doubtful that the German Social Democratic Party will follow the Third Way. Even Blair's policies in use today to reduce unemployment in Europe are closer to Aznar's than to Jospin's or even Gerhard Schröder's. Blair's looking to Clintonomics as an inspiration for his economic and social policies concerns and alarms his fellow social democrats across the channel. *Social democracy needs a process for reform, but not in the Third Way direction.*

Social democracy as the major instrument of the European labor movement established the welfare state in western continental Europe. The U.K. welfare state, with the exception of the National Health Service, is underdeveloped. Most social transfers are quite low by European standards and frequently are means-tested. What seems to be needed is not for social democracy to learn from the Third Way, but rather the Third Way to learn from what Giddens derisively calls "classical" social democracy. Its "break" with the latter condemns the Third Way to becoming a step back rather than a progressive step in the proper direction.

Note — This chapter is based on a paper presented at the Contemporary Politics Seminar at the International Center for International Studies of the Johns Hopkins University, Washington, D.C., on March 15, 1999.

REFERENCES

1. Giddens, A. *The Third Way: The Renewal of Social Democracy.* Blackwell, Oxford, 1999.
2. Huber, E., and Stephens, J. D. Internationalization and the social democratic model: Crisis and future prospects. *Comp. Polit. Stud.* 13(3): 353–397, 1998.
3. Merkell, W. *¿Final de la Social Democracia?* Editorial Alfons el Magnanim, Alencia, Spain, 1989.
4. Navarro, V. The political economy of the welfare state in developed capitalist countries. *Int. J. Health Serv.* 29(1): 1–50, 1999.
5. Therborn, G. *European Modernity and Beyond: The Trajectory of European Societies,* 1945–2000. Sage, London, 1995.
6. Korpi, W. Eurosclerosis and the sclerosis of objectivity: On the role of values among economic experts. *Econ. J.* 106: 1727, November 1996.
7. Walker, R. The Americanization of British welfare: A case study of policy transfer. *Int. J. Health Serv.* 29(4): 679-697, 1999.
8. Giddens, A. *New Statesman,* February 26, 1999.

CHAPTER 19

TOWARD AN ECOSOCIAL VIEW OF HEALTH

Richard Levins and Cynthia Lopez

An examination of the changing health patterns in this century justifies both celebration and dismay. We can celebrate the increase in life expectancy at birth, the disappearance of smallpox, and the decline of other diseases. We can marvel at technical advances such as the development of reliable heart surgery, molecular methods for diagnosis, sophisticated electronic imaging. But we also have to recognize that diseases we thought were on their way out have returned with a vengeance (tuberculosis, cholera, malaria), that apparently new diseases have arisen (AIDS, Legionnaires' disease, ebola, hepatitis C, cryptosporidiosis, *E. coli* 0157, Lassa fever, hanta virus), while microorganisms have shown remarkable flexibility in thwarting our therapies. Agricultural productivity has risen greatly, but without eliminating hunger. The gap between rich and poor in life expectancy and morbidity has remained robust for more than a century despite changes in the details of class structure and substitutions of specific causes of death.

When we examine the pattern of success and failure, it seems as if the successes occur in the solution of narrow, highly specific problems (smallpox) amenable to molecular and technical solutions, while the dramatic failures (wide disparities in health) appear at the level of whole systems, where factors that were not taken into account can overwhelm the expected results deduced from simple logic.

Solutions designed to solve isolated problems can exacerbate or give rise to new ones. Pesticides can increase pest problems and poison people, antibiotics give rise to new pathogens, hospitals are a focus of infection, agricultural development can lead to hunger, and flood control may make us more vulnerable to floods. Therefore a public health community better prepared for surprise has to include the perspectives of evolution, biogeography, and ecology as well as social science, and deal not only with current problems but also with those that might arise.

FOUR HYPOTHESES

The U.S. paradox is that although we spend more on health care than any other country we rank in the lowest quartile among the 25 industrialized countries for infant mortality, life expectancy, and other health indicators. We offer four hypotheses for this dismal datum:

1. *We do not get more health care, it only costs more* (Figures 1 and 2).
2. *We do get more health care, but a significant fraction of it is inappropriate, ineffective, or even harmful.*
   - 120,000 deaths per year are caused by medical error (including iatrogenic disease, nosocomial infection, and unnecessary medical intervention).
   - 80 percent of cases referred for second opinion on cardiac bypass do not need the surgery.

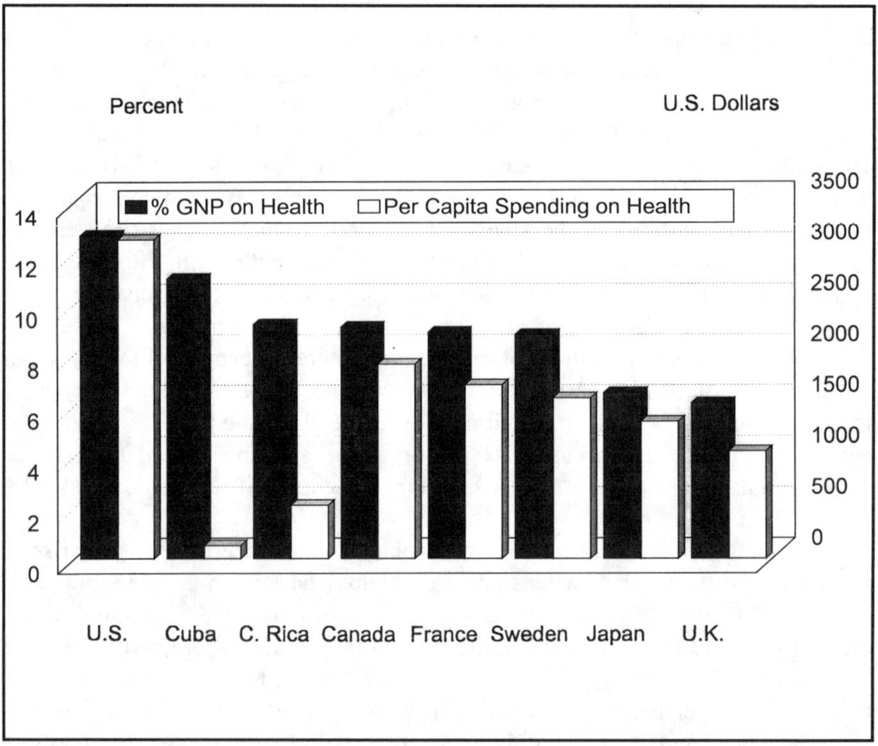

Figure 1. Spending on health care in various countries: of all nations, the United States spends the most. Data from the United Nations and national ministries.

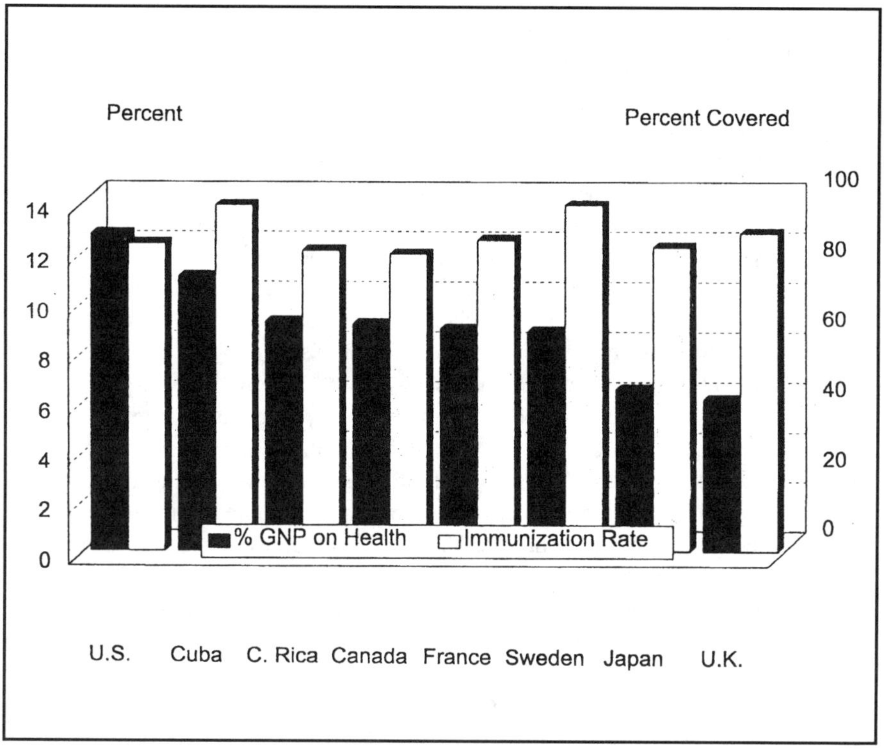

Figure 2. Spending on health care compared with immunization rate: the United States does not get better coverage for the extra paid for health care. Data from the United Nations and national ministries.

3. *Only some of us get more health care.* Inequalities along class, race, and geographic lines in access to health care result in neglect of many and over-treatment of the few.
   - Black women are 35 percent less likely than white women to receive a mammogram.
   - White seniors are 2.5 times more likely to receive bypass surgery and 2.2 times more likely to receive angioplasty than black seniors.
   - The uninsured poor are twice as likely as those with private insurance to report a delay of hospital care. Among those whose care is delayed, hospital stays are longer and death rates higher (1).
4. *Our way of life makes us sick, and then we invest more in repairing the damage.*

Our research program examines each of these not mutually exclusive hypotheses, but with emphasis on the last because the others are more familiar.

It is at the level of complex interactions that our science has been least successful. Fragmentation of knowledge prevents us from seeing the whole, and methodologies encourage explanations within the confines of single disciplines, assigning relative weights to "factors" rather than elucidating their interactions.

Several important movements and intellectual currents have arisen that together offer a more holistic view of the complexities of health at the population level. They include: Ecosystem Health, Environmental Justice, Social Determination, and Health Care for All. Each of these four currents is on the cutting edge of a breakaway from the classical microbiological or single-factor epidemiology that has proven so vulnerable to surprises.

Ecosystem Health sees the human species as one among many in an environment that is changing as a result of human activity: land use patterns, climate change, population growth, resource depletion, pollution, urbanization, loss of biodiversity, and other local and global processes all disrupt the natural self-regulation of the biosphere. These changes harm people, domestic animals, wildlife, the oceans, and the forests. The crucial response has to be to redesign our relations with the rest of nature.

Environmental Justice points out that "we" are not undifferentiated "we." Polluters pour thousands of kinds of historically new organic compounds into our rivers, clear cut our forests, dirty our skies, and protect these activities from criticism. Environmental destruction, internationally and domestically within countries, often imposes health burdens unevenly, as the environmental justice movement points out: with greater exposure at home and at work, the less well-off suffer higher disease rates as a consequence. The priorities have to be: stop spoiling the environment, minimize the trade-offs between economic development and toxicity, and eliminate the differential exposure of population subgroups to environmental hazards.

The Social Determination Movement studies the inequality of health within a nation or among nations. It sees steep gradients of education, income, and social position as adversely affecting the health of a population, not only at the bottom but throughout the entire range of the social structure, from the bottom throughout the middle and into the upper, even of people who are far removed from the abject poverty of Calcutta. This field holds that inequality per se rather than absolute privation in developed economies undermines the capacity of people to resist disease. The psychological concomitants of steep social positioning are emphasized both at the individual (self-esteem, hopefulness) and collective (community efficacy, social capital) levels (3, 4).

The Health Care for All Movement focuses on the inequality of access to health care as a major deterrent to health improvement. This movement advocates universal access to health care as a basic right of membership in the human species. It evaluates the quality of health care only insofar as it is unequal and therefore does not touch on fundamental questions of the generation of health and disease.

Each of these four intellectual currents opens up areas that have been ignored by traditional epidemiology. Each is supported by both theory and observation. And each, in emphasizing the importance of ignored phenomena in its field, tends to ignore the advantages of including perspectives from other fields.

But these four currents should not be intellectual competitors. When we move from a model that assigns relative weights to isolable influences ("factors" or "independent variables") to a model of whole-system determination, we can see the absolute importance of each of them because:

- All theory is wrong that limits concern to just our species and pushes the rest of nature into the background.
- All theory is flawed that sees our species as an undifferentiated whole and ignores injustice that we inflict upon each other.
- All theory is too narrow that looks only at the individual confronting an "environment" and fails to see that individual as a unique "particle" formed in an ecosocial field.
- All theory is wrong that separates mind from body, that sees the psychological impact of social location but dismisses the intricate, criss-crossing pathways by which a hierarchical society creates adverse health outcomes and undermines people's capacity to prevent or ameliorate them.
- All methodology is wrong that pits quantitative against qualitative methods or looks only at undirectional causation from "independent" to "dependent" variables without taking into account the feedbacks between them.
- Finally, all policy derived from theory is hopelessly biased if "policy" is seen as the allocation of resources and the drafting of regulations by those who control the resources and make the regulations; if real conflict of interest is denied and the boundary conditions within which policy is formed are simply accepted as "life"; and if researchers are not at the disposal of all affected parties.

Our task, then, is to integrate the insights of these most perceptive efforts and to confront health, society, and habitat as a whole, in their full complexity.

THE PRODUCTION OF KNOWLEDGE ABOUT HEALTH

Gaining an understanding of the health of even a single region is a daunting task. We have adopted an approach to health in Kansas that depends on the convergence of three sources of knowledge: theoretical, data-driven, and experiential. Our strategy is to integrate these three sources of knowledge and understanding, each with its particular insights, gaps, and biases. A starting point is to recognize the strengths and weaknesses of each.

1. *A general theoretical framework.* We apply to public health problems the theoretical perspectives from ecology, geography, systems theory, philosophy of science, policy studies, and various social sciences. Our emphasis is on wholeness and process in complexly connected networks of causes that cross the boundaries of disciplines. This demands a critical stance toward the familiar dichotomies—such as social/biological, environment/lifestyle, physical/psychological, individual responsibility/social determination of health—that have fragmented our discipline and pitted half-truths against half-truths. We are actively interested in a number of policy questions that lie outside the normal domain of public health, in fields such as environmental protection and agriculture.

We also use a comparative approach. If Kansas comparisons are made to fairly similar places such as neighboring states, it is easier to explain any observed differences against a background of shared conditions. When we compare very different places, the explanation for observed differences may be less accessible. But by showing that patterns that hold in one place are not necessarily universal, the comparisons broaden the range of possible alternatives. When very different conditions show similar patterns we are identifying robust properties of human health. We try to work with both kinds of comparisons, selected in part for degrees of difference and similarity, and partly through chance access to information.[1]

2. *Kansas public and private health research and data.* A great wealth of data has been collected by a number of Kansas agencies at the statewide and county level, which provide the core material for our analysis.

3. *Interviews with Kansans outside the formal public health system who have special insights into a particular kind of phenomenon or local conditions.* Here we have made use of informal contacts through our associates, the children of one of us, friends of friends, and people we meet after we lecture on various topics around the state. They help us interpret anomalies in the data, call our attention to very local situations that do not affect county-level data, and provide historical background.

The approach to knowledge production outlined above is supported by past experience and also reflects two theoretical commitments on our part: the need for a self-reflective looking at our own scientific practice as a social process, and the democratic commitment that makes research a community effort combining professional and nonprofessional inputs.

[1] In the full study we are using comparisons with selected Canadian provinces, Mexican and Brazilian states, Israeli health districts, and Cuban provinces. At the time of this writing, only the Cuban data were available.

WHOLENESS: A WHOLE-SYSTEM APPROACH

Hegel warned that the truth is the whole (5). Of course we cannot really see "The Whole." But we can recognize the following.

1. *A problem has to be posed big enough to accommodate an answer.* In an atomic world, the laws of conservation of matter and conservation of energy are too small and have to be united in the larger conservation of matter/energy. If we fail to define the problem big enough, then many important impacts on a variable come from outside the domain of the problem and are treated as "random" or "error." When we control away the heterogeneity of social life in order to plot levels of cholesterol against rates of heart disease, we have lost most of the determinations and are left with a statistically significant but weak explanation. Contrary to common sense, big problems are often more soluble than small ones.

2. *The relevant systems are bigger and more complex than our tradition acknowledges.* In order to understand the upsurge in infectious disease we cannot limit ourselves to diseases of humans. Similar patterns of resurgent and emerging diseases can be seen in wild and domestic animals and in crop plants. When we include them, we can begin to see parasitism as a universal phenomenon of evolutionary ecology and can pose questions such as, How wide a host range do diseases have? Do they mostly affect similar hosts? When do pathogens extend their host range? Are diseases with many hosts more or less severe than those with few hosts? How do nutrition and environmental stress affect vulnerability to disease? Most infections fail to take, so what makes some successful?

3. *There will always be an "outside."* After we have expanded our model to include much more than was formerly included, there is still an outside impinging on the system and capable of overwhelming the processes on which we have chosen to focus.

The systems are bigger than we expected in another sense: the objects of analysis are not individuals but populations. Concepts such as vulnerability or health apply also to population subgroups such as classes, occupations, communities, genders, races, and ethnic groups. Health is generated in households, neighborhoods, workplaces, communities, nations, and the whole world. Individuals are imbedded in several kinds of larger units, each with its own unique impact on health. Within the same community, people may breathe the same air and drink the same water but experience different environments at work or school and while going to and from work or school; may walk the same pot-holed streets and swelter in the same heatwaves, but some have and others lack air conditioning; may fear the same dangers but have different histories of knowledge about facing them. They may be immersed in different cultural and dietary and religious worlds, and may be represented quite differently by the same elected representatives.

From the perspective of an organized community, the people are simply who they are, the givens to be taken into account in any effort at change. From the perspective of individuals, their overlapping communities (home, neighborhood, workplace, town) are the givens within which life unfolds and health is created and undermined. When we study the community, we see a collection of individuals and treat their uniqueness statistically to identify community characteristics or structurally to understand and influence community processes of change. When we work with individuals, we have to see each one as a special point of intersection of many current and past influences. Units at different levels determine each other mutually, and a reliable theory cannot reduce one to the other or rank them in a hierarchy of relative fundamentalness. After emphasizing the unique properties of each community, we then have to recognize their connectedness. Although each subpopulation has its unique health problems, these cannot be contained just within its boundaries, but spill over to other populations and become problems of the whole society (6).

Therefore, programs aimed at helping individuals to escape from their communities while leaving the impoverishment intact do not really address the problem: if every person earned a Ph.D. we would hear great seminars at the soup kitchens unless homelessness was also addressed. In the long run our "patient" is the species, suffering from an ecosocial distress syndrome that links the daunting problems of resource depletion, resurgent disease, pollution, inequality, oppression, climate change, and alienation.

Once we argue the need for a more inclusive, complex frame of reference for the study of health, we have to confront an awesome, daunting complexity that can overwhelm us. How is it possible to face such complexity?

We claim that the study of complexity is not so much difficult as unfamiliar, and that the task of theoretical work is to make obvious what is initially obscure. This has happened in the past. For example, while medieval monks could add, subtract, and even multiply, division remained a mystery that required specialists. The simple shift from Roman to Arabic numbers made division accessible to all literate people. Now we have to shift from the reductionist notion that to understand the world it is sufficient to study its smallest pieces. Instead, we must adopt a holistic dynamic approach informed by philosophy and systems theory that can reeducate our intuitions until such notions as feedback, interpenetration, sinks and sources, connectivity, bifurcations and phase transitions, self-damping and system memory become as familiar to us as the independent variable, correlation coefficient, or regression line. Below are three principles for taking a more complex whole-system view of health problems.

1. *Challenge the false dichotomies that plague science.* Replace these by the principles that human biology is a socialized biology, that we can choose to

change our environments, but recognize that all our choices are constrained choices; that our beliefs and feelings affect our immune, detoxification, and endocrine systems, while the state of our bodies affects our thinking and feeling; and that genes may influence how we relate to our environments, while society can determine which environments we face, and these environments can then determine which genetic differences are trivial and which are significant. A particularly important dichotomy is that between individual responsibility and social determination of health.

Separately false, jointly true: Consider the two propositions (*a*) we are each responsible for our own health, and (*b*) health is socially determined. Both are claims about reality, and about the causes of disease. Both are also normative: each person should take responsibility for her or his own health, or our society should take collective responsibility for the health of all of us. Each proposition is separately false, but together they are jointly true.

When stated by policymakers, the first proposition blames the sick (or their parents) for being sick and justifies the denial of public resources for health improvement. The second, accepting social responsibility, would propose actions to improve health care, make it more available, or reduce environmental insults to our health such as pollution, but it leaves the individual out of the equation or as a passive onlooker.

When the sick (or the potentially sick) receive these propositions, the impact depends upon these people's power to act. If someone is without the resources, knowledge, skill, and energy to act, the first proposition leads to guilt and makes health problems worse. The second proposition also leads to helplessness: "this world is making me sick and I can't help it no matter what I do."

But when stated by someone able to act, the first proposition can be interpreted to mean "I have been harmed, but I won't let it defeat me." The individual can become better informed, make decisions about lifestyle within the limits of his or her social location, and demand the necessary care. The second proposition would lead to collective action such as identification and publication of pollution sources, demands for health insurance or free care, or introduction of health-protective measures into collective agreements. In the long run, individual action can achieve significant but still limited results, while action at the community level may reduce future damage but perhaps not help the actors themselves very much.

Therefore, taken separately each proposition is false and harmful, but taken together they are true and can be empowering.

2. *Respect the spontaneous activity of nature.* Organisms—and infectious agents are organisms—evolve in response to their own circumstances and to our attempts to control them. Pathogens are always navigating among opposing demands of natural selection for a good meal, protection from the body's defenses, and an exit to new hospitable hosts. They change when they encounter

the new environments we create for them or when our therapies make drug resistance an overwhelming survival requirement.

Species are always probing the boundaries of their ecological niches and geographic extensions, and invading new territories when opportunities permit. We sometimes create the opportunities. *Legionella* is a bacterium found all over the world, but rarely and in small numbers. These bacteria are poor competitors and have finicky nutritional requirements, but they do tolerate higher temperatures than most bacteria and can resist chlorine. Therefore, when we remove the natural enemies of the *Legionella* bacteria by our usually effective purification techniques, they will thrive in the heated and chlorinated water pipes of hotels and conference centers. Lately several cases of Legionnaires' disease have occurred among truck drivers who have used the showers at truck-stops on the interstate highways.

If climate fluctuations increase natural production of mouse food, or if we clear the natural vegetation to plant grain while the harvest is left in the field or barn when prices are too low, and if we kill the predators of mice—the coyotes, snakes, and owls—mouse populations will explode on the newly available food and, according to the location, offer us hanta virus or plague. These diseases are current threats in the southwestern United States. In other countries current threats include Venezuelan hemorrhagic fever, Bolivian hemorrhagic fever, and other novelties.

If malaria spreads in the United States it will be a result not so much of invasion by exotic mosquitoes as of economic hardship that forces people to sleep outdoors without protection from mosquitoes. If global temperature continues to rise we can expect heat waves. Those who lack access to air conditioning and who are elderly or already sick will be most vulnerable to heat death. If *Salmonella* or *Cryptosporidium* contaminate our food or water, it will be because technical changes in industry have not been matched by corresponding changes in our surveillance and regulation, or because we fail to know that all systems, no matter how up-to-date, break down sometimes.

It may seem too much to ask that we put effort into studying diseases that have not happened yet when there is enough to do with present health problems, but unless we prepare for change and uncertainty we will face many unpleasant surprises.

A seeming detour is needed here to examine how other organisms confront uncertain environments. There are really only four modalities available: detection and response, long- and short-range prediction, tolerance of a broad range of conditions, and prevention.

Of course these are not mutually exclusive modalities and must be combined. Even after we have done our best guessing what might happen and have made our best preparations, we have to accept that the world still can surprise us, and we always have to ask the questions, "but what if we're wrong?" Here is where we need to combine the most promising approaches selected by scientific consensus with some proportion of unpopular ideas that may seem way out, just in case these ideas prove correct (7).

3. *Respect the systemic nature of health-related phenomena.* The variables that affect our health are linked in reciprocal feedback loops rather than by one-way causal chains separating independent from dependent variables. The causal pathways cross disciplinary boundaries and loop back and forth in positive and negative feedbacks (Figure 3).

Negative feedback loops can be protective: an outbreak of a disease can lead to immunization programs that reduce that disease. An uncomfortably high temperature can increase sweating or the use of air conditioning, in either case reducing the discomfort. An infection may call forth the macrophages and other anti-infection responses. But negative feedback can also thwart interventions. Antibiotics result in drug resistance. Pesticides lead to pesticide resistance. Increased policing can lead to increased alienation. Food distribution may lower the price of food to the point where farmers stop producing food. Too much health-promoting exhortation can provoke boredom, resentment, disconnection, and reduced effectiveness of health promotion.

Negative feedbacks may lead to either positive or negative correlations among the variables that are linked, depending on whether outside influences spread along the positive or negative branch of the loop. Since they may spread along both pathways, this can give rise to inconsistency across epidemiological studies. Carcinogens in the blood can lead to tumors, generating a positive correlation between these two variables. But tumors have a higher affinity for carcinogens, removing them from the blood and generating a negative correlation. Doctors treat disease, creating a negative correlation between medical service and disease prevalence. But high disease rates among insured populations attract doctors, creating a positive correlation.

Positive feedbacks reinforce any initial deviation of a variable. If a child is held back from her or his studies by the sequelae of poverty, that child may be labeled a poor learner and tracked toward dead-end occupations and more poverty; a child in an enriched program will be offered more opportunity. A youngster's first foray into petty crime may be greeted by rejection in the home, expulsion from school, and harassment by the police, but may be praised and supported by gang brothers and guided toward further crime in the subculture that is welcoming. Thus positive feedbacks can create the illusion of irreversible determination at an early age (Figure 3).

When multiple causes affect health, the same variable may produce opposite effects by different pathways that may cancel each other. For example, crowding is harmful to us because of increased contagion, but multi-generational households, particularly in immigrant or marginalized populations, provide support. This paradox can cause us to underestimate the negative effects of crowding and isolation, and the positive effects of family support. Our task then is not to choose

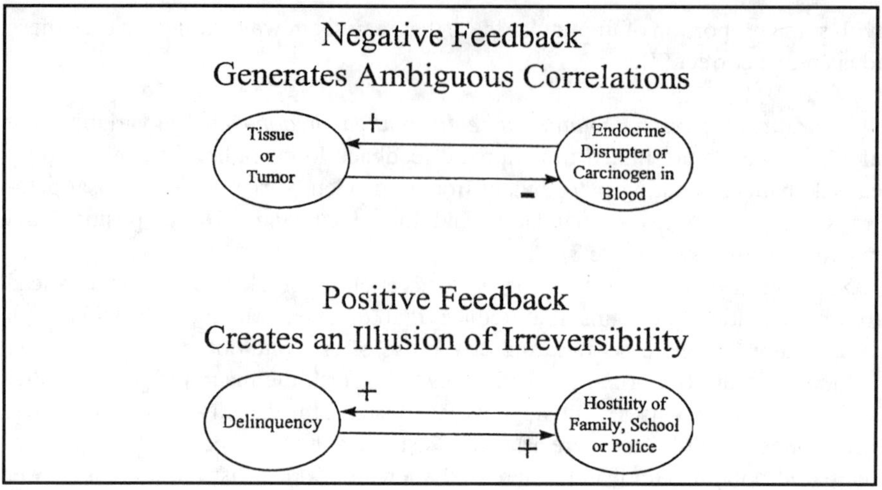

Figure 3. Feedback loops: negative and positive.

some optimum density, but to ask what arrangements would permit the transmission of support without the transmission of infection.

One way that poverty is harmful is through insufficient access to medical care, but the affluent might be unnecessarily exposed to excessive and costly interventions. In a statistical analysis of the health impact of access to medical care, a gradient by income would obscure the harmfulness of both unavailable and excessive medical intervention. Our task is not to give everyone the care the affluent get but to improve the quality of care, eliminate clinical decisions made for nonmedical reasons, and make the improved care equitably available to all.

Unemployment can undermine health. Unemployment reduces access to medical treatment and sometimes to potable water, disrupts social networks, can cause depression and excessive alcohol consumption with attendant cirrhosis, and forces skimping on food or home heating. But Singh and colleagues (8) found that Kansas counties with high unemployment rates showed lower overall crude death rates and rates of death from cancer and heart disease. Unemployment is bad for your health, but under certain conditions so is working. The death rates from cancer and heart disease are higher in some occupational groupings. For example, "Kansas farmers are at a significantly elevated risk of death for non-Hodgkin's lymphoma, leukemia, and cancers of the prostate and brain" (9). There is a positive association between counties with a large amount of agricultural activity and the cancer death rate for all residents; and in industries such as meat packing more than one worker in four is injured or made ill each year from work-related causes. Once again, an aggregated comparison of the health of employed and unemployed would obscure the health impacts of both conditions.

Reducing unemployment would not improve health unless jobs are also made safer. Table 1 shows the differential effects on health of being in counties in the highest or lowest quartiles for some social indicators.

Note that above 75 years of age, the social indicators have less effect on the death rate than for the general population or youth. This does not mean that older people are insensitive to social conditions. Across counties, the range for death rate of the over 75 group is 43 percent of the mean, only slightly less than the 56 percent for the general population. The appreciable variation across counties, although not across the selected indicators, suggests that elders are sensitive to different aspects of their social environment that were not captured in the indicators used. Median household income and percentage with available health care (Medicaid card) seem to be the best predictors of outcome disparities. For all indicators, heart disease is more responsive than cancer, but the two show a nearly perfect correlation of more than .97 over indicators. This suggests that they are sensitive to identical social conditions, but that heart disease is more sensitive than cancer to these factors. Both chronic obstructive pulmonary disease and pneumonia/influenza are strongly correlated with heart disease and cancer, and this whole cluster is less strongly responsive to the same indicators as cirrhosis, infectious disease, or motor vehicle accidents.

Table 1

Ratio of outcomes of lowest to highest quartiles for social indicators across Kansas counties, 1988–1993[a,b]

Social indicator	CDR	Deaths >75	Deaths 15–24	IHD	Cancer	COPD	Cirr.	Inf.	P & I
High school	1.83	1.03	1.62	1.67	1.40	1.38	1.39	1.41	1.65
Median income	1.89	1.02	1.40	2.38	1.68	1.73	1.29	1.21	2.31
Poverty rate	1.23	1.02	1.25	1.28	1.17	1.14	1.34	1.27	1.26
200% Poverty rate	1.36	1.02	1.22	1.63	1.24	1.23	1.18	0.97	1.65
Medicaid card	1.68	1.06	1.99	1.85	1.52	1.66	1.88	1.66	1.71
Unemployment	0.80	1.08	0.89	0.79	0.83	0.84	2.04	1.08	0.64
No car	1.37	1.06	1.37	1.42	1.26	1.38	1.82	1.61	1.48
Average	1.41	1.04	1.39	1.57	1.30	1.34	1.56	1.32	1.53

[a]Source: computed from reference 8.

[b]The *social indicators* are proportion of the population with at least a high school diploma, median income, poverty rate, 200 percent of poverty rate, a Medicaid card, unemployment rate, and households without a vehicle. The *numbers in the table* are the ratio of outcomes in the first to last quartile of Kansas counties for percentage having at least a high school education, median household income, poverty rate, 200 percent of poverty rate, absence of Medicaid card, and households with no vehicle. The *outcomes* are crude death rate (CDR), death rate for people 75 and older, deaths for ages 15–24, and deaths from ischemic heart disease (IHD), cancer, chronic obstructive pulmonary disease (COPD), cirrhosis of the liver (Cirr.), infectious diseases (Inf.), pneumonia and influenza (P & I).

Table 2 shows the correlations among the highest to lowest quartiles of social indicator ratios of the causes of death, indicating the similarity of their responses to different indicators. The nearly perfect correlation between cirrhosis deaths and deaths over age 75 is not remarkable since cirrhosis deaths do tend to occur late in life. But the nearly perfect correlations among heart disease, cancer, chronic pulmonary obstruction, and pneumonia and influenza show their very similar sensitivities to the indicated social factors. The social indicators themselves are also intercorrelated as manifestations of undesirable conditions, but all social indicators do not create their health effects in exactly the same way.

The Importance of Variability

Traditional public health is interested in estimating the average effect of something, and treats the variance as noise, to be reduced to a minimum by skillful selection of data sets so as to minimize the confidence interval. An ecologically informed approach would examine the variabilities of phenomena as objects of interest in their own right.

For example, the stability of physiological measures such as blood pressure indicate the effectiveness of homeostasis, while increasing variability with age or deprivation attests to its erosion. We have found (10) that the variance of blood pressure and some other traits increases with age, decreases with income, and is greater for African Americans than for whites. Here we do not see age as a "risk factor" but rather see homeostasis being undermined at different rates according

Table 2

Correlations among causes of death over socioeconomic quartiles[a]

	Deaths >75	Deaths 15–24	IHD	Cancer	COPD	Cirr.	Inf.	P & I
Deaths >75	1	–.09	–.56	–.49	–.32	.99	.32	–.62
Deaths 15–24		1	.61	.75	.79	.00	.76	.58
IHD			1	.97	.93	–.51	.20	.99
Cancer				1	.98	–.42	.40	.96
COPD					1	–.25	.53	.92
Cirr.						1	.43	–.58
Inf.							1	.20
P & I								1

[a]The strong correlation between death rate for people over 75 and cirrhosis (Cirr.) reflects the fact that cirrhosis deaths usually occur at a more advanced age than deaths from the other causes. All the causes of death respond to social conditions prevailing in the different counties, but heart disease (IHD), cancer, chronic obstructive pulmonary disease (COPD), and pneumonia and influenza (P & I) show an almost perfect correlation among themselves, while cirrhosis and infectious disease (Inf.) are more loosely connected to the others.

to people's life situations. Thus African Americans age faster than whites, and the variance of their blood pressure is greater.

Schmalhausen's law generalizes the undermining of homeostasis under stress. It states that a system at the boundary of its tolerance along any dimension of its existence is more vulnerable to small differences of circumstance along any dimension. Thus, under conditions of poverty, individual differences in shopping skill can have a big effect on well-being. Someone who clips all the coupons, saves all the green stamps, and takes the time to track down bargains and preserve left-overs may get by where someone who does not have the available time, child care, mobility, energy, or skill would suffer from malnutrition. But in an affluent household these differences will have trivial effects. A child with poor visual acuity in a crowded classroom with overworked teachers may be shunted out of academic study as a slow learner, but in a better school system might simply get eye glasses.

Suppose that a person is subject to many life circumstances that could cause illness or injury, but has defenses that buffer their effects. Suppose that the probability of successful protection is p, which is close to 1 (after all, most people do not get sick with every exposure to pathogens and most cancerous cells do not develop into cancer). By and large our defenses are pretty effective. So, if p is equal to .99 (or 99 percent), 1 percent of the time the defenses will fail and we will see harmful outcomes. Now suppose that in another community or household or subgroup p is equal to .98 (or 98 percent). This reflects only a 1 percent change in the defenses, but the rate of harmful outcome has doubled to 2 percent. The big differences in outcome among individuals or households could be associated with changes in their parameters (behavioral, physical, skills, history) that are too small to measure.

We can ask the question, why is it that not everyone in a poor community loses children, or turns to crime, or is frequently ill? When we observe that misfortunes tend to cluster, it is often more important to ask why some people are so vulnerable in that circumstance, rather than attempt to identify the particular precipitating factors in each case that make for heightened vulnerability in those circumstances.

Variability in Space

The differential variability of health outcomes across regions is also rich in information and is a research tool imported from our ecological work. Those causes of death or morbidity that vary geographically are by definition sensitive to conditions, and therefore more likely to be amenable to change. We can use the pattern of variation to set ameliorative goals, for instance raising the life expectancy of all districts at least to the state average or to that of its top five counties.

Geographic variation takes place on different scales, and we can use this to interpret the pattern. First, suppose that the variation is caused by some geographic gradient, say elevation or rainfall. Since the midpoints of states are farther apart than those of counties or zip codes, there should be more variation among states than within them.

On the other hand, suppose that very local conditions determine the local health outcomes. Then the variation among different localities within a state would tend to cancel out. The variance among states would be local variance divided by the number of counties. Now suppose that local outcomes are not independent, that affluence leads to affluence and attracts doctors, and rich areas create adjacent poor ones to serve them. Then there would be large local variance and smaller county or regional variances. But if deliberate efforts were made to equalize conditions, the variances might be much smaller and decrease over time.

Unemployment in Kansas counties is usually in the single digit range. It varied by less than 20 percent among the three metropolitan areas, about 142 percent across counties, but as much as threefold from zip code to zip code within Wichita alone.

For Kansan African Americans the unemployment rate was 12.3 percent in 1996. For zip code regions in northeast Wichita, composed predominantly of an African American population, the rate was 36 percent. The range of personal income is 30 percent of the average across states in the United States, 70 percent across counties in Kansas, and much higher (but not easily calculated) across zip codes. From the 12 counties with more than 200 African Americans, per capita income was 53 percent of that of whites. In those same counties, African Americans were only 38 percent as likely as whites to own their own homes; the same income does not go as far for blacks as for whites. Health outcomes show a similar pattern. Thus, in Sedgwick County total infant mortality was 10.9 deaths per 1,000 live births, compared to 7 per 1,000 for the state as a whole. For African Americans, infant mortality is about double that of whites, as are the rates of perinatal death and low birth weight. The county infant mortality rates are higher for African Americans than for whites (28.6 and 10.9 per 1,000 live births, respectively). Both these rates are above Havana's rate of 7.9 per 1,000 (11). The rate for the whole county is slightly above that of Isla de la Juventud (Cuba's worst province). In 1994, African American men died an average of 14.1 years earlier than whites, and African American women died 10.3 years earlier. African Americans are the largest minority in Kansas, and therefore the easiest to study, but we have the impression that similar patterns occur for Hispanic, Native American, and some of the Asian populations. Minorities suffer from a systematic structure of unequal power and disadvantage in addition to prejudice. These discrepancies then remain a problem in Kansas, as well as in the rest of the United States.

In the course of travel in Kansas we were sometimes told of local disease clusters such as multiple sclerosis or cancer that were discovered when old friends got together and discussed "whatever happened to . . . ?" Although clusters may sometimes be the random events that inevitably show up in small samples, a pattern of local clustering may indicate the focal distribution of insults and therefore has to be examined as a pattern rather than case by case. In this work, nonprofessional neighborhood groups are especially important in observing anomalies and tracing their sources.

Different diseases show different degrees of variability. Consider the major causes of death across counties in Kansas and provinces in Cuba (Table 3). Heart disease varies geographically more than does cancer in both countries. This difference also is seen in comparing the responsiveness of the two diseases to socioeconomic indicators (Table 2) and even over time. In Cuba, the economy experienced abrupt changes in the late 1980s with the sudden loss of favorable and stable prices and long-term trade relations with the Soviet bloc. This affected all health indicators, but particularly heart disease, and diabetes more than cancer.

The average values of the death rates are comparable for the two countries except for cancer, but the variabilities are strikingly different. Until we have obtained the data for other states and nations we are unable to assign the differences in variability to general economic and social conditions or the uniform availability of health care in Cuba.

A second aspect of geographic variation is the correlations of disease prevalences among Kansas counties across regions. Gopal Singh and colleagues (8) have found that the major causes of death showed positive correlations among them, averaging .47 (Table 4). The same thing holds for hospital admissions for different causes. There are counties where the risk of hospitalization is consistently above that for the state for almost all causes of admission. These are diseases that are not closely related in terms of medical "cause." The correlation

Table 3

Mean values and range/mean for causes of death over Kansas counties, 1988–1993, and Cuban provinces, 1995[a,b]

	Kansas		Cuba	
Cause of death	Mean	Range/mean	Mean	Range/mean
IHD	208.3	2.19	200.9	0.63
Cancer	203	1.35	132.9	0.51
COPD	40	2.37	9[c]	1.57
Cirr.	6.6	4.09	8.2	0.95
Inf.	14.4	3.40	13.4	0.83
P & I	36.6	4.29	34.1	1.21

[a]Source: data for Cuba from reference 11.

[b]The death rates in Kansas and Cuba are comparable except for a lower cancer rate in Cuba, but the variabilities differ. Abbreviations as in Table 1.

[c]The Cuban data are for bronchitis, emphysema, and asthma.

Table 4

Correlations matrix for major causes of death, Kansas[a,b]

	IHD	Cancer	COPD	Cirr.	Inf.	P & I
IHD		.86	.70	.27	.13	.79
Cancer			.77	.34	.37	.77
COPD				.36	.34	.65
Cirr.					.44	.29
Inf.						.26
Average	.55	.62	.57	.34	.30	.55

[a]Source: Singh (1997, unpublished data).

[b]The average is the average correlation between a given disease and all the others. Infectious diseases are least correlated with the other diseases, and cancer is most strongly connected to the others. Abbreviations as in Table 1.

may have two explanations. First, the precipitating factors may be correlated. For instance, poor household water sources may both be contaminated with pesticides and carry intestinal bacteria. The second explanation is that despite a large number of possible insults to the body, we confront them with relatively few kinds of defenses: the integrity of the epithelium of the digestive, reproductive, and respiratory systems; cellular and humoral immunity; sympathetic/parasympathetic balance; the inflammation response; perhaps half a dozen pathways of detoxification in the liver; excretion by the kidneys of solubilized toxins. Social-environmental factors concentrated by poverty, relative privation, or other conditions that undermine any of these defenses will make people more vulnerable to different kinds of precipitating factors, whether infectious or not. Then diseases might be classified by the bodily defenses required to fight an insult rather than by the precipitating agent or the organ affected.

Consider the correlations among causes of death across Kansas counties and Cuban provinces (Table 5). The correlations look remarkably similar for heart disease with cancer, respiratory disease, and cirrhosis and for cancer with respiratory disease, but correlations with influenza are strikingly different. Kansas partakes of the U.S. influenza immunization program, while Cuba has no such program. Therefore any correlations that depend on uneven medical access, with more flu shots in the same counties having more available treatment of other diseases, would disappear in Cuba. We do not yet know why the correlation between cancer and liver disease is different in the two countries. One possibility is that in Kansas, evangelical Christian churches that prohibit smoking also prohibit drinking alcohol, risk factors for cancer and liver disease, respectively. This connection may be weaker in Cuba.

Table 5

Correlations among causes of death across Kansas counties and Cuban provinces[a]

	Kansas	Cuba
Heart/cancer	.86	.65
Heart/respiratory	.70	.58
Heart/liver	.27	.28
Heart/influenza	.79	.04
Cancer/respiratory	.77	.78
Cancer/liver	.34	.07
Cancer/influenza	.77	0.0
Respiratory/liver	.36	.78
Respiratory/influenza	.65	.08

[a]The association between diseases that are not medically related indicates either a social correlation of the exposures or that our body depends on similar defenses to confront both. Heart disease, cancer, and respiratory disease form one cluster in both Kansas and Cuba, and the other conditions (liver disease, influenza) are more loosely associated with these. The big discrepancy between Kansas and Cuba in the correlations of influenza with other diseases may reflect the absence of an annual flu immunization program in Cuba.

As the social determinants of disease are likely to have different patterns in the two countries (for instance, education is less linked to income and varies much less in Cuba than in Kansas) (12), this would lead us to expect different correlations among diseases although some correlations are similar. The close correlations among heart disease and cancer also hold up across social indicators in Kansas and over time in Cuba. This finding may give support to the idea that certain social circumstances undermine the same defense systems even for very different diseases in quite different societies. At this stage, we have only the first hints derived from this new research tool analyzing multiple disease rates and correlations in widely disparate societies.

The Reality of History

People, like all systems, respond to their experiences and are changed thereby. But these changes take place at different rates. We are familiar with the use of a child's weight-for-height to measure acute malnutrition because this measure changes on a scale of weeks to months, whereas height-for-age measures the accumulated nutrition over a life time. The risk of lung cancer responds over months to years when someone stops smoking. People's situations therefore reflect different aspects of their past with different rates of erasure.

If history is important in determining health, then the direction and amount of change in a county should be relevant for predicting outcomes as well as the present state. In collaboration with Gopal Singh at the Kansas Health Institute, we have prepared an index of decline which measures the loss of population and farms, growing poverty, increased school dropout rate, and other aspects of a region in decline. The health implications of this index have not yet been analyzed, but the index identifies counties mostly in the southeastern and central parts of Kansas that are in serious decline. We hypothesize that high rates of decline are correlated with high prevalence of disease.

For behavior too, we should look not only at someone's present social location but also whether that person is moving upward or downward or sideways. Behavior depends on different time horizons. Only when people have had the experience that what they do now affects what happens to them later can they make long-term health-promoting decisions. But this time horizon of efficacy is itself socially influenced, linked to socioeconomic position, gender, and race. If we aim to affect health behavior, we have to examine the circumstances that generate behavior and understand the relation of choice to non-choice. Choices are always made from among alternatives presented by the social environment, or by circumstances that were themselves not chosen. Choice depends on the tools for making choices, the outer edge of people's aspirations as they have been encouraged or dampened by past experience. When we recognize the elements of non-choice in choice,.we can escape from the contradiction between social causation and individual responsibility and understand the interactiveness of the two, and thus see the individual as a unique particle in a social field.

The Significance of the Material Environment

While emphasizing the neglected domain of social determination of health, we do not reject or ignore ecological and physical factors that interpenetrate with them. It is necessary to restate that health is created and eroded in an ecosocial/physical world, and that the artificial separation of "environmental" from social aspects of these processes can only weaken our understanding and interfere with efforts to reduce health-undermining conditions in our lives.

In this context, we mean by "environment" all conditions that arise outside the body, whether these reach us inadvertently, despite our efforts, or through choices we or others make. At the most elementary level, the case for environmental determination of health and disease includes the following observations.

1. *The geography of cancer, as related to the location of industry and agriculture.* The highest rates of cancer mortality in the United States are in the

"rust belt" of the midwest, the lower Mississippi valley, and the northeast. The high rates of cancer mortality occur across all age groups. In Kansas, cancer rates tend to be higher in counties with more agricultural activity. Other studies have shown that farmers exposed to the herbicide atrazine suffer elevated rates of several cancers. These geographic areas are not distinguishable from the rest of the country in their degree of social inequality, poverty levels, or less tangible indicators.

2. *The history of disease, with cancer rates following industrialization and the chemicalization of agriculture.* The increases in cancer occur across all age groups.

3. *Changes in disease rates among immigrant groups in the generations following immigration.* The changes are shifts from the rates in the country of origin toward the rates in the immigrants' new locations.

4. *The association of diseases with occupations as well as with ranks within an occupation.*

5. *The distribution of cancer across species:*

• Geographically, concentrating in areas where human cancers are most common.

• Across ecological guilds, with bottom-feeding fish and predators (eating the detritus where the pollutants concentrate or prey that have already concentrated pollutants) showing higher rates than open ocean feeders.

• In laboratory studies with animals exposed to specific chemicals. Although all species have their own unique sensitivities, which may prevent us from attributing specific cancers in humans to specific chemicals, the fact of differential sensitivity among species does not make us systematically less vulnerable than others. The case for chemical carcinogenesis is strong even where a direct one-to-one linking of specific chemical concentrations to disease prevalence is not possible.

Water quality is the primary environmental threat to Kansas health. Almost half the private drinking water wells are contaminated with coliform bacteria, and 17 percent with the herbicide atrazine (13) which is associated with non-Hodgkin's lymphoma in farmers (14). Atrazine is also suspected of disrupting the human endocrine system.

Despite a strong inferential case for the role of the environment in causing major diseases, classical epidemiological studies are inconsistent with each other or often inconclusive. This paradox is not a good reason to dismiss environmental causation but rather urges us to examine why epidemiological studies are so often inconsistent or inconclusive. Among the problems are the failure to take feedback into account in the modeling, frequent omission of women and minorities in the studies, and the inability to disentangle multiple causes and their interactions in causing illness.

But the recognition of physical environmental factors does not detract in any way from the importance of social determination. The outstanding conclusion of this area of study is that social stratification, by education and income, and injustice are the critical factors that detract from the health of our population. Variations in health within a population are an epidemiological issue. When we look more closely we see that the relationship between the social and physical environments has several nuances:

(*a*) Populations that are poor, marginalized and discriminated against have higher exposures to pollutants, lower-quality food, and more dangerous jobs. The regulatory agencies are slower to identify the exposures in these communities and are more tolerant in the corrective measures they impose (15).

(*b*) Poor people are already more vulnerable to disease due to marginal diets, higher stress, hopelessness, the anxiety of dangerous neighborhood, the basic insecurity of life. Those of us who have never lived in marginal circumstances, or have forgotten the experience after escaping, often oversimplify the pervasiveness of deprived and subordinate social condition. At the margin of their tolerance, all species are more vulnerable to almost all perturbations.

(*c*) Cigarettes, alcohol, fatty and sweet foods, and sedentary activities are embedded in our culture and aggressively promoted by advertising so that they become powerful "environmental" factors. Stressful circumstances make these habits attractive for short-term relief.

(*d*) Diet is "chosen." But the choice is constrained by prices, availability in neighborhoods, the shortage of time for food preparation or for meals, and the shortened time horizon of control over one's life that poor people experience. The distancing from dietary health information is a response to just one more exhortation to do something additional that is difficult.

(*e*) Attitudes of hopelessness, anxiety, a short time horizon, and so forth, are derived from real experience, including the experience of frequent illness, chronic poor health, and little power to plan what happens later. Although not everybody in adverse circumstances exhibits these characteristics, they are stronger if reinforced by experience. Focusing on why some individuals respond to adversity in more productive or less productive ways can divert us from asking the bigger question about the adversity itself and ways to change it.

(*f*) Collective action could and sometimes does remedy environmental exposures, but disadvantaged neighborhoods also have less political influence and fewer resources for organizing (15).

None of these nuances negates the importance of social factors. Society creates the exposures to physical factors both by producing them and by directing them at particular populations. Social conditions produce the differential vulnerability of communities and provide the resources, knowledge, and confidence to affect exposures. In run-down neighborhoods, the ugliness, noise, and smell affect people's sense of well-being, which in turn affects health and creates a consciousness of despair, irrelevance, and impotence.

Organisms select, transform, and define their environments; the environments thus created form the organisms and therefore the next round of selecting, transforming, and defining processes. The inseparability of social, ecological, physical, chemical, and biotic environments is a crucial framework for a whole-system approach to health.

Looking Critically at Our Own Science

Public health is a historically evolving system with its own agenda and preferred solutions to problems. The principle that things are the way they are because they got that way has to be applied to public health as well. Then we can see the ways in which the present pattern of knowledge and ignorance is not a spontaneous consequence of some problems being harder than others, but rather a consequence of intellectual choices encouraged by the fragmentation of disciplines and institutions, the structures of reward and recognition, the financing of research in order to find marketable commodities, and unacknowledged constraints on the investigations, conditions that are accepted as givens without question.

The effect of recent economic changes on research should be a major concern of our community since it will determine the "self-evident" truths of the next decades. We also look at our own sciences and institutions when we ask: "Can this really be done? Can we adopt a whole-system approach?"

We can only answer this question by looking at the opposing processes at work. On the one hand, the internal intellectual needs of science move us increasingly toward the greater inclusiveness of our problems and our theoretical frameworks. This is expressed through conferences, books, and programs that emphasize inter-, multi- or trans-disciplinary frameworks. On the other hand, the economic changes in the knowledge industry promote fragmentation of knowledge, jealousy about boundaries, an emphasis on short-term results that are easily commodified, a shift of accountability from the horizontal to the vertical, diminishing job security for researchers, a business-type structure of rewards and recognition, and the growing corporate influence in university life. All these factors work against the kind of whole-system approach discussed here.

A Note on Children

Children share the same needs as adults as well as having unique needs. The same needs include food and shelter, and poverty is the major obstacle here. Poverty affects children even before birth, as shown by the association of poverty with birth defects, low birth weight, and infant mortality, and after birth at all ages. Children are more vulnerable than adults to external insult.

1. Their immune systems are not yet developed.
2. Vulnerability to insults of many kinds is usually greatest for tissues that are actively differentiating or growing, have a rapid throughput of nutrients and toxins, and have a large surface to volume ratio.
3. Children lack many of the behavioral options for avoiding harm, because of physical strength and stature and their limited knowledge and experience.

One way of describing variability is to subtract the minimum value from the maximum and divide by the average value (Table 6).[2] Infant mortality varies by about 145 percent across U.S. states and 264 percent across Kansas counties (Table 7 on p. 452). Child mortality (ages 0–14) varies across counties by 180 percent, mortality for ages 15–24 varies 350 percent, but total age-adjusted death rates vary by only 73 percent across states and 59 percent across counties. And, for people over 75 years, the death rate varies by only 43 percent. We look at the variability because it tells us that some conditions that cause this mortality are varying geographically and therefore can be ameliorated with a substantial improvement in health. All of these variations are associated with social and economic conditions, but a small difference in economic resources has a bigger impact on children (Table 7).

While social conditions vary and affect children, state-organized efforts to protect children are allocated more equitably and therefore show less variation. For example, the immunization rate for children across counties varies by 86 percent. In the more thorough Cuban immunization program there is almost no variation; the centralized reporting and absence of private physicians make for reliable data.

Although the average outcomes are comparable in Kansas and in Cuba, the variability is much greater in Kansas so that 51 Kansas counties have higher infant mortality than Cuba, and 27 of them do more poorly than Cuba's worst-off province of Isla de la Juventud. Furthermore, the variability has been increasing for Kansas and the United States as a whole but remaining steady for Cuba.

About a fourth of the private wells in Kansas are contaminated with nitrate. Nitrates are a particular risk to children, causing blue baby syndrome when a child is deprived of oxygen by nitrates in the blood. Nitrates are also associated with risks of spontaneous abortion and gastric cancer (16, 17). We cannot determine how many children are affected since physicians are not required to report cases to any data center. However, water quality seems to be an urgent environmental health issue in Kansas.

[2] For technical reasons, the coefficient of variation, equal to the standard deviation divided by the average, is a more appropriate measure for statistical testing since it is not sensitive to the sample size. But for a nontechnical audience, the relative range has a more intuitive meaning. Table 6 shows that the qualitative conclusions are similar for both measures.

Table 6

Age-adjusted mean values, range/mean, and coefficients of variation (CV) for selected causes of death and low birth weight, Kansas and Cuba[a]

	Kansas			Cuba		
	Mean	Range/mean	CV	Mean	Range/mean	CV
IHD	167.8	0.85	13.8	159.8	0.34	12
Cancer	120.4	0.70	13.6	111.0	0.36	9.0
Cirrhosis	4.85	3.28	58.7	6.8	1.02	32.5
Diabetes	10.78	2.44	41.2	18.8	1.84	43.2
IMR[b]	7.81	2.91	63.2	7.9	0.60	18.2
LBW[b]	5.87	1.72	28.1	7.0	0.56	13.8

[a]Kansas data for 1988–95 (except as noted) from Singh (unpublished), unweighted (that is, each county given equal weight in averaging). Cuban data for 1996 from reference 11, age adjusted. Means for Cuba are the national means, but variation was calculated using the unweighted means over provinces. The differences are small. IHD, ischemic heart disease; IMR, infant mortality rate; LBW, low birth weight.

[b]Kansas data for 1989–93.

As mammals, we are born partly formed. Our development depends on regularly occurring environmental factors that have become incorporated into our developmental biology. The development of vision requires light. The development of muscles and bone requires exercise. Brain development requires stimulation. Intellectual development needs challenge. Emotional and social development require touch, attention, and loving care. Light is almost always available. The other influences reach the child first through the immediate caregivers, then through increasingly widening concentric circles of more numerous but less intense contacts with other people. Many children do not have these needs met.

Therefore, a childhood program must first address inequity and inadequate income. Without such efforts, attempts to mitigate consequences of inadequate income, such as low parental education levels, will be thwarted. We have to support the caregivers in their homes with the skills, knowledge, and social support to provide effective early care. In an economy that increasingly requires two wage earners to barely keep up with a family's survival needs, and certainly to strive for some advancement in life, we have to reduce the contradiction between the demands of home and paid work, invent ways of making work child-friendly so that parents can jointly attend to their children at those times when it is especially necessary, and allow for the special needs of individual children. Finally, we have to improve organized care in daycare enrichment facilities and schools, providing material resources, training for caregivers, and the remuneration, autonomy, and respect that qualified and committed professional caregivers deserve and that can assure the quality of the care.

Table 7

Geographic variation in infant mortality rate and low birth weight rate, United States, Kansas, and Cuba[a]

	Mean IMR or LBW over regions	Minimum	Maximum	Range/ mean
U.S. states				
IMR, 1980	12.6	9.2 Maine	25 Washington, D.C.	125%
IMR, 1995	7.6	5.2 Mass.	16.2 Washington, D.C.	145%
LBW, 1970	7.9	5.7 N. Dakota	12.5 Washington, D.C.	86%
LBW, 1995	7.3	5.3 Alaska, N. Dakota	13.4 Washington, D.C.	111%
Kansas counties				
IMR, 1966–70	19.0	3.1 Decatur	51.5 Hamilton	255%
IMR, 1989–93	8.6	0 Several counties	22.7 Chautaqua	264%
LBW, 1981–83	6.2	1.9 Phillips, Republic	9.6 Clark	124%
LBW, 1991–93	6.4	1.9 Republic	12.0 Wallace	158%
Cuba provinces				
IMR, 1975	27.5	18.8 Villa Clara	35.1 Ciego de Avila	59%
IMR, 1996	7.9	5.4 Cienfuegos	10.3 Isla de la Juventud	60%
LBW, 1977	10.6	7.3 Sancti Spiritus	11.9 Granma	43%
LBW, 1996	7.0	4.9 Havana	8.9 Guantanamo	54%

[a]IMR = infant mortality rate; LBW = low birth weight (less than 2,500 grams). The range is maximum – minimum value.

TOWARD A SYNTHESIS

Health is produced and eroded in a natural and social environment that varies in time and space and according to the social locations of people in various hierarchical, cooperative, and competitive relationships. External influences—chemical, physical, and microbial—impinge on us in a pattern that depends on how we produce and consume goods and use our time. What happens next depends on the coping mechanisms that we develop in the course of a lifetime. The external becomes part of the internal; previous experience alters our body and mind and our behavior in ways that influence how we respond to the next encounter. Our own physiological and psychological processes erase these impacts, some of them rapidly, some slowly, and some so slowly that they have permanent effects on us. But the internal also becomes external, as our own activity selects, transforms, and even defines our environment. For the most part, this pattern was not constructed with health in mind. The health consequences are essentially random, side effects of economic and social processes. But their consequences have become so powerful and pervasive that we now have to intervene in social development with health and well-being in mind.

The chain of events leading to disease includes four major contexts.

1. *The precipitating factors.* These are the familiar microorganisms, chemicals, and stressors, often referred to carelessly as the "causes" of disease. They tend to be highly specific, respond to particular climatic and ecological conditions, fluctuate with changing technologies and economic activity, and, in the case of microorganisms, adapt to what we do. Thus these factors are responsible for the ways in which different diseases have very individual distributions. Most research has been directed toward these factors and has provided some of our most dramatic successes. But the research is mostly on a case-by-case, disease-by-disease basis that does not see the whole pattern of our relations to the rest of nature, or prepare us for surprises. Here the most urgent task is to broaden research to consider the evolutionary ecology of disease. An analysis of health impacts must be incorporated into the design of technology so that the engineers prioritize health improvement as a goal—"If we don't need it and we can't get rid of it, don't make it!"

2. *The context of exposure.* These factors have intermediate specificity. The exposures to pesticides and toxins, to poor diet, to food poisoning, and to high-stress occupations are unevenly distributed across class and racial lines, with marginalized and disadvantaged communities having worse health outcomes for pretty much everything. Here the major tasks are tasks of promoting community action for equity and the consideration of the health impact of land use, urban planning, sanitation, and food-processing technologies.

3. *The context of vulnerability.* The factors of vulnerability are more generic because they depend on the same relatively small number of protective mechanisms in the body and in society: poverty and toxic exposures undermine health in general, a heart-friendly diet is also preventive of cancer, a sense of control over one's own life can help to avoid cirrhosis and lung cancer, racism can raise blood pressure and depress the immune system. These conditions give rise to correlated distributions among diseases that are not related medically and can be studied comparatively. This is a domain where individual and collective responsibilities interpenetrate most strongly, where empowerment and education can be most effective, and where the democratization of public health is most urgent.

4. *Context of therapy.* Medical care is not relevant to all disease and cannot claim credit for most of the expansion of life expectancy. Sometimes ignorance prevents effective therapy. Then we have to examine how the political economy of research and the culture of the research community created the present pattern

of knowledge and ignorance. Sometimes medical decisions are influenced by nonmedical considerations or are guided more by custom and fashion than by validated research. Sometimes effective practices such as prenatal care and childhood immunization are simply not available to everyone. Current changes in health care delivery and the deskilling of the health professions threaten to undermine both the quality of care and its availability.

SOME CONCLUSIONS AND PROVISIONAL RECOMMENDATIONS

Among the U.S. states, Kansas health occupies a middling position. The United States as a whole does rather poorly among the developed countries and in some ways even compared to some developing countries. And the whole world does more poorly, and is less prepared to face inevitable change, than any lack of material or intellectual resources could excuse.

This preliminary report maps out some of the dimensions of health problems in Kansas and begins to develop an approach for looking at the whole. We have some firm conclusions, some plausible inferences, and some mere hints. Therefore our recommendations include suggestions for how to think about the issues, some specific proposals for implementing these ideas, and a perspective on future research.

There are several things we can do to correct this situation and to take seriously the international goals of the Alma-Ata conference on health for all.

First, think big. We have to pose a question big enough to accommodate an answer. For public health this means seeing the system in the large, including areas that are outside its traditional boundaries but have major effects on us: agriculture, environmental protection, industrial design, urban development, and education. A first step would be a consultative conference and continuing group drawn from public and private agencies in all these fields. Our research program would move on to integrate analyses in these separate fields into a whole-systems model of Kansas health. Its goal would be a coherent policy to make Kansas a more healthful place.

Second, the variability of health outcomes across geographic areas, social groups, and occupations means that conditions that vary within Kansas affect health in major ways. Therefore we can set as preliminary goals the raising of health outcomes within the state to the level of the best achieved anywhere in the state:

- All counties can be as healthy as the five healthiest counties.
- Minorities can aim at health indicators equal to the health status of the majority white population.
- All occupations can aim at the health levels of the safest jobs.
- All people could have their risk profiles improved to the level of those with average income.

The more variable a health outcome over geographic areas or social indicators, the more can be gained by bringing the whole state up to the level of its best. When this is achieved, death rates will be reduced by some 20 percent.

This would be only a first step: we could also aim to reach the levels of the healthiest states in the Union and help our country rise to the level of the healthiest countries in Europe.

Our country is now rich enough to aspire to a rising standard of living, not so much through increased consumption of energy and materials as through investing in healthful habitats and even in designing production, not to minimize damage, but in such a way that work is fulfilling and health enhancing and even joyful.

One way to contribute to this process is to place rising and equitable health on the national and state agendas and to make it impossible for any candidates for public office to ignore the health needs of the population. Our research would pursue the analysis of the variability of health outcomes to identify possible areas of intervention. It would look at geographic patterns to answer such questions as why relative risks of hospitalization for many causes are greater, and deaths from specific diseases are earlier, in the southwest part of the state. Clusters of health problems below the county level will be examined in detail.

Third, all diseases are unique but also similar. Each has its own precipitating agent, its etiology and possible therapy. Traditional medicine and public health epidemiology emphasize the uniqueness of each disease at the expense of the generality. But we have shown that there are strong correlations among diseases that are not related medically. These correlations hold over geographic regions in very different societies, across time when conditions change rapidly, and over social indicators. Similar factors affect our exposure or vulnerability to the major causes of death. The study of these patterns is a powerful research tool. It also suggests that health-enhancing measures that improve our resistance to one disease also improve our resistance to other diseases. We will develop comparative and correlational analyses to find out why the prevalences of medically unrelated diseases are often closely associated, and what measures might ameliorate multiple risks at the same time.

Therefore, taking on the bigger problem of improving health is not simply adding to a growing list of things to do for a growing list of problems. The problems of poverty, inequity, pollution, poor diet, unhealthful work and rest regimens, and inadequate health education affect health as a whole. Their improvement would improve health as a whole. And the inclusion of the other agencies with responsibilities in other areas of life increases the resources available.

An effective policy requires good theory. In order to have a valid theory of public health we have to challenge the traditional boundaries. We have to recognize inequality, class hierarchy, racism, regional decline, and social fragmentation as pathogenic agents central to our analysis. This requires a revision of our conceptualization, data collecting, and methods of interpretation.

We have to expand the way we analyze data, sometimes in exquisite microscopic detail, sometimes stepping back to see global patterns, always taking into account that the system is an integrated whole, with feedbacks, time lags, multilevel connections, sinks and sources. Our research will develop the mathematical methodology for interpreting this. We especially have to examine why so many epidemiological studies are inconclusive or inconsistent with each other.

We not only have to examine present-day health problems but also anticipate what might happen; instead of waiting for surprises, we need a program to prepare for uncertainty as a permanent fact of life. Our research will identify potential problems of disease emergence and resurgence, and strategies for confronting the specific emergencies that Kansas health might have to face.

We have to democratize health research and policy so that professional technical skill and theoretical structures can be combined with people's detailed, intimate, and intricate knowledge about their own circumstances. Our research will focus on the mobilization of untapped intelligence in our communities so that policies jointly arrived at can be jointly implemented. We need to encourage mechanisms such as town meetings, conferences of community groups, surveys, focus groups, and after-school clubs, to explore problems, develop solutions, and carry them out so that every Kansas county can be as healthy as the best counties.

Acknowledgments — This work (supported by the Kansas Health Foundation) reports on a preliminary scouting of the needs of public health in Kansas and more broadly. It reflects the joint work of a group of investigators—Jarvis Chen, Department of Health and Social Behavior, Harvard School of Public Health; Rae Lewis, University of New Mexico; and Katherine Worster, The Land Institute, based in Salina, Kansas. We had the cooperation of many people in public and private institutions in Kansas. We are especially indebted to Dr. Gopal Singh and Dr. Elizabeth Saadi, with whom interviews developed into full collaborations on aspects of our research.

Note — This chapter is adapted from the 1998 Robert H. Ebert Lecture, published by the Kansas Health Foundation, Wichita, Kansas, 1998.

REFERENCES

1. Himmelstein, D. U., and Woolhandler, S. *The National Health Program Book.* Common Courage Press, Monroe, Me., 1994.
2. Rapport, D., et al. *Ecosystem Health.* Blackwell Science Publishers, London, 1998.
3. Amick, B. C. *Society and Health.* Oxford University Press, New York, 1995.
4. Wilkinson, R. G. *Unhealthy Societies: The Afflictions of Inequality.* Routledge, London, 1996.
5. Hegel, G. W. F. *Hegel's Philosophy of Right.* G. Bell, London, 1896.

6. Wallace, R., and Wallace, D. Community marginalization and the diffusion of disease and disorder in the United States. *BMJ* 314: 1341–1345, 1997.
7. Levins, R. Preparing for uncertainty. *Ecosystem Health* 1(1): 47–57, 1995.
8. Singh G., et al. *Health and Social Factors in Kansas: A Data and Chartbook 1997–1998.* Kansas Health Institute, Topeka, 1998.
9. Frey, R. S. Cancer mortality in Kansas farmers. *Trans. Kansas Acad. Sci.* 99(1–2), 1996.
10. Himmelstein, D. U., Levins, R., and Woolhandler, S. Beyond our means: Patterns of variability of physiological traits. *Int. J. Health Serv.* 20(1): 115–124, 1990.
11. Ministerio de Salud Publica, Republica de Cuba. *Anuario Estadistico.* 1996.
12. Diaz, B. Cuba: modelo de desarrollo equitativo. In *Sistemas Politicas, Poder y Sociedad (Estudios de Casos en America Latina).* Nueva Sociedad, Caracas, 1992.
13. *Kansas Environmental Almanac.* 1996.
14. Zahm, S. H., et al. Role of the herbicide atrazine in the development of non-Hodgkins' lymphoma. *Scand. J. Work Environ. Health* 19: 108, 1993.
15. Gerrard, M. B. *Whose Backyard, Whose Risk? Fear and Fairness in Toxic and Nuclear Waste Siting.* Massachusetts Institute of Technology Press, Cambridge, Mass., 1994.
16. Lee, Y. W., Dahab, M. F., and Bogardi, I. Nitrate risk management under uncertainty. *J. Water Resources Plann. Manage.* 118(2): 151, 1992.
17. Spontaneous abortions possibly related to ingestion of nitrate-contaminated well water—Lagrange County Indiana, 1991–94. *Morb. Mortal. Wkly. Rep.,* 1996.

ADDITIONAL SOURCES

Ewald, P. Cultural vectors, virulence and the emergence of evolutionary epidemiology. *Oxf. Surv. Evolutionary Biol.* 5: 215–245, 1988.

Kansas Department of Health and Environment. *Occupational Injury and Illness.* Topeka, 1995.

Levins, R. Toward an integrated epidemiology. *Trends Ecol. Evolution,* 1997.

McMichael, A. J. *Planetary Overload.* Cambridge University Press, Cambridge, England, 1993.

CHAPTER 20

DEVELOPMENT AND QUALITY OF LIFE: A CRITIQUE OF AMARTYA SEN'S *DEVELOPMENT AS FREEDOM*

Vicente Navarro

WHAT IS THE GOAL OF DEVELOPMENT?

Thank you so much for inviting me to discuss Amartya Sen's *Development As Freedom* (1). As a researcher who has worked for many years on the relationship between development and well being, I read this book with great pleasure. It centers on some of the issues I have been working on most of my life. The pleasure of reading the book was accompanied by the enjoyment of being exposed to a very well-thought-out argument that goes against the major position upheld by some of the most influential and powerful institutions working on development today. Indeed, Sen's main objective is to dismantle the widely held position, constantly reproduced by the World Bank, the International Monetary Fund, the U.S. White House, the U.S. State Department, the U.S. Agency for International Development, and many other international and U.S. agencies, that the best way for a country to develop is to increase its rate of economic growth. I am aware of the growing differences among these institutions on the question of how development policies should be realized. I am also particularly aware of the growing distance between the World Bank and the International Monetary Fund on the means of achieving development; but these two institutions share the basic assumption that, in a fast-growing economy, whatever is produced at the top trickles down to all members of society, improving the lot of the majority of a country's people. This position, which has reached the level of dogma, is what Amartya Sen calls—accurately, I believe—"conventional wisdom among the economic developmentalists" (1, p. 6).

I should indicate right away that this conventional wisdom had its share of critics from its very beginning, I being one of them. Actually, the first investigation I carried out in my academic career, back in the 1960s, was on the impact of what was then called the "economic miracle" of Brazil on the quality of life of that country's people (2). As you may recall, the economic literature on development was full of articles highly laudatory of the Brazilian economy during the period 1968–1981, when that country had a very high rate of economic growth. The Brazilian economy seemed to be doing very well indeed—but what about the Brazilian people? The data I studied and published showed that while the economy was indeed doing very well, the people were not doing so well. In fact, infant mortality was growing rather than declining, as one would have expected if economic growth were benefiting all Brazilians. The infant mortality increased quite dramatically during that period, from 70 infant deaths per 1,000 live births at the beginning of the "miracle" to 92 per 1,000 at the end. That increase could not be explained by improvements in the system of collecting vital statistics in Brazil. I checked on this possibility; no major changes had occurred on that front. The reason for the spectacular increase in infant mortality had to be sought elsewhere—that is, in the general deterioration in the standard of living (as measured by available disposable income) of the majority of the Brazilian population, accompanied by a very significant reduction in social public expenditures during that period. These two sets of variables were the root of the problem: a most substantial redistribution of wealth and income in Brazil during the economic "miracle," a redistribution not from the top down but from the bottom up. For the top 5 percent of the Brazilian population, the percentage of national consumption increased from 20 percent at the beginning of the "miracle" to 48 percent by the end; for the bottom 50 percent of the Brazilian population, consumption declined from 20 to 12 percent over this period. This is why infant mortality was increasing.

The detailed analysis I conducted showed what was actually happening: the top income groups were doing very well; their incomes were increasing so rapidly that even though the income of the majority was declining, Brazil's average GNP per capita was growing dramatically. Rather than a trickle down of resources, Brazil was experiencing a sucking up of resources from the bottom to the top, impoverishing and lowering the quality of life of Brazilians at the bottom, as indicated by the growth of infant mortality. While my report did have some impact in Latin America (where I was working as a consultant to the U.N. Socioeconomic Planning Council at that time, on leave from Hopkins), it had no impact whatsoever in the United States. In fact, not one U.S. academic journal to which I submitted the article wanted to publish it.

With this biographical note, you can understand why I was so pleased that the Nobel Memorial Prize in Economic Science was finally awarded (in 1998) to a person who was saying, in a far more elegant and convincing way than I ever could, what I had been saying for over 35 years: that measuring the rate of economic growth is different from measuring development. I was, I repeat, delighted that the committee granting the Nobel Prize in economics was finally acknowledging that the primary objective of development is not to stimulate and facilitate economic growth and, equally important, that economic growth does not necessarily lead to better development. These two fairly basic propositions represent a break and a confrontation with the dominant developmentalist thesis, which, as I noted earlier, has been very influential in the major international and national development agencies and, if I may add, in the committee that grants the Nobel Prize in Economic Science—until recently, that is, when a leading neoliberal Swedish economist, Professor Lindbek, resigned from the committee, which was no doubt a key factor in Sen's being granted the award.

Let me finish this introduction with a personal remark. I recently had the pleasure of meeting and debating with Professor Sen in a splendid setting, the Bocaccio Palace in Bologna, where we had been invited to a Seminar on Development by the Municipality of that city. Professor Sen is an extremely pleasant gentleman; it was a joy to talk and debate with him. I was very favorably impressed by his openness and willingness to debate, an attitude one rarely finds among recipients of the Nobel Prize in economics.

THE MAIN THESIS OF AMARTYA SEN

Let me now focus on Sen's thesis. He stresses in many parts of his book, in very strong terms, that the main objective of development is freedom: freedom is the goal of development (what he calls the *constitutive* role of freedom), by which he means the capability to develop one's own potential, unrestrained by circumstances outside one's control. Freedom is thus understood as developing one's own capabilities. But for Sen, freedom is even more than the objective of development; it is also the means of achieving that development. He thus considers freedom as instrumental in, or an instrument of, development, and he designates as *instrumental* freedoms the following five freedoms:

1. *Political freedom,* which refers to "the opportunity that people have to determine who should govern and on what principles and also includes the possibility to scrutinize and criticize authorities, to have freedom of political expression and an uncensored press, to enjoy the freedom to choose between different political parties and so on" (1, p. 38).
2. *Economic facilities,* which refer to the ability to have, to own, and to use economic resources for the purpose of consumption, production, or exchange. In this freedom, Sen includes also the freedom to be involved in the market, by selling or buying labor or labor power and property. In this respect, Sen is a strong advocate of the market, not only as an instrument to generate information, but also as a human right in itself; he cites Adam Smith approvingly and extensively on this point (1, p. 39).
3. *Social opportunities,* which include education, health care, and other types of services and interventions important for allowing people to lead better lives and to participate effectively in economic and political activities (1, p. 39).

4. *Transparent guarantees,* by which Sen means openness and transparency in economic and political life, preventing corruption, financial irresponsibility, and underhanded dealings (1, p. 40).
5. *Protective security,* which is the social safety net that prevents people falling into misery, starvation, and even death, as well as preventing social exclusion (1, p. 40).

In reading Sen's description of these five freedoms, I recalled the famous five freedoms articulated by President Franklin Roosevelt in his address summoning the nation to a better future with the New Deal. You will recall President Roosevelt's five freedoms: freedom from hunger, freedom from ignorance and disease, freedom to organize and vote, freedom to choose among political options, and freedom from want and need. These freedoms were later written into the Universal Declaration of Human Rights of the United Nations, which explicitly refers to the right to life and liberty (understanding liberty as the right to freedom of organization and of opinion) as well as social and economic rights (including the right to work and to a fair wage, the right to health and health care, the right to education, and the right of secure retirement).

A major difference, however, between Roosevelt's five freedoms and Sen's five instrumental freedoms is that Roosevelt had a distinct priority in the ordering of the five freedoms. It was clear to Roosevelt (in his message to Congress on January 11, 1944) that "necessitous men are not free men," meaning that socioeconomic rights were a prerequisite for full realization of civil and political rights.

There is no such ordering of priorities in Sen's list, however. Sen refers frequently to the relationship among his five freedoms but never establishes a scale of relationships among them. He rightly criticizes those who see civil and political rights as independent of socioeconomic rights. And he also questions those who believe that the suspension of civil and political rights may be needed in developing countries in order to advance socioeconomic rights. But, having established the need for and interdependence among these rights, he nowhere explains the nature of the relationship or the reason for the interdependency. Only once does he explicitly state that basic needs such as the right to the minimum resources required to live take precedence over liberty. Sen does establish such a priority when he criticizes John Rawls for holding to the position that individual liberty is the most important norm in a just society. He rightly questions that priority by raising the obvious point—nowhere considered by Rawls—that in order to be free, you first need to be alive. But apart from this observation, made in passing, Sen never establishes the relationship among his five freedoms or the motor that moves all of them.

As I discuss shortly, I believe this is one of the major flaws of Sen's work. But it is not the only one. Another major weakness, related to the first, is the absence of a theory that could relate his five freedoms. In this respect, Sen moves within the classical economic tradition, based on Adam Smith, in which the individual is the subject and object of analysis; collective agents and subjects such as social classes do not appear, nor does any analysis of what articulates these collective agents such as exploitation or domination.

For Sen, the market is the major motor for change and improvement—subject, of course, to the active intervention and regulation of the state, which must correct the imperfections of the market and invest in people to enrich human capital and increase the power and ability to succeed in the market. But issues of power and how that power is reproduced are rarely, if ever, touched on. What I find surprising is that a work in which freedom and democracy play such a key role lacks an analysis of the political context of development. Sen's definition of democracy is therefore rather generic and his definition of dictatorship rather sketchy. For example, one of his key positions in favor of democracy, repeated in many parts of his book, is that "no democratic country has ever suffered famine," because democratic governments are afraid of the wide mobilizations that famine would awaken, which could topple them. The sustainability of such a position may depend on how we define the terms "democratic country" and "famine." But using Sen's definitions (which I will come back to later), we have to conclude that, even on empirical grounds, the position is not sustainable. Take just one example: Bangladesh, which happens to be Sen's country of birth, has had famines despite being, by Sen's definition, a democratic country. But before I present the empirical information, let me focus on what I consider the major problem of Sen's thesis: its limited conceptualization.

THE MAJOR PROBLEMS WITH SEN'S CONCEPTUALIZATION

Listing the five instrumental freedoms without explaining the frame in which the matrix of those freedoms is positioned seriously weakens Sen's analysis. This weakness is based on his reluctance to focus on the sources of power in a society and how that power is reproduced. Let me quickly say that I believe the sources of power in our societies are multiple. We constantly see expressions of class power, gender power, race power, national and regional power, and so forth. But this multiple focus of power does not mean that structurally, under capitalism, some powers are not more important than others. I believe that class power is the frame within which the power matrices operate. And class power is based primarily, as my good friend Eric Olin Wright has indicated, on ownership of resources, be they means of production, knowledge, or organization (3). Another point that merits clarification is that while class power is reproduced in many different spheres, the public sphere—that is, the state—plays a critical role. Actually, it was none other than Adam Smith, a major point of reference for Sen, who wrote in an infrequently cited passage of the *Wealth of Nations* "Civil government, so far as it is instituted for the security of property, is in reality instituted for the defense of the rich against the poor or of those who have some property against those who have none at all" (4, p. 149).

I believe Adam Smith's statement is too sketchy and simplistic. It has an instrumental view of the state reminiscent of Marx's famous dictum that the "state is the executive committee of the bourgeoisie." But, though reality is more complex than that, since the state is a synthesis of power relations, understanding class power relations is essential to an understanding of the nature of the state. And the state plays a critical role in reproducing class relations in any society. Adam Smith and Marx were not completely wrong after all; they were partly right.

State power and class power are not unrelated. Power, and thus class power, is what gives meaning to the freedoms Sen describes. When property such as land, or knowledge, or organization is highly concentrated, we can predict a serious limitation of civil and political rights and also of socioeconomic rights. Class power is also realized through the expression of political projects—and the absence of any discussion of this is the other great omission in Sen's work, an omission that is particularly odd given the enormous importance he gives to democracy as an instrument and an end of development. Democracy, liberty, and freedom are, like love, highly subjective categories; their meaning is in the eye of the beholder. Let me quote from one of the United States' greatest presidents, Abraham Lincoln (5, p. 12):

> We all declared for liberty; but in using the same word, we do not all mean the same thing. With some, the word liberty may mean for each to do as he pleases with himself, and the product of his labor; while with others the same word may mean for some men to do as they please with other men, and the product of other men's labor. Here are two, not only different, but incompatible things, called the same name, liberty. And it follows that the respective parties call each of the things by two different and incompatible names—liberty and tyranny.
>
> The shepherd drives the wolf from the sheep's throat, for which the sheep thanks the shepherd as his liberator, while the wolf denounces him for the same act, as the destroyer of liberty . . . plainly the sheep and the wolf are not agreed upon the definition of the word liberty.

Sen constantly refers to liberty and freedom without once making reference to the political context that gives them meaning. One cannot equate Fidel Castro's dictatorial regime, for example, with Augusto Pinochet's dictatorial regime. Both regimes are dictatorships. But the first is run by a political party with a social base, historical rooting, and political context completely different from that of the second. To put them both in the same box is not fair to either. The Cuban regime is based on a solidaristic project historically rooted in the peasantry and large sectors of the working class, the majority of the Cuban population; it allows for the expression of direct forces of democracy, even though the absence of representative and indirect democracy has been a serious flaw of that political system, which is leading—as happened in the former USSR—to the establishment of a new dominant class based on the state and party apparatuses. Pinochet's regime in Chile, on the other hand, was a dictatorship of a class alliance between the landowners, industrial bourgeoisie, and upper middle classes against the working class; its political project was not solidaristic with the interests of the majority of Chileans. We can call the first system Leninist socialism, the second fascist capitalism. Let me stress that I am not in the business of name-calling. All I intend to do here is introduce political categories in order to add some rigor to a political typology that offers only two major categories, dictatorships or democracies. Dictatorships and democracies exist in different forms, depending on their political contexts. Thus there is an urgent need in Sen's project to include political categories such as socialism, Christian democracy, liberalism, fascism, and other political traditions responding to different forces and collective agents that shape the nature of these political systems—besides, of course, other influences such as culture and religion. Liberal democracies such as the United States are very different from social democracies such as those of the Scandinavian countries, for example, and the differences have important consequences for the quality of life of populations living in those democracies. Similarly, in the world of underdevelopment, fascist dictatorships are very different from Leninist dictatorships, with different consequences for the quality of life of their populations.

When we analyze the reality of development through these political categories, we see the typology of countries differently and more accurately than does Sen. In a research project carried out several years ago I showed that, contrary to what is claimed today, socialism did not fail in the 20th century (6). In both the developed and the underdeveloped countries of the world—and with the sole exception of the countries of eastern Europe—nations governed by political forces based in the socialist tradition (whether social democratic or communist) have done much better in improving the quality of life of their populations than have those governed by non-socialist forces. Table 1, for example, shows how infant mortality improved more rapidly in China than in India during the period 1940–1987. A similar situation occurred for mortality rates in children under five from 1960 to 1983 (Table 2) and in one- to four-year-olds from 1960 to 1981 (Table 3): China did a much better job than India in preventing deaths among children. The decline of mortality among the most vulnerable group in any population, young children, was a consequence primarily of better nutrition and better education. The data in Tables 4, 5, and 6 show how China was also more successful than India in improving literacy rates, school enrollment, and nutritional levels from 1960 to the early 1980s.

In summary, from 1940 to 1987 (Table 1) and from 1960 to 1980 (Tables 2–6), China, governed by a socialist party of the Leninist tradition, did much better than India in most quality of life indicators, even though China started out at a much worse level. The reason was not that China had a better distribution of resources

Table 1

Infant mortality rate (per 1,000 live births) in China and India, 1940–1987[a]

	China	India
1940–45	290	192 (1941–50)
1945–50	265	
1950–55	236	140 (1951–60)
1955–60	229	
1965–70	137	
1970–75	96	135 (1972)
1975–80	65	126 (1977)
1985	36	105
1987	32	99

[a]Sources: For China, 1940–1980: World Bank estimates based on officially available data; and Hill, K., *China: An Evaluation of Demographic Trends—1950–82,* PHN Technical Note DEM 4. For India, 1940–1970: Halstead, S., Walsh, J., and Warren, K. (eds.), The impact of social and economic development on mortality. In *Good Health at Low Cost,* The Rockefeller Foundation, New York, 1985. Remaining years (except 1985), for India and China: World Bank, *World Tables,* 1989–1990 Ed., unless otherwise noted. For 1985: UNICEF, *Statistics on Children in UNICEF Assisted Countries,* New York, 1987.

and paid more attention to human capital (as Sen seems to believe), but that China was governed by a socialist project and India was not. The better distribution of resources and the emphasis on human capital were the symptoms, not the causes, of China's success. I find it necessary to clarify this point because the importance of the political context is rarely expressed in economic analyses or by international agencies. Ignoring the importance of the political context, however, can lead to authentic disasters. Let me share with you one of the most obvious examples.

Twenty-five years ago, the Chinese regime developed a program of "barefoot doctors," peasants trained in basic medical skills, which proved extremely effective. This development occurred within a political context, beautifully explained in my friend Joshua Horn's book *Away with All Pests* (7), that responded to a clear mandate of what the Chinese government called "serving the people." The World Health Organization was impressed by China's experience and wanted to export the barefoot doctors program to many other developing countries. As is typical of WHO, however, it saw this as a technological and programmatical breakthrough without realizing that it was primarily a political development.

Table 2

Under-five mortality rate (per 1,000 live births) in China and India, 1960 and 1983[a]

	China	India
1960	340	300
1983	55	165

[a]Sources: UNICEF, *World Statistics on Children: UNICEF Statistical Pocketbook,* New York, 1986.

Table 3

Child (age one to four years) death rates (per 1,000) in China and India, various years, 1960 and 1981[a]

	China	India
1960	26.1 (1964–65)	26.2
1965	17.7	23.2
1970	10.7	20.7
1975	10.3	19.0
1977	9.0	18.6
1979	7.4	17.8
1981	7.2	17.0

[a]Sources: World Bank, *World Bank Tables,* Ed. 3, New York, 1983.

Table 4

Literacy rate, school enrollment, and nutritional levels in China and India, various years[a]

	China	India
Percent of adults who are literate, male/female, 1985	82/56	57/29
Percent enrolled in primary school, male/female, 1982–84	100/93	100/68
Daily per capita calorie supply as percent of requirements, 1983	111	96

[a]Sources: UNICEF publications: *World Statistics on Children: UNICEF Statistical Pocketbook,* New York, 1986; *Statistics on Children in UNICEF Assisted Countries,* New York, 1987; and *The State of the World's Children,* Oxford University Press, New York, 1985.

Table 5

Calorie supply per capita (as percent of requirements) in China and India, various years, 1960–1983[a]

	China	India
1960	78.8 (1964–65)	95.6 (1961–65)
1965	N.A.	N.A.
1970	88.7	90.4
1975	94.3	81.8
1977	96.6	88.7
1979	104.9	94.2
1981	107.0	87.5
1983	111.0	96.0

[a]Sources: For 1960–1981: World Bank, *World Bank Tables,* Ed. 3, 1983, unless otherwise noted. For 1983: UNICEF, *Statistics on Children in UNICEF Assisted Countries,* New York, 1987.

Table 6

Protein supply per capita (grams per day) in China and India, various years, 1960–1980[a]

	China	India
1960	49.6 (1964–65)	53.6 (1961–65)
1965	N.A.	N.A.
1970	53	49.7
1975	58.1	45
1977	59.7	48.3
1979	65.5	50.6
1980	66.8	46.6

[a]Sources: World Bank, *World Bank Tables,* Ed. 3, 1983.

Needless to say, the barefoot doctors program failed miserably in Iran and many other countries where the political situation was very different indeed.

A somewhat similar depoliticization appears in Sen's analysis of what he rightly considers successful countries—that is, countries that have combined economic growth with distribution and human development. Sen repeatedly refers to China, Kerala State in India, and Costa Rica as points of reference, success stories worth emulating. But nowhere does he state that these countries or states have been governed by socialist parties of the Leninist tradition (in the case of China and Kerala) and of the social democratic tradition (in the case of Costa Rica); actually, terms such as "socialism" and "capitalism" rarely appear in Sen's book. The paradox of this silence is even more apparent when Sen compares China with India. He recognizes that China did a better job than India in training its labor force and keeping it healthy. And he also indicates that because of this situation, China was better able to take advantage of the market than was India, since it had a better-educated labor force. The book almost reads as if Sen's position is that socialism, an expression he never uses, is the best condition for introducing capitalism. Many people will question whether introduction of the market has been a good thing for China's quality of life. In fact, since introduction of the market, China's rate of improvement of mortality indicators by age group (such as infant mortality (Table 1)) has slowed dramatically and mortality differentials have markedly increased. But even if we assume (which I do not) that market reforms have been good for the quality of life of most Chinese people, the better preparation of China for the market, including its better education and health, was the outcome of the dominance of a political project that at least theoretically claims alliance with socialism. And in my opinion, the worsening of the situation in China since the mid-1980s has resulted primarily from its distancing itself from the political project that governed China for over 40 years.

The only time Sen explicitly refers to political variables is when he indicates that dictatorships are bad for quality of life because they cannot detect and respond to acute problems such as famines. This is why he comments, as noted earlier, that no democratic country has ever faced famine and the only countries that have faced famine have been dictatorships. When I first came across this position in an article by Sen published in *Scientific American* (8), I sent a clarification to that journal describing how some of the greatest successes in fighting hunger have occurred in countries that Sen would define as dictatorships (9). In his reply, Sen said there was a difference between hunger, even chronic hunger, and famine (10). I must admit I was not convinced. Even defining famine as an acute rise of hunger, the two are, in my opinion, related. A condition for famine is a population in which hunger is chronic, except in times of conflicts, wars, or national disasters.

But even accepting Sen's definition, we have to analyze the occurrence of famine in Bangladesh, which he would define as a democracy. Let me expand on this case, because I believe it touches on a key weakness in Sen's typology of countries as dictatorships or democracies, defining them more by the symptoms of democracy than by the causes. And let me quote from an instrument one would not suspect of being skeptical of liberal democracy, the *New York Times*.

In a study of hunger and famine in Bangladesh (one of the poorest countries in today's world), the *New York Times* goes directly to the root of the problem: the type of land ownership. Let me quote (11):

> The wealthiest 16.7 per cent of the rural population controls two-thirds of the land and almost 60 per cent of the rural population hold less than one acre of property, up from 38 per cent in 1975. This growing multitude of 45 million people—fully half of the population of Bangladesh—is as vulnerable to famine as it was in the mid-1970s.

The article mentions that new technologies are not going to solve the problems of hunger and famine; let me quote again: "And the new agricultural technologies being introduced have tended to favor the larger farmers, putting them in a better position to buy out their less fortunate neighbors." The *Times* notes that Bangladesh has democratic institutions, with a plurality of parties, and the other major characteristics Sen includes in his definition of democracy. And yet, as the article indicates, "since the Government and the Parliament are basically dominated by land owners—about 75 per cent of members of Parliament own land—no one foresees any official support for fundamental changes in the system." Hunger is endemic and famine is a frequent occurrence in Bangladesh, stimulating international aid in the form of food donations. But, again, according to the *Times* article:

> Food aid officials here privately concede that only a fraction of the millions of tons of food aid sent to Bangladesh has reached the poor and the hungry in the villages. The food is given to the Government, which in turn sells it at subsidized prices to the military, the police and the middle class inhabitants of the cities.

There is a clear pattern of class dominance in the state institutions that reproduces this situation; the expression of democracy takes places within a clear set of parameters established by the set of property relations in Bangladesh. The problem, therefore, is not a lack of resources but who has control over these resources. As the *New York Times* article concludes:

> Bangladesh is producing enough food to provide an adequate diet for every man, woman and child in the country. And the agricultural potential of this lush green land is such that even the inevitable population growth of the next twenty years could be fed by the resources of Bangladesh alone. American diplomats here tend to prefer the explanation that Bangladesh is the victim of a cataclysmic combination of exploding population and recurring disasters. But most of the longtime aid officials in Dacca strongly believe that hunger would not exist (and famine would not appear) in Bangladesh except for an inefficient, still largely feudal economic and social structure.

The only observation worth making here is that, unfortunately, Bangladesh is rather representative of many so-called democracies in the underdeveloped world. What passes as a democracy may be highly discredited, as recent events in

Venezuela show. Democracy is indeed necessary to guarantee development, but the specific types of property relations in those democracies are a major handicap to democratic and human development. This is why I started my presentation with the intention of focusing on understanding the matrix of power relations in each country and in the world, framed primarily but not exclusively by property relations. This is the context in which we need to evaluate the credibility of democracy and the validity and usefulness of economic institutions such as the market. And this is also why understanding the political context of economic development is so important to fully understanding human development. The absence of such political sensibility, when not silencing political analysis and discourse, very seriously weakens Sen's scholarly project.

Let me finish this address to a group of human development experts by expressing a major concern. The international agencies are masters of depoliticizing what is profoundly political. And the same is true of the academic cultures of such countries as the United States and the United Kingdom. One can take a course on human rights in the United States today without once hearing about exploitation and domination and their reproduction through political institutions. I believe the technocratic practice and discourse in current analyses of inequalities is just another example of what I am saying. We see this situation, for example, in the United Nations' annual Human Development reports, a source of inspiration for Sen. These excellent reports analyze in great detail the consequences of the growth of inequalities while meticulously avoiding any analysis of the causes of that growth. Not surprisingly, the list of recommendations about how to address this growth of inequalities is not only extremely generic but also very disappointing. Not even the regulation of financial flows is suggested.

I assure you I am not naive. Just as the funding of academia in the United States explains the silence on these topics in American universities, so the funding of the U.N. Human Development reports, mostly by the U.S. government, explains the silence in the reports. But the reality is that this silence (and discrimination) reproduces an extremely ideological culture in which the roots of these problems and, equally important, the correct solutions to these problems are actually avoided. Let me therefore conclude by saying that Sen's work is a major step toward challenging the conventional wisdom in human development studies. But it does not go far enough. It leaves untouched the core of this conventional wisdom, without penetrating the question of how power is produced and reproduced in the world today. And that is the question we need to ask.

Note — This chapter is adapted from a presentation to the Human Development Seminar of The Johns Hopkins University, Baltimore, February 11, 2000.

REFERENCES

1. Sen, A. *Development As Freedom.* Knopf, New York, 1999.
2. Navarro, V. Un Analisis del Milagro Brasileno. *Revista de Economia Politica* 34(5): 23–34, 1968.
3. Wright, E. O. *Classes,* Verso Classics 16. Verso, London, 1998.
4. Smith, A. *An Inquiry into the Nature and Causes of the Wealth of Nations.* Clarendon Press, London, 1976.
5. Lincoln, A. *Collected Papers,* Vol. VII, No. 35. 1958.
6. Navarro, V. Has socialism failed? An analysis of health indicators under socialism. *Int. J. Health Serv.* 22(4): 583–601, 1992.
7. Horn, J. *Away with All Pests: An English Surgeon in People's China, 1954–1969.* Monthly Review Press, New York, 1971.
8. Sen, A. The economics of life and death. *Sci. Am.,* May 1993.
9. Navarro, V. Vital priorities (letter to the editor). *Sci. Am.,* October 1993, p. 8.
10. Sen, A. Sen replies (letter to the editor). *Sci. Am.,* October 1993, p. 8.
11. Bangladesh hunger. *New York Times,* November 24, 1981.

CHAPTER 21

ARE PRO–WELFARE STATE AND FULL-EMPLOYMENT POLICIES POSSIBLE IN THE ERA OF GLOBALIZATION?

Vicente Navarro

THE ASSUMED END OF EXPANSIONIST AND FULL-EMPLOYMENT POLICIES

According to a widely held belief in major economic, financial, political, and academic circles in the western developed world, the globalization of the world economy has considerably weakened the power of states, making it practically impossible for them to carry out the expansionist and full-employment policies that have characterized social democratic policies during the post–World War II period. According to this belief, governments that expand their public and social expenditures and try to follow full-employment policies will be penalized by the international markets that drive the process of economic globalization. A most recent example of this position is John Gray's *False Dawn,* which argues that social democracy is impossible today owing to the globalization of the economy, because "social democracy presupposed a closed economy" (1, p. 88). Accordingly, the welfare states have had "to progressively dismantle themselves, so that they can compete on more equal terms with economies in which environmental social and labor costs are lowest" (1, p. 92).

This belief has also permeated large sectors of the leadership of the social democratic parties (and the intellectuals related to them), traditionally identified with expansionist and full-employment policies. Oscar Solchaga, Minister of Finance of the Spanish socialist government (1982–1996), starts his memoirs with the statement that today, a country cannot successfully carry out full-employment policies. Spain's unemployment rate increased from 9 percent of the labor force in 1982, when the socialist party was elected, to 22 percent in 1996, when it was defeated by the Conservative party. Solchaga's book starts with an extract from Eric Hobsbawn's *Age of Extremes,* in which the British historian writes, "the most important characteristic of today's capitalism has been that the state has lost all its economic powers" (2). More recently, Anthony Giddens (3) notes in his *Third Way* that Keynesian policies, assumed to be the economic base of social democratic policies, cannot be carried out in today's globalized world. Moreover, in his 1999 Reith Lectures (on the BBC), Giddens stated "that nations have lost most of the sovereignty they once had, and politicians have lost most of their capacity to influence events" (4). He thus concludes that the only way to carry out such policies is at the multinational level, establishing what he calls "institutions of cosmopolitan global governance" yet to be envisaged. Others, like Jacques Delors (5), in his Social Agenda for Europe, while agreeing on the impossibility of carrying out social democratic policies at the state level, support the need to develop them at the continental level. This last opinion has become widely held by European members of the Socialist International, who conclude that to follow social democratic policies at the state level is a practical impossibility and that the focus should shift to carrying out these policies at the continental, multistate, or multinational level, the only level where policies of this type are still considered possible.

It is important to stress that the acceptance of this interpretation of the impact of globalization on state power leads progressive governments to carry out public policies not very different from those carried out by other political traditions, because there is not much space to do differently. This lack of differentiation leads to a depoliticization of democratic institutions, justifying the disenchantment of the electoral base of the social democratic parties with their governments' failure to carry out social democratic policies (see 6 for a review of the undemocratic consequences of Giddens's position).

Actually, the weakening of social democratic parties' commitment to expansionist and full-employment policies at the state level is also frequently seen as exacerbated by the decline of their social base—the labor movement—which has traditionally been the main force behind the development of these policies (3). The assumption is that there has been a shift of the sphere of production from developed to developing countries as a consequence of the process of globalization that—side-by-side with the introduction of new labor-saving technologies—has been responsible for the decline of the traditional instruments of western labor movements, such as the labor unions and the social democratic parties. It is not a mere coincidence that the disappearance of the working class in the discourse of many social democratic leaders is accompanied by a reference to the middle class as their new basic constituency, replacing the former by the latter. This chapter provides empirical information that questions each of these theses.

EMPIRICAL FACTORS USUALLY IGNORED IN GLOBALIZATION THEORY[1]

Table 1 shows the evolution of one key indicator of globalization: the percentage of gross national product (GNP) represented by exports plus imports for selected OECD countries from 1960 to the early 1990s. This table groups the countries of the OECD according to the political tradition that has governed each country (either alone or in coalition) for the majority of the period 1960–1990. I have explained in Chapter 4 the criteria used to develop such groupings (11; this typology follows that of Huber and Stephens (12)). Here I limit myself to listing them. Sweden, Norway, Denmark, Finland, and Austria are included in the social democratic tradition; Belgium, Germany, France, the Netherlands, and Italy in the conservative tradition (of Christian influence); the United States, Great Britain, Ireland, and Canada in the Anglo-Saxon liberal tradition; and Spain, Greece, and Portugal as countries in the conservative tradition that suffered right-wing dictatorships during the majority of the period 1960–1990.

Table 1 illustrates several points. *First, the internationalization of commerce (and its importance for each country, measured by the size of exports and imports as percentage of GNP) grew far more rapidly in the 1960s than in the 1970s or 1980s.* From 1960 to 1974, imports plus exports as percentage of GNP grew from 56.7 to 68.5 percent in the social democratic countries; from 51.0 to 71.2 percent in the conservative countries; from 38.7 to 56.0 percent in the Anglo-Saxon liberal countries; and from 24.7 to 43.0 percent in the conservative southern European countries governed by authoritarian right-wing regimes. No postwar period saw a faster integration into the international economy (what is now called the process of economic globalization) than 1960–1974.[2]

The second point that merits special attention in Table 1 is that *during the 1960s the social democratic countries were already the countries best integrated into the international economy.* In 1960, for example, their exports plus imports as percentage of GNP were on average 56.7 percent, larger than in the conservative countries (51 percent), liberal countries (38.7 percent), and southern European authoritarian right-wing countries (24.7 percent). *And during the entire period 1960–1990, the social democratic countries remained among the most internationally integrated economies.* As we see later in this chapter (see Table 4), it

[1] It is not the purpose of this chapter to discuss whether globalization of the world economy is as new or extended as is claimed. I discuss this in Chapter 5 of my book *Neoliberalismo y Estado del Bienestar* (7). See also 8–10 for critiques of globalization.

[2] While this chapter focuses on commerce, another of my publications focuses on foreign investment, which is of lesser importance in quantitative terms than the imports and exports of goods and services. The percentage of GNP involved in foreign investment is much lower than that for imports and exports (7).

Table 1

Imports and exports as percentage of GNP, OECD countries, 1960 to early 1990s[a, b]

	1960	1974	Early 1990s
Social democratic countries			
Sweden	46.0	64.4	61.8
Norway	76.9	86.9	70.3
Denmark	65.6	66.5	61.6
Finland	45.7	58.7	60.8
Austria	49.3	66.4	73.4
Average	*56.7*	*68.5*	*65.5*
Conservative countries			
Germany	29.9	45.3	43.8
Belgium	77.7	122.0	132.0
The Netherlands	90.9	102.0	95.3
Italy	26.5	44.5	43.0
France	30.1	42.4	41.8
Average	*51.0*	*71.2*	*70.7*
Liberal countries			
United States	9.6	17.3	21.9
Canada	35.6	49.8	59.8
Great Britain	43.2	61.0	52.2
Ireland	66.5	96.1	122.7
Average	*38.7*	*56.0*	*64.1*
Southern Europe			
Spain	16.2	33.6	39.4
Portugal	36.1	60.5	60.4
Greece	21.8	35.1	44.0
Average	*24.7*	*43.0*	*47.9*

[a]Sources: OECD Historical Statistics, Table 2.3 in Castles, F. G., *Comparative Public Policy: Patterns of Post War Transformation,* p. 39, Edward Elgar, 1998; and own calculations.

[b]In this chapter I consider foreign commerce an indicator of globalization. The flow of investments is of less quantitative importance in the process of globalization (see 7, Chap. 5).

was during the period of maximum growth of international economic integration (1960–1974) that all these countries (except the southern European countries) underwent their largest growth of public expenditures, with most growth in precisely those countries—the social democratic countries—where growth of international economic integration was largest.

Based on this empirical evidence, the thesis that globalization forces governments to diminish their expansionist policies is unsustainable. *On the contrary, the countries that became integrated into the international economy most rapidly were those that followed expansionist policies most actively.* I am not making the point that in order for those countries to follow social democratic policies they needed to be globalized. What I am indicating is that globalization was not an obstacle to their following social democratic policies. In fact, following such policies was a condition for their successful integration in the global markets, a point also made by Darin Rodrick (13), although he erroneously reduces the social democratic project to a mere collaborative strategy among government, employers, and labor. The social democratic project is based on a social pact between capital and labor, developed under the supervision of the social democratic government. That social pact is a necessary but not sufficient condition for developing the social democratic project (see Chapter 4 for a discussion of the characteristics of the social democratic project).

An identical situation occurred regarding unemployment, also discussed in a later section. All the selected countries had, on average, lower unemployment during the period of faster international economic integration than in subsequent periods of slower economic integration. And the social democratic countries—those undergoing faster international economic integration and having greater internationalization of their economies—were also the ones with the lowest unemployment. Given these data, it is difficult to sustain the position that (*a*) unemployment in all these countries was and continues to be a result of the process of globalization, or (*b*) globalization requires a growth of unemployment. Globalization may create unemployment. But it does not *need* to create unemployment if there is a social pact that facilitates the country's integration into the world economy (with the need to increase competitiveness) without labor bearing the costs of that integration. This situation explains why globalization, rather than weakening the state, requires a strengthening of the state to better respond to the challenge of globalization—precisely the opposite of what Gray and others are claiming. This strengthening of the state facilitates the social pact, which calls for employer-employee collaboration to better face competition (14). It is only in the absence of these arrangements that globalization creates unemployment. Not surprisingly, then, unemployment during the post–World War II period has, in general, been higher in the liberal and Christian democratic countries than in the social democratic countries.

Let me clarify that until now, I have carried the terms of the debate into the terrain of those I am engaging in debate—the theorists of globalization, ranging from Gray to Habermas (15), to mention just the two poles of globalization theory. But I want to repeat what I have stated elsewhere, and what others in the economic and political science literature have stated more extensively and elegantly, that what we see in today's world is not globalization but internationalization of commerce and production around the major economies—the United States, Germany, and Japan, which have dominated the three major regional blocs, North America, Europe, and Asia. Most international trade and capital flows (productive and finance) move between and within these three blocs, shaped and determined by the relationship among these states (16).

A further clarification is that nothing I have said should preempt the thesis that there is a need to coordinate economic and fiscal policies at the E.U. level so as to better develop social democratic expansionist and full-employment policies along the lines suggested by Oskar Lafontaine and Crista Müller (17). But the point that needs to be made is that in today's Europe, a country can follow social democratic policies, and could do so even at a time (as in the 1980s) when the majority of governments in the European Union were conservative. As I mentioned earlier, to think otherwise paralyzes those countries that have elected left-of-center or left governments, forcing them to develop policies indistinguishable from conservative and liberal policies, creating an enormous disenchantment among their electorates. The globalization argument reproduces the famous Trotskyite principle that unless there is a continental or worldwide revolution, a country cannot control its own destiny. Paradoxically, we are now witnessing right-wing sectors within the social democratic tradition that accept this extremist Trotskyite policy to justify the development of proposals for neoliberal policies in their own countries.

THE ASSUMED DISAPPEARANCE OF THE LABOR MOVEMENT AS A CONSEQUENCE OF GLOBALIZATION: THE CASE OF THE TRADE UNIONS

Table 2 shows the evolution of the rate of unionization in the same OECD countries from 1960 to the early 1990s. A great variability in the evolution of unionization rates is evident during that period, a variability that corresponds primarily to political rather than economic forces such as globalization. We can see, for example, a significant growth in the percentage of the active population unionized during that period in all social democratic countries (with the exception of Austria), as well as in Belgium, Italy, Portugal, Spain, and Greece during periods of social democratic participation in government. We also have seen an increase in the rate of unionization during the same period in Canada, which was due to legislative interventions (established by the less conservative of the two major parties) that facilitated unionization.

Thus, there has not been a general process of decline in the rate of unionization, and where a decline has occurred, it has been due more to political causes than to globalization. Moreover, another indicator of union and working-class strength (an even more potent indicator than the rate of unionization), the percentage of the labor force covered by collective agreements negotiated by the unions, shows that unions' influence increased rather than declined in most of those countries from 1960 to the early 1990s. Only in the liberal countries was there a decline in coverage; a decline did not occur in the majority of countries, either social democratic or conservative (7, pp. 87–92).

Table 2

Percentage of the labor force that is unionized, OECD countries, 1960 to early 1990s[a]

	1960	1974	Early 1990s
Social democratic countries			
Sweden	73.0	67.7	82.5
Norway	62.0	51.4	56.0
Denmark	69.0	60.0	71.4
Finland	33.0	51.4	56.0
Austria	72.0	62.2	46.2
Average	*61.8*	*58.5*	*62.4*
Conservative countries			
Germany	39.0	33.0	32.9
Belgium	58.0	45.5	51.2
The Netherlands	44.0	38.0	25.5
Italy	61.0	36.3	38.8
France	17.0	22.3	9.8
Average	*43.8*	*35.0*	*31.6*
Liberal countries			
United States	31.0	23.2	15.6
Canada	31.0	31.0	35.8
Great Britain	45.0	44.8	39.1
Ireland	50.0	53.1	49.7
Average	*39.2*	*38.0*	*35.0*
Southern Europe			
Spain	0	0	11
Portugal	0	0	31.8
Greece	0	0	34.1
Average	*0*	*0*	*25.6*

[a]Sources: Stephens, J. D., *The Transition from Capitalism to Socialism,* Macmillan, New York, 1979; *OECD Employment Outlook,* 1994; Castles, F. G., *Comparative Public Policy: Patterns of Post War Transformation,* p. 68, Edward Elgar, 1998; and own calculations.

A DECLINE OF SOCIAL DEMOCRACY?

Here I need to clarify that I define as social democratic parties all parties from the center left or left that, independent of their self-identification and denomination—socialists, social democrats, labor, communists, or whatever—support, at least rhetorically, the application of expansionist policies that are universal (rather than assistential) and have redistributive effects and full employment as a political objective. (The only exception among socialist parties in the European Union is the Spanish Socialist Party (PSOE), which did not claim full employment as a political objective during the years that it governed, 1982–1996.)

Table 3 shows the number of social democratic ministers in the OECD countries during the periods 1960–1973 and 1974 to early 1990s. We can see a clear growth in the number of social democratic members of central governments during that entire period in the majority of OECD countries. Social democratic power (measured as the number of social democratic ministers in government) increased (*a*) in all social democratic countries; (*b*) in the Netherlands, Italy, and France, countries in the conservative tradition; (*c*) in Ireland, a country in the liberal tradition; and (*d*) in all countries in southern Europe. Today, the majority of governments in the European Union are social democratic. And half of the 132 parties of the Socialist International are in government.

The evidence against the decline of social democracy is so overwhelming that the claim of its demise because of globalization has lost all credibility. This argument has been recycled recently, however, indicating that, while it is true that social democracy has grown considerably, its growth has been a consequence of the adaptation to the process of globalization, with social democratic parties giving up or considerably diluting their commitment to traditional expansionist and full-employment policies. The new version of the globalization theory is that the electoral successes of social democratic parties are based on their abandonment of social democratic policies.

EMPIRICAL EVIDENCE THAT QUESTIONS THE GLOBALIZATION THESIS

The problem with this and other globalization theories is that they are not supported by readily available empirical information. Let's look at the facts, which can speak for themselves. If the globalization thesis were correct, we should see that the larger the scope and the faster the rate of globalization, the smaller the percentage of GNP spent in the public and social sectors and the slower the rate of growth of both types of expenditures (as percentages of GNP). We should also see a decline in public and social expenditures (as percentages of GNP) or a decline in the rate of growth of these expenditures with the growth of the globalization process. Moreover, such declines should be more accentuated in countries that are more globalized.

Table 4, however, tells a different story. We have already seen that the social democratic countries were among the most globalized countries during the period 1974–1995; Table 4 shows that they also had the largest public expenditures and (except for the southern European countries) the fastest growth of those expenditures. We can also see from the data in Table 4 that there was a continuous

Table 3

Percentage of social democratic ministers in governments, OECD countries, 1960–1973 and 1974 to early 1990s[a]

	1960–1973	1974 to early 1990s
Social democratic countries		
Sweden	100	59
Norway	54	73
Denmark	61	52
Finland	33	36
Average	*59.4*	*59.6*
Conservative countries		
Germany	33	31
Belgium	33	26
The Netherlands	5	21
Italy	12	19
France	0	46
Average	*16.6*	*28.6*
Liberal countries		
United States	0	0
Canada	0	0
Great Britain	41	25
Ireland	2	15
Average	*10.7*	*10*
Southern Europe		
Spain	0	55
Portugal	0	21
Greece	0	46
Average	*0*	*40.6*

[a]Sources: Table 3.3 in Castles, F. G., *Comparative Public Policy: Patterns of Post War Transformation,* p. 72, Edward Elgar, 1998; and own calculations.

growth of public expenditures for all the OECD countries, along with a growth in globalization. The only exceptions are the United Kingdom and Ireland, where public expenditures (as percentage of GNP) declined during the period 1974–1995. This was due to the very aggressive neoliberal policies carried out by the British and Irish governments during the majority of that period. Otherwise, the social democratic parties did not dilute or weaken their commitment to expansionist policy measures in the size and rate of growth of their public expenditures.

Table 4

Public expenses as percentage of GNP, OECD countries, 1960–1995[a]

	1960	1974	1995
Social democratic countries			
Sweden	31.0	48.1	66.2
Norway	29.9	44.6	47.4
Denmark	24.8	45.9	62.4
Finland	26.6	32.0	57.6
Austria	35.7	41.9	52.8
Average	*29.6*	*42.5*	*57.28*
Conservative countries			
Germany	32.4	44.6	49.5
Belgium	43.6	45.6	54.9
The Netherlands	33.7	47.9	50.9
Italy	30.1	37.9	51.9
France	34.6	45.6	54.9
Average	*33.0*	*44.3*	*52.42*
Liberal countries			
United States	27.2	32.1	33.3
Canada	28.6	36.8	46.2
Great Britain	32.2	44.8	43.4
Ireland	28.0	43.0	42.0
Average	*29.0*	*39.1*	*41.0*
Southern Europe			
Spain	10	23.1	44.3
Portugal	17	24.7	43.1
Greece	17.4	25.0	46.0
Average	*17.2*	*24.2*	*44.0*

[a]Source: OECD Statistical Series, Table 4.1 in Castles, F. G., *Comparative Public Policy: Patterns of Post War Transformation,* p. 101, Edward Elgar, 1998.

Nor did they dilute or weaken their commitment to full-employment policies. Data in Table 6 of Chapter 4 show how the social democratic governments, during the entire period, were the most successful in reducing unemployment, with the lowest rates of unemployment in the OECD. That table also shows that it was during the period of fastest integration of their economies into the international markets (1960–1973) that the social democratic countries had the lowest unemployment.

This relationship also applied in the majority of conservative and liberal countries: it was during the period of fastest globalization that they had the lowest unemployment. As indicated earlier, the thesis that unemployment is a result of globalization cannot be sustained: it is plainly wrong. Unemployment responds more to political than to economic causes such as globalization. This reality must be fully understood when considering the consequence of globalization for unemployment. Unemployment is basically a political not an economic indicator (18).

THE SUPPOSED FAILURE OF SOCIAL DEMOCRACY IN REDUCING UNEMPLOYMENT

As shown in Chapter 4, Table 6, the only period when social democratic countries had, on average, higher unemployment than the conservative and liberal countries was at the beginning of the 1990s. The primary cause was the dramatic increase of unemployment in Sweden, which went from a very low 1.6 percent in 1990 to a very high 8.2 percent in 1993. A similar situation occurred in Finland, whose unemployment rate rose from a low 3.6 percent in 1990 to an extremely high 17.9 percent in 1993. These increases in unemployment have been presented by defenders of the globalization thesis as proof that even social democratic countries finally have to succumb to the globalization forces and give up their full-employment policies. John Gray, for example, writes "that the extensive Swedish welfare state has rendered Sweden internationally uncompetitive, explaining its high unemployment (1, p. 82). Those who hold this view, however, should explain why this growth of unemployment took place in the 1990s rather than in the 1980s or the 1970s, when the degree of globalization was even higher.

Actually, the sudden growth of unemployment in both countries was due primarily to political interventions, related to changes in the power relations within those countries and to the collapse of the Soviet Union and the unification of Germany, events that occurred during a very short time period and were unrelated to globalization. In Sweden, the social democratic government deregulated the financial markets, implementing policies that were expanded by the right-wing parties (which in Sweden call themselves the bourgeois parties), which governed for most years during that period. This deregulation of the financial markets, a consequence of the growing political influence of banking and insurance companies over the economic and political institutions of Sweden, dramatically weakened one of the classical instruments in the social democratic armamentarium: the control of credit and monetary policies. This deregulation of the financial market caused a large increase in interest rates that was responsible for slowing down economic growth and increasing unemployment. This phenomenon was made even worse by the government's decision to fix the value of the Swedish crown to the German mark (as a way of strengthening financial capital), at a time when the German mark was clearly overvalued as a result of the Bundesbank having imposed policies of high interest as a response to German unification. The deregulation of financial markets in Sweden at a time of very high interest rates in

Germany, together with the fixing of the Swedish crown to the German mark, delivered an enormous shock to the Swedish economy, creating a sudden and dramatic slowing down.

Similar policies were carried out in Finland by the right-wing government, with similar consequences—consequences further aggravated by the collapse of the Soviet Union, which used to absorb 32 percent of all Finnish exports. As noted by Geoffrey Garret, "very few countries have seen their exports decline so dramatically in such a short period of time as Finland" (19, p. 143). In both cases—Sweden and Finland—the growth of unemployment cannot be explained by the process of globalization; rather, it can be explained only with reference to political events and political decisions that bear very little relationship to globalization. In the case of Sweden, other economic and fiscal policies could have been applied that would have avoided unemployment. Actually, the reversal of some of those policies explains the impressive decline in unemployment that occurred in the rest of the 1990s, placing Sweden, once again, among the countries with lowest unemployment and fastest growth in the European Union. The economic correspondent of the *New York Times,* Mr. Andrews, was forced to report in the *Herald Tribune* on the Swedish "miracle," expressing surprise "that those countries that have followed more closely the social democratic strategy, i.e., the Northern Scandinavian countries and Jospin's French government have been the most successful ones" (20, p. 1). A similar change has taken place in Finland, where exports have improved significantly as a result of the Finnish adaptation to new economic partners.

It is important to mention that those social democratic governments that have most weakened their commitment to social democratic policies, such as Blair's and Schroeder's governments, have also been the ones most castigated by the electorate, and are responsible for the European Socialist Party losing its majority in the European Parliament.

ECONOMIC AND FISCAL CHANGES NECESSITATED BY DEREGULATION OF WORLDWIDE FINANCIAL MARKETS

The information provided in the previous sections questions the widely held position that economic globalization has made it practically impossible for states to carry out expansionist and full-employment policies. *However, such information does not question the need of states to adapt these policies to the changes occurring in the world economy and in particular to the internationalization of financial markets,* the only new element in the globalization process that has indeed forced states to make some changes to these policies. In other words, internationalization of the financial markets has forced states committed to expansionist and full-employment policies to adapt those policies without, however, abandoning their objectives.

As shown in Table 5, during the period 1991–1995, the social democratic countries continued to be the countries with the largest public expenditures and the fastest growth of those expenditures. The same table shows that, in general, these countries did not have larger public deficits than the conservative or liberal countries, although the rate of growth of their public deficits during the 1990s was larger than in the conservative and liberal countries. This faster growth in public deficits was a result, as I have shown in Chapter 4, of their having had historically (since World War II) very low public deficits and even public surpluses (11). The growth of the public deficits in the social democratic countries has not produced larger public debt than in the conservative or liberal countries (Table 6).

The most significant change in these countries during the 1990s, however, was in their fiscal policies and, very much in particular, in their taxing policies with respect to capital. Table 5 shows how in all the countries—social democratic, conservative, and liberal—there has been a reduction of taxes on capital (corporate taxes), particularly accentuated in the social democratic countries. In these countries, the reduction of corporate taxes was, on average, 16.4 points, compared with reductions of 1.4 points in the conservative and 4.0 points in the liberal countries. This dramatic reduction of corporate taxes in the social democratic countries was due to the high corporate taxes formerly imposed by those countries. The reduction of corporate taxes in the high-taxing social democratic countries has led to a certain convergence of capital taxation policies, a convergence that has narrowed the former difference in the taxing rates of capital between the social democratic countries and the conservative and liberal countries. This convergence is a direct consequence of the deregulation of financial markets in the social democratic countries in response to the internationalization of financial markets and in particular to their integration (except Norway) into the European Union. Another characteristic of the changes in fiscal policies of the social democratic countries has been the reduction in their rate of progressivity (Table 5).

These two changes in the fiscal policies of the social democratic countries—the reduced taxes on capital and the reduced progressivity of their tax policies—could indeed represent a clear threat to their expansionist and full-employment policies. But the revenues that the state requires to follow these expansionist and full-employment policies can be obtained from other sources, as consumption taxes. Consumption taxes have always been a very important source of state revenue in the social democratic countries, as shown in Table 7. The consumption taxes in these countries (as percentage of GNP) are, on average, 14.5 percent, similar to (although lower than) the percentage of revenues derived from income taxes, 16.9 percent. In social democratic countries, consumption taxes are designed in such a way that their regressivity is moderated by, for example, excluding items of popular consumption, such as food and clothes. These consumption taxes have increased at a higher rate in the social democratic countries than in the conservative and liberal countries (19).

Table 5

Fiscal policies in the OECD countries in the 1990s, given as percentage of GNP[a]

	Public expenditures, 1991–95	Change[b]	Public deficit, 1991–95	Change[c]	Differential tax rate, 1990[d]	Change[e]	Corporate taxes, 1992[f]	Change[g]
Social democratic countries								
Sweden	67.3	1.5	8.0	6.9	20.0	–31.5	30.0	–19.6
Norway	49.6	4.9	1.0	5.5	17.0	–5.5	28.0	–22.8
Denmark	61.8	2.7	3.0	0.3	18.0	–5.0	38.0	–7
Finland	58.0	15.5	5.4	8.6	—	—	—	—
Austria	51.5	1.5	3.89	0.9	40.0	–3	—	—
Average	*57.6*	*5.16*	*4.24*	*4.4*	*23.0*	*–11.25*	*32*	*–16.4*
Conservative countries								
Germany	48.9	1.9	3.0	0.9	34.0	—	51.9	–3.5
Belgium	56.2	–4.0	6.0	–3.0	30.0	14.5	39.0	–0.4
The Netherlands	53.8	–3.3	3.3	–1.8	30.0	–24.0	35.0	1.0
Italy	54.1	5.0	9.1	–1.9	40.0	–11.0	55.2	10.8
France	53.2	4.1	4.6	3.6	51.0	–2.0	34.0	–9.3
Average	*53.2*	*0.7*	*5.2*	*–2.2*	*37.0*	*–10.3*	*43.0*	*–1.4*

Liberal countries								
United States	34.1	4.1	2.9	3.4	16.0	–20.0	34.0	–2.8
Canada	48.5	5.0	6.2	1.8	12.0	–13.0	39.0	–0.9
United Kingdom	42.5	0.3	5.6	3.6	15.0	–21.5	33.0	–8.5
Average	*41.7*	*3.1*	*4.9*	*2.9*	*14.3*	*–18.1*	*35.3*	*–4.0*

[a]Source: Adapted from reference 19, Table 6.1, p. 137.

[b]Average public expense for 1991–1995 minus annual average public expense for 1980–1990. The number is the increase or decline, in points, of public expenses during the 1990s versus the 1980s. Sweden, for example, spent 1.5 points more in the public sector in 1991–1995 than in 1980–1990.

[c]Change in the public deficit, in points, from 1980–1991 to 1991–1995.

[d]Difference in nominal tax rates between top and bottom income groups. In general, the higher the number, the more progressive the tax code. This does not include, however, the actual tax rate, which can differ from the nominal rate, particularly in the conservative countries where tax fraud is prevalent.

[e]Reduction, in points, in tax differentials between top and bottom income groups from 1980–1990 to 1991–1995.

[f]Nominal rate for corporate taxes

[g]Change in nominal rate of corporate taxes from 1980–1991 to 1990–1995.

Table 6

Accumulated public debt, OECD countries, 1999, as percentage of GNP[a]

	Public debt
Social democratic countries	
Sweden	81.8
Norway	36.5
Denmark	78.3
Finland	63.0
Austria	69.4
Average	*65.8*
Conservative countries	
Germany	61.6
Belgium	131.1
The Netherlands	79.1
Italy	123.0
France	57.9
Average	*90.5*
Liberal countries	
United States	64.5
Canada	99.1
Great Britain	57.6
Average	*73.7*

[a]Sources: Adapted from *Gross Financial Liabilities of General Governments,* OECD, 1996; reference 19, p. 138.

In summary, the internationalization of capital has forced a change in public finance, with reductions in taxation of capital (the moveable input on production) and increases in the taxation of private consumption and increases in user fees for public consumption. The latter taxes have the indirect effect of penalizing labor over capital. Also, the employer component of social security taxes has declined in most countries, a decline implemented with the avowed purpose of increasing employment, though the empirical information establishing a relationship between level of social security taxes and employment is not very convincing. Denmark had the lowest social security taxes—0.6 percent of GNP (Table 7) and the highest unemployment rate in the social democratic bloc for the period 1970–1990 (see Chapter 4, Table 6).

As a consequence of these changes in fiscal policies, we have seen a redistribution of national income in favor of capital over labor during the 1980s and 1990s in most E.U. countries. Labor income as a share of GDP has decreased for the

Table 7

State revenue, OECD countries, 1985–1990, as percentage of GNP[a]

	Taxes	Income taxes	Consumption taxes	Corporate taxes	Social security taxes
Social democratic countries					
Sweden	54.4	20.5	13.1	2.2	13.2
Norway	47.5	12.1	17.0	4.5	7.6
Denmark	50.1	25.5	16.2	2.3	0.6
Finland	37.5	17.5	13.8	1.6	3.1
Austria	42.1	9.3	12.8	1.4	6.7
Average	*46.3*	*16.9*	*14.5*	*2.4*	*6.2*
Conservative countries					
Germany	38.4	10.9	9.5	2.1	7.2
Belgium	45.4	14.6	10.4	3.0	9.5
The Netherlands	46.3	10.1	11.0	3.4	7.0
Italy	37.4	10.0	9.3	3.7	8.8
France	44.2	5.5	12.3	2.3	12.1
Average	*42.3*	*10.2*	*10.5*	*2.9*	*8.9*
Liberal countries					
United States	29.2	10.4	4.3	2.3	5.0
Canada	35.5	13.6	9.0	2.8	3.1
Great Britain	37.3	10.2	11.0	4.2	3.5
Average	*33.9*	*11.2*	*8.1*	*3.1*	*3.8*

[a]Source: reference 19, Appendix 4.2, p. 105.

15 E.U. member states, on average, from 55.3 percent in 1980 to 50.1 percent in 1996, while operating profits as a share of GDP increased from 9.7 to 13 percent over the same time (21, 22). This redistribution has been a major cause of the increased income inequalities in the majority of E.U. countries. Another important cause of the growth in income inequalities has been the changes in the level of progressivity in income taxation, a phenomenon that is difficult to attribute to the process of globalization, unless one could prove that upper-income groups are more mobile internationally than lower-income groups—a thesis disproved by the fact that in continental Europe, most migration has been of unskilled rather than skilled labor. In Spain, almost one-fifth of the labor force migrated to central and northern Europe in the 1970s; these were primarily

unskilled workers from the rural sectors, where agricultural jobs were being rapidly destroyed.

The only justification for fiscal policies that benefit the upper income groups would be unrelated to the process of globalization—that is, the oft-used argument that the rich are the ones who save most. I will not repeat here the arguments against this justification, explored extensively in another forum (7). Suffice it to say that the problem of slow economic growth in the European Union is not due to lack of savings. The implementation of these regressive policies is, again, a response to political rather than globalization forces. In this respect, the globalization thesis has constantly been put forward by governments to justify highly unpopular public policies that respond to specific rather than general interests. As Garret writes, "Governments have promoted this association in the eyes of citizens—playing on inherent fears about international entanglements—when real problems facing the revised economies of the OECD have little to do with international market integration" (23).

CONCLUSION

The data presented in this chapter show that, given the political will, expansionist and full-employment policies are possible today, both in the European Union and in the globalized world. Needless to say, some elements of globalization (and in the European Union, some elements of economic and monetary integration) have forced changes in these policies. The deregulation of financial markets in the 1970s (as a consequence of the collapse of the Bretton Woods accords) forced changes in full-employment and expansionist public policies and in the fiscal policies required to achieve them. Similarly, the requirements set up to achieve monetary policies (requirements I have criticized elsewhere as unnecessarily stringent, arbitrary, and even harmful) can indeed be balanced by changes in fiscal policies that would allow a continuation of expansionist and full-employment policies.

The answer to the question "are social democratic policies possible in the European Union today?" is in the affirmative. And the best proof is that, as this chapter shows, there are countries, both within and outside the European Union, that are following these policies today. Whether a country follows these policies depends on the correlation of forces within the country (of which class forces continue to be of great importance) and the presence of political and social institutions that enable the development of such policies. Among the latter institutions, a key element is the existence of a social pact between employers and unions and the government. This pact requires strong trade unions, representative employers' association (for both large and medium-sized employers), and a government clearly committed to full-employment and expansionist policies. These are the key political ingredients for the implementation of such policies.

This national policy in western Europe should be accompanied by European-wide policies, including, within the European Union, coordination of national economic policies and harmonization of fiscal and social policies, leading to establishment of European social rights—which will not be developed unless the enormous democratic deficit is resolved with full development of fully accountable, European-wide political institutions. It is within this broader political context that European-wide expansionist policies will occur. Until then, however, there is much that each country can do to improve people's lives by expanding the welfare state and implementing full-employment policies.

Note — This chapter is modified from a paper presented at the Plenary Session of the Conference "Welfare State and Employment," sponsored by *Qualita Equita: Revista del Welfare Futuro* and by the Italian Ministry of Labor, Rome, September 9, 1999.

REFERENCES

1. Gray, J. *False Dawn: The Delusions of Global Capitalism.* Granta Books, London, 1998.
2. Hobsbawn, E. *Age of Extremes: The Short Twentieth Century, 1914–1992.* Abacus, London, 1995.
3. Giddens, A. *The Third Way.* Polity, London, 1998.
4. Giddens, A. 1999 Reith Lectures. Transcript, p. 9. BBC, London, 1999.
5. Delors, J. *The European Social Agenda.* European Commission, The Hague, 1993.
6. Hayes, C., and Watson, M. Globalization: Skeptical notes on the 1999 Reith Lectures. *Polit. Q.* 70(4): 418–425, October-December 1999.
7. Navarro, V. *Neoliberalismo y Estado del Bienestar,* Ed. 2. Ariel Economica, Barcelona, 1998.
8. Hirst, P., and Thomson, G. *Globalization in Question.* Polity, London, 1996.
9. Boyer, R., and Drache, D. (eds.). *States Against Markets: The Limits of Globalization.* Routledge, London, 1996.
10. Hay, C., and Marsch, D. (eds.). *Demystifying Globalization.* Macmillan, New York, 1999.
11. Navarro, V. The political economy of the welfare state in developed capitalist countries. *Int. J. Health Serv.* 29(1): 1–50, 1999.
12. Huber, E., and Stephens, J. D. *Political Choice in Global Markets.* 2000, in press.
13. Rodrick, D. *Has Globalization Gone Too Far?* Institute of International Economics, Washington, D.C., 1997.
14. Thelen, K., and Kume, I. The effect of globalization on labor revisited: Lessons from Germany and Japan. *Politics and Society* 27(4): 471, December 1999.
15. Habermas, R. Europe and globalization. *New Left Review* 235, 1999.
16. Hirst, P. Has globalization killed social democracy? In *The New Social Democracy* (special issue of The Political Quarterly), edited by A. Gamble and T. Wright, pp. 84–96. Blackwell, Oxford, 1999.
17. Lafontaine, O., and Müller, C. *No hay que temer a la globalization.* Bibliotica Nueva, 1999 [English version to be published by Verso, 2000].

18. Therborn, G. *Why Some Countries Have More Unemployment Than Others.* Verso, London, 1987.
19. Garret, G. *Partisan Politics in the Global Economy.* Cambridge University Press, Cambridge, 1998.
20. Sweden bounces back: Welfare and entrepreneurs combine powerful transformation of the economy. *Herald Tribune,* October 9–10, 1999.
21. Kramer, H. Economic aspects of tax coordination in the E.U. In *Conference Proceedings: Tax Competition and Coordination of Tax Policy in the European Union, Vienna, 13–14 July 1998.* Austrian Federal Ministry of Finance, Vienna, 1998.
22. Schulze, G. G., and Urspjorung, H. W. Globalization of the economy and the national state. *The World Economy* 22(3), May 1999.
23. Garret, G. Global markets and national politics: Collision course, or virtuous circle? *International Organization* 52, 1998.

CONTRIBUTORS

DEBABAR BANERJI is a professor at the Centre of Social Medicine and Community Health, Jawaharlal Nehru University, New Delhi. After he graduated from the Medical College, Calcutta, in 1953, he worked as a physician in western Tibet and in the interior Himalayan tribal regions, in order to relate the practice of Western medicine to the conditions in these regions. He has continued this line of work at the National Tuberculosis Institute, Bangalore (1959–1964), at the National Institute of Health Administration and Education, New Delhi (1964–1971), and in his present position. Dr. Banerji's publications cover a number of facets of the relationships between health technology and people, and the formulation of people-oriented health technologies and programs for India. A study of this relationship in 19 villages in different parts of India for a period of 16 years (1972–1988) has been one of his major research contributions, and is reported in part in *Poverty, Class and Health Culture in India* (1982). Dr. Banerji is also the author of *Health and Family Planning Services in India: An Epidemiological, Socio-cultural and Political Analysis and a Perspective* (1985); *The Making of Health Services of a Country: Postulates and a Theory* (1985); and *Social Sciences and Health Service Department in India: Sociology of Formation of an Alternative Paradigm* (1986).

RICHARD B. DU BOFF is Samuel and Etta Wexler Professor of Economic History at Bryn Mawr College in Pennsylvania. He received his A.B. from Dartmouth College, and his Ph.D. from the University of Pennsylvania in 1964. He has written an economic history of the U.S. public sector and has revised his book *Accumulation and Power,* a macroeconomic history of the United States. Since 1993 some of his attention has been taken up by the assault on social security systems in the United States and elsewhere.

RAY KIELY is a senior lecturer in development studies and media studies in the Department of Cultural Studies at the University of East London, England. He studied politics and political sociology at the B.A. (1985) and M.A. (1987) level at the University of Leeds, and completed his Ph.D. at Warwick University in 1991. His books include *Sociology and Development: The Impasse and Beyond* (1995), *The Politics of Labour and Development in Trinidad* (1996), *Industrialization and Development: A Comparative Analysis* (1998), and, most recently, an edited collection entitled *Globalization and The Third World.*

GABRIEL KOLKO is Distinguished Research Professor of History, Emeritus, at York University in Toronto. He has published 11 books, including studies of the Third World, economics, and economic history. His book *Vietnam: Anatomy of a Peace* was published in 1997.

ASA CRISTINA LAURELL is a professor of social medicine at the Autonomous Metropolitan University–Xochimilco in Mexico City and a member of the Mexican National Research System. Her basic training was in medicine at the University of Lund, Sweden; she obtained her M.P.H. at the School of Public Health, University of California, Berkeley, and her Ph.D. in sociology at the National Autonomous University of Mexico, Mexico City. Dr. Laurell has published articles and books on social epidemiology, the labor process and workers' health, and social and health policy.

RICHARD LEVINS is an ex-farmer turned ecologist working in evolutionary ecology, mathematical biology, and philosophy of science, and he applies these perspectives to ecological agriculture and public health ecology. He teaches human ecology at the Harvard School of Public Health in Boston and leads the Working Group on New and Resurgent Disease. He is the author of *Evolution in Changing Environments,* co-author of *The Dialectical Biologist, Humanity and Nature* and *Qualitative Analysis of Complex Systems,* and co-editor of *Ecosystem Health and Disease in Evolution.*

CYNTHIA LOPEZ is an assistant professor at the University of New Mexico School of Medicine in Albuquerque. From September 1997 to December 1998 she was a visiting scientist at the Harvard School of Public Health, and from March to December 1998 was a research consultant at the New England Medical Center in Boston. She received her D.P.H. from Harvard in June 1997. Her dissertation was entitled "The Human and Political Ecology of the U.S.-Mexican Border Colonia: An Elucidation of Relationships between Environmental Contamination, Disease, and the Political Agenda." Dr. Lopez has published a number of articles and made conference presentations on water quality and water monitoring programs, ecosystem health, and effects on human health.

OLIVA LÓPEZ ARELLANO is a professor of social medicine at the Autonomous Metropolitan University–Xochimilco in Mexico City and a member of the Mexican National Research System. Her basic training was in medicine at the Metropolitan University–Xochimilco, where she also obtained her Master of Social Medicine. She has published articles and books on health policy and urban health.

JOHN LYNCH, Ph.D., is an assistant research scientist in the Department of Epidemiology at the School of Public Health, University of Michigan, Ann Arbor, and is affiliated with the Institute for Social Research. He conducts research in the area of social inequalities in health, including studies of social stratification over the lifecourse, working conditions, and cumulative economic deprivation.

CARLES MUNTANER, M.D., Ph.D., is an assistant professor at the Institute of Occupational and Environmental Health, School of Medicine, West Virginia

University. He conducts research on class analysis, race relations, the labor process, and mental health in cooperation with unions.

VICENTE NAVARRO is a professor of health and public policy, sociology, and policy studies at the Johns Hopkins University in Baltimore and professor of political and social sciences at the Universitat Pompeu Fabra in Spain. A founder and past president of the International Association of Health Policy and founder and editor-in-chief of the *International Journal of Health Services,* he has written extensively on health and public policy themes. Dr. Navarro is the author of many books and articles on these subjects, including, most recently, *The Politics of Health Policy* (Blackwell, 1996) and *Neoliberalismo y Estado del Bienestar* (Ariel, 1997).

GARY L. OATES is an assistant professor in the Department of Sociology at the University of Connecticut. He obtained his Ph.D. in sociology from the University of Maryland in 1993 and was a postdoctoral fellow at the laboratory of Socio-environmental Studies, National Institute of Mental Health. His area of specialization is social psychology. Dr. Oates has recently published an article on self-esteem, fertility, and social class in the *American Sociological Review.*

JONATHAN OBERLANDER is an assistant professor of social medicine at the medical school of the University of North Carolina at Chapel Hill. He was previously a visiting scholar and Robert Wood Johnson scholar in health policy at the University of California, Berkeley. He received his Ph.D. in political science from Yale University in 1995. Dr. Oberlander's research interests include Medicare policy, health care politics, and the welfare state.

ADRIANA PUIGGRÓS is professor of the History of Argentine and Latin-American Education in the Faculty of Philosophy and Language at the University of Buenos Aires, Argentina. She is also a researcher at the National Council of Technical and Scientific Research, a member of the government's Technical Commission of the Federal Council of Education, and a representative of the Confederation of Educational Workers of the Argentine Republic. She graduated as a teacher in Educational Sciences at the University of Buenos Aires in 1969, and received a Master's Degree in Education at CINVESTAV, Mexico, in 1980, and a Ph.D. in pedagogy at the National University of Mexico in 1983. Dr. Puiggrós has published 20 books, including *Volver a educar: el desafío de la ensenanza argentina a finales del siglo XX* (Ariel, 1995).

LEIYU SHI, Dr.P.H., M.B.A., M.P.A., is an associate professor at the Johns Hopkins School of Hygiene and Public Health and associate director of the Johns Hopkins Primary Care Policy Center for the Underserved. His research contributions concern primary care, with particular emphasis on vulnerable and underserved populations. Dr. Shi is the author of *Health Services Research Methods; Delivering Healthcare in the U.S.: A Systems Perspective;* and *Physician Recruitment and Retention,* and he has published numerous papers evaluating various aspects of health services provision.

PILAR VERGARA is a senior researcher at the Latin American Faculty of Social Sciences (FLACSO) in Santiago, Chile. From 1975 to 1981 she was senior researcher at the Corporación de Investigaciones Económicas para América latina (CIEPLAN). She did advanced studies in sociology at the Catholic University of Santiago and received her M.S. in economic sciences at the Chilean University of Santiago. Ms. Vergara has taught at the Catholic University, held numerous visiting appointments, and served as a consultant to the International Development Bank. She is the author of numerous books and articles on economics, social policy, the state, and the authoritarian regime in Chile, including *Auge y Caída del Neoliberalismo en Chile* (Santiago, 1985) and *Políticas hacia la extrema pobreza en Chile 1973–1988* (FLACSO, 1988).

RICHARD G. WILKINSON is a professorial research fellow at the Trafford Centre for Medical Research at the University of Sussex and visiting professor at the International Centre for Health and Society at University College, London. After several years of manual work and a first degree in economic history, he trained in epidemiology and worked for some years in Britain's National Health Service. For almost 20 years he has been engaged in research on health inequalities and the social and economic determinants of health. His book *Unhealthy Societies: The Afflictions of Inequality* (Routledge, 1996) explains why more egalitarian societies tend to be healthier than less egalitarian ones.

ACKNOWLEDGMENTS

It is a pleasure to acknowledge the assistance of Linda Strange and Jean McMahon, Technical Editor and Managing Editor of the *International Journal of Health Services,* in preparing this book. It could not have been done without them. My thanks also to Stuart Cohen, President of Baywood Publishing, for his encouragement and support.

Vicente Navarro

Index

Page numbers in *italics* indicate figures; those followed by "t" indicate tables; those followed by "n" indicate footnotes.